Progress in
Cancer Research and Therapy
Volume 22

THE POTENTIAL ROLE OF T CELLS IN CANCER THERAPY

Progress in Cancer Research and Therapy

Progress in
Cancer Research and Therapy
Volume 22

The Potential Role of T Cells in Cancer Therapy

Editors

Alexander Fefer, M.D.
*Department of Medicine
Division of Oncology
University of Washington and Fred
Hutchinson Cancer Research Center
Seattle, Washington*

Allan L. Goldstein, Ph.D.
*Chairman, Department of Biochemistry
The George Washington University
School of Medicine
Washington, D.C.*

Raven Press ■ New York

Raven Press, 1140 Avenue of the Americas, New York, New York 10036

Great care has been taken to maintain the accuracy of the information contained in the volume. However, Raven Press cannot be held responsible for errors or for any consequences arising from the use of the information contained herein.

Materials appearing in this book prepared by individuals as part of their official duties as U.S. Government employees are not covered by the above-mentioned copyright.

Library of Congress Cataloging in Publication Data
Main entry under title:

The Potential role of T cells in cancer
    therapy.

    (Progress in cancer research and therapy;
v. 22)
        Bibliography: p.
        Includes index.
        1. T cells—Therapeutic use.   2. Cancer—
Treatment.   3. Immunotherapy.   4. Cellular
therapy.   I. Fefer, Alexander.   II. Goldstein,
Allan L.   III. Series.   [DNLM: 1. Neoplasms—
Therapy.   2. Neoplasms—Immunology.
3. T-Lymphocytes—Immunology.   W1 PR667M
v.22 / QZ 266 P861]
RC271.T15P67   616.99'4079   80-5901
ISBN 0-89004-747-2   AACR2

Preface

The past decade has seen a veritable revolution in cellular immunology in animals and man. Recent studies indicate that T cells are likely to have a major role in cancer therapy. Consequently, the Subcommittee on Biological Response Modifiers of the Board of Scientific Counselors to the Division of Cancer Treatment of the National Cancer Institute organized a workshop to explore the potential role of T cell subpopulations in cancer therapeutics.

This volume contains the work of experts in fundamental cellular immunology—especially as it relates to cancer therapy—and their discussion of the interaction between T cell subsets in immunity, the generation and maintenance of reactive T cells *in vitro* in long-term culture, and the positive or negative influences of T cells on tumor activity *in vivo*.

Several major areas are covered herein, often with data not previously published. The development of tumor immunity *in vivo* and *in vitro* (whether to tumor-specific antigens, tumor-associated antigens, differentiation antigens, or pooled alloantigens) and the limitations on such development are reviewed. Animal models are presented in which progressively growing fatal tumors were eradicated by lymphocytes used alone or as an adjunct to other antitumor therapies. The prerequisites for such therapy, the identity of the effector cell(s), and the host contribution are discussed. Also covered are specific or nonspecific suppressor cells that interfere with effector function *in vitro* or with therapy *in vivo*.

The need for large quantities of effector cells led to the inclusion in the volume of a review of the role of Interleukin 2 and Interleukin 3 in the differentiation and proliferation of T cells. Efforts to maintain lymphocytes in culture with Interleukin 2 and to study their characteristics and function *in vitro* are described. Moreover, new, previously unpublished, encouraging data about the therapeutic antitumor efficacy of cells maintained with IL 2 are presented. Finally, the need for T cell clones for studies of cellular interactions, immune regulation, and therapy is recognized and discussed, as are the specificity and function of cloned T cells and their potential use for therapy.

This volume serves as a state-of-the-art review, and identifies some of the major areas that require increased investigative attention and some of the problems that must be resolved to facilitate eventual recognition of the optimal role for T cells in cancer therapy. The results presented herein clearly demonstrate that T cells can be therapeutically effective against disseminated advanced tumors in animal models, that the requisite cells are being characterized and identified, and that they can be generated and maintained in long-term culture. It is also shown that T cells might be cloned, and that they are subject to various positive and negative influences which can be identified and manipulated.

These developments increase the likelihood that T cells will eventually play a significant role in cancer therapy. This volume will thus be of considerable interest to basic scientists and clinicians interested in cellular immunology and tumor immunology, especially as it relates to experimental and clinical oncology.

Acknowledgments

The editors of this volume wish to express their gratitude to Dr. V. T. DeVita, Jr., Director of the National Cancer Institute and Dr. R. K. Oldham, Director of the Biological Response Modifiers Program, Division of Cancer Treatment, National Cancer Institute, and their staff for their invaluable support that made this Workshop possible, and to the members of the Biological Response Modifiers Subcommittee: Drs. E. Mihich, E. Hersh, M. J. Mastrangelo, H. Oettgen, M. Krim, M. Mitchell, J. Whisnant, J. Betram, M. Chirigos, and A. Goldin for their encouragement and suggestions. Special thanks is due to M. Lund for the typing and collation of this volume.

Contents

Contributors

Barbara J. Alter
Mayo Memorial Building
Immunobiology Research Center
University of Minnesota at Minneapolis
Minneapolis, Minnesota 55455

J. A. Alvarez
Laboratory of Immunodiagnosis
National Cancer Institute
National Institutes of Health
Bethesda, Maryland 20205

Fritz H. Bach
Mayo Memorial Building
Immunology Research Center
University of Minnesota at Minneapolis
Minneapolis, Minnesota 55455

R. Chris Bleackley
Department of Biochemistry
University of Alberta
Edmonton, Alberta, Canada T6G 2H7

Guy D. Bonnard
Laboratory of Immunodiagnosis
National Cancer Institute
National Institutes of Health
Bethesda, Maryland 20205

Mortimer M. Bortin
May and Sigmund Winter Research Laboratory
Mount Sinai Medical Center
PO Box 342
Milwaukee, Wisconsin 53201

Johathan S. Bromberg
Department of Pathology
Harvard Medical School
25 Shattuck Street
Boston, Massachusetts 02115

Hartwig Bunzendahl
Box 724 Mayo Memorial Building
Immunobiology Research Center
University of Minnesota at Minneapolis
Minneapolis, Minnesota 55455

Martin A. Cheever
Division of Oncology RK-25
BB1015 Health Sciences
University of Washington
Seattle, Washington 98195

M. Cianfriglia
Genetics Unit
Swiss Institute for Experimental Cancer
Research
1066 Epalinges, Switzerland

Paul J. Conlon
The Fred Hutchinson Cancer Research Center
Program in Basic Immunology
1124 Columbia Street
Seattle, Washington 98104

A. Conzelmann
Genetics Unit
Swiss Institute for Experimental Cancer
Research
1066 Epalinges, Switzerland

Gunther Dennert
Department of Cancer Biology
The Salk Institute for Biological Studies
PO Box 85800
San Diego, California 92138

Deno P. Dialynas
The Committee on Immunology and
The Department of Pathology
The University of Chicago
Chicago, Illinois 60637

Earl S. Dye
The Trudeau Institute
Saranac Lake, New York 12983

T. Eberlein
Surgery Branch
National Cancer Institute
National Institutes of Health
Bethesda, Maryland 20205

John M. Ely
The Committee on Immunology and
The Department of Pathology
The University of Chicago
Chicago, Illinois 60637

C. G. Fathman
Department of Medicine
Division of Immunology
Stanford University School of Medicine
Stanford, California 94305

Alexander Fefer
Division of Oncology
BB1015 Health Sciences
University of Washington
Seattle, Washington 98195

J. D. Feldman
Department of Immunopathology
Scripps Clinic and Research Foundation
La Jolla, California 92037

E. Fernandez-Cruz
Department of Immunopathology
Scripps Clinic and Research Foundation
La Jolla, California 92037

Frank W. Fitch
The Committee on Immunology and
The Department of Pathology
The University of Chicago
Chicago, Illinois 60637

L. S. Fonseca
Laboratory of Immunobiology
National Cancer Institute
National Institutes of Health
Bethesda, Maryland 20205

Steven Gillis
The Fred Hutchinson Cancer Research Center
Program in Basic Immunology
1124 Columbia Street
Seattle, Washington 98104

Janis V. Giorgi
Transplantation Unit
Department of Surgery
Massachusetts General Hospital
Boston, Massachusetts 02114

Andrew L. Glasebrook
The Swiss Institute for Experimental Cancer
    Research
1066 Epalinges, Switzerland

Eliezer Gorelik
Laboratory of Immunodiagnosis
National Cancer Institute
National Institutes of Health
Bethesda, Maryland 20205

Douglas R. Green
Department of Pathology
Yale University School of Medicine
310 Cedar Street
New Haven, Connecticut 06510

Mark I. Greene
Department of Pathology
Harvard Medical School
25 Shattuck Street
Boston, Massachusetts 02115

Philip D. Greenberg
Division of Oncology
BB1015 Health Sciences
University of Washington
Seattle, Washington 98195

Joel Greenberger
Sidney Farber Cancer Center
44 Binney Street
Boston, Massachusetts 02115

E. Grimm
Surgery Branch
National Cancer Institute
National Institutes of Health
Bethesda, Maryland 20205

Andrew Hapel
Biological Carcinogenesis Program
Frederick Cancer Research Center
Frederick, Maryland 21701

Steven H. Hefeneider
The Fred Hutchinson Cancer Research Center
Program in Basic Immunology
1124 Columbia Street
Seattle, Washington 98104

Christopher S. Henney
The Fred Hutchinson Cancer Research Center
Program in Basic Immunology
1124 Columbia Street
Seattle, Washington 98104

Ronald B. Herberman
Laboratory of Immunodiagnosis
National Cancer Institute
National Institutes of Health
Bethesda, Maryland 20205

J. T. Hunter
Laboratory of Immunobiology
National Cancer Institute
National Institutes of Health
Bethesda, Maryland 20205

James N. Ihle
Biological Carcinogenesis Program
Frederick Cancer Research Center
Frederick, Maryland 21701

Eli Kedar
Hadassah Medical School
Jerusalem, Israel

Oded J. Kuperman
Mayo Memorial Building
Immunobiology Research Center
University of Minnesota at Minneapolis
Minneapolis, Minnesota 55455

John C. Lee
Biological Carcinogenesis Program
Frederick Cancer Research Center
Frederick, Maryland 21701

Benney Leshem ,
Mayo Memorial Building
Immunobiology Research Center
University of Minnesota at Minneapolis
Minneapolis, Minnesota 55455

A. Mazumder
Surgery Branch
National Cancer Institute
National Institutes of Health
Bethesda, Maryland 20205

Charles D. Mills
The Trudeau Institute
Saranac Lake, New York 12983

Gordon B. Mills
Department of Biochemistry
University of Alberta
Edmonton, Alberta, Canada T6G 2H7

M. Nabholz
Genetics Unit
Swiss Institute for Experimental Cancer
    Research
1066 Epalinges, Switzerland

Nicanor Navarro
Laboratory of Immunodiagnosis
National Cancer Institute
National Institutes of Health
Bethesda, Maryland 20205

Robert J. North
The Trudeau Institute
Saranac Lake, New York 12983

J. R. Ortaldo
Laboratory of Immunodiagnosis
National Cancer Institute
National Institutes of Health
Bethesda, Maryland 20205

Verner Paetkau
Department of Biochemistry
University of Alberta
Edmonton, Alberta, Canada T6G 2H7

Linda Perry
Department of Pathology
Harvard Medical School
25 Shattuck Street
Boston, Massachusetts 02115

Michael B. Prystowsky
The Committee on Immunology and
The Department of Pathology
The University of Chicago
Chicago, Illinois 60637

H. J. Rapp
Laboratory of Immunobiology
National Cancer Institute
National Institutes of Health
Bethesda, Maryland 20205

Alan Rein
Biological Carcinogenesis Program
Frederick Cancer Research Center
Frederick, Maryland 21701

Ellis L. Reinherz
Division of Tumor Immunology
Sidney Farber Cancer Institute and the
    Department of Medicine
Harvard Medical School
Boston, Massachusetts 02115

Alfred A. Rimm
The Section of Biostatistics
The Medical College of Wisconsin
Milwaukee, Wisconsin 53226

Lee K. Roberts
Department of Pathology
Immunobiology Laboratories
University of Mexico
School of Medicine
Albuquerque, New Mexico 87131

S. A. Rosenberg
Surgery Branch
National Cancer Institute
National Institutes of Health
Bethesda, Maryland 20205

M. Rosenstein
Surgery Branch
National Cancer Institute
National Institutes of Health
Bethesda, Maryland 20205

Stuart F. Schlossman
Division of Tumor Immunology
Sidney Farber Cancer Institute and the
    Department of Medicine
Harvard Medical School
Boston, Massachusetts 02115

Chiu-Yang Shih
May and Sigmund Winter Research Laboratory
Mount Sinai Medical Center
Milwaukee, Wisconsin 53201

S. Shu
Laboratory of Immunobiology
National Cancer Institute
National Institutes of Health
Bethesda, Maryland 20205

Craig W. Spellman
Department of Pathology
Immunobiology Laboratories
University of New Mexico
School of Medicine
Albuquerque, New Mexico 87131

Benjamin Sredni
Laboratory of Immunology
National Institute of Allergy and Infectious
   Diseases
National Institutes of Health
Bethesda, Maryland 20205

ManSun Sy
Department of Pathology
Harvard Medical School
25 Shattuck Street
Boston, Massachusetts 02115

Anna Tai
Department of Pathology
Immunobiology Laboratories
University of New Mexico
School of Medicine
Albuquerque, New Mexico 87131

Muneo Takaoki
Department of Pathology
Harvard Medical School
25 Shattuck Street
Boston, Massachusetts 02115

T. T. Timonen
Laboratory of Immunodiagnosis
National Cancer Institute
National Institutes of Health
Bethesda, Maryland 20205

Laurence D. Tempelis
Department of Medicine
Hematology/ Oncology Section
University of Wisconsin Medical School
Milwaukee, Wisconsin 53201

Akira Tominaga
Department of Pathology
Harvard Medical School
25 Shattuck Street
Boston, Massachusetts 02115

Robert L. Truitt
May and Sigmund Winter Research Laboratory
Mount Sinai Medical Center
Milwaukee, Wisconsin 53201

B. M. Vose
Laboratory of Immunodiagnosis
National Cancer Institute
National Institutes of Health
Bethesda, Maryland 20205

John F. Warner
Department of Cancer Biology
The Salk Institute for Biological Studies
PO Box 85800
San Diego, California 92138

Noel L. Warner
Monoclonal Antibody Laboratory
Becton Dickinson and Company
509 Clyde Avenue
Mountain View, California 94043

Joyce M. Zarling
Mayo Memorial Building
Immunobiology Research Center
University of Minnesota at Minneapolis
Minneapolis, Minnesota 55455

The Potential Role of T Cells in Cancer Therapy,
edited by A. Fefer and A. Goldstein,
Raven Press, New York © 1982.

Overview of Prospects and Problems of Lymphocyte Transfer for Cancer Therapy

A. Fefer, M. A. Cheever, and P. D. Greenberg

*Division of Oncology, BB1015 Health Sciences RK-25, University of Washington,
Seattle, Washington 98195*

Present at this workshop are investigators whose interest is chiefly
in fundamental cellular immunology -- regardless of its relevance to
cancer -- and others whose primary interest is in cancer and for whom
immunology provides the tools and a context for studying cancer biology
and therapy.

The plan for this workshop is to review some of the basic information about T cells and their interactions in the immunologic network,
about the generation and maintenance of T cell subsets in vitro, and
about the use of T cells for therapy in vivo, in the hope that some
direction will be provided for developing models for maximal therapeutic
efficacy in animals and for identifying areas which must be explored
before such therapy can be applied to man.

Several of the assumptions which form the basis for lymphocyte
transfer as potential cancer therapy are listed in Table 1. Their
validity will be discussed at this workshop.

TABLE 1. Assumptions underlying lymphocyte transer for cancer therapy

1. Tumor possesses antigens which can serve as targets
2. The critical anti-tumor reaction is mediated by the type of
   lymphocyte(s)
3. Tumor growth reflects inadequate, defective or deleterious host
   response
4. Infused cells will overcome the problem and cure the host

About 10 years ago, a number of animal models were developed and,
prematurely, a number of clinical trials of lymphocyte transfer in man
were begun, with inconclusive results (9,19). Recently there has been a
resurgence of interest in this approach due to several developments
which make it more likely that T cells will indeed have a role in cancer
therapy. Those developments are listed in Table 2. Progress in maintaining reactive T cells in culture with Interleukin 2 (15) and in cloning the requisite effector cell (21) for potential therapy (17) represent

the most relevant technologic advances.

TABLE 2. <u>Basis for increased interest in T cells and cancer therapy</u>

1. Increased number of models for effective therapy
2. T cells can be sensitized <u>in vitro</u> and used <u>in vivo</u>
3. Sensitized T cells can be maintained in large number in long term culture
4. Increased knowledge of T cell subsets and their interactions
5. Allogeneic marrow has anti-leukemic effect in man

Although immune syngeneic lymphocytes can affect tumor growth in animals when given shortly before or after tumor inoculation (9), with rare exceptions (2,8,17), lymphocytes alone are not effective against a normal host bearing a tumor which has already become established. The limiting factor may be in part the large tumor load and/or the development of host immunosuppressive factors which interfere with the efficacy of infused donor cells (12). Accordingly, in more recent models, syngeneic immune donor T cells were shown to be more effective when used in hosts whose suppressive factors have been depleted by pre-irradiation of the host and/or by T cell depletion of the host (1,13,14,18) -- as will be presented at this workshop. Moreover, immune T cells are predictably more effective in animal models when used as an <u>adjunct</u> to other forms of therapy, such as tumoricidal chemotherapy, radiation, and surgery -- all of which reduce the tumor load and concurrently can decrease some of the immunosuppressive factors (10,12). Thus, a number of effective syngeneic adoptive therapy models have been developed against the tumors listed in Table 3, all involving the transfer of syngeneic lymphocytes immune to tumor to a host bearing an advanced growing tumor (12). A number of the apparent prerequisites for therapeutic efficacy of immune syngeneic cells in these models will be discussed during this workshop. Additional therapy models are needed, especially using tumors of more recent origin and of lesser immunogenicity so as to confirm the general validity of the approach.

TABLE 3. <u>Targets for models of effective syngeneic adoptive therapy</u>

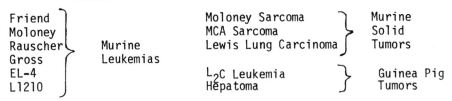

Friend		Moloney Sarcoma	Murine
Moloney		MCA Sarcoma	Solid
Rauscher	Murine	Lewis Lung Carcinoma	Tumors
Gross	Leukemias		
EL-4		L_2C Leukemia	Guinea Pig
L1210		Hepatoma	Tumors

Many studies have been and are being performed in <u>in vivo</u> therapy models with T cells generated <u>in vitro</u> (3-6,12-14,17,18) and, increasingly, with cells maintained in long-term culture (7) -- with promising results. The factors which determine whether such <u>in vitro</u>-generated cells will or will not be therapeutically effective have also not yet been identified. Indeed, cells generated <u>in vitro</u> can actually interfere with the therapeutic efficacy of infused T cells (16).

Unfortunately, therapeutic efficacy in vivo is not predictable from test results in vitro (4). Knowledge about immune networks and the various cells and cell products that are generated in vitro and in vivo should be used to determine how best to manipulate or modify the network in vitro, in vivo and in the tumor-bearing host so as to facilitate the therapeutic efficacy of infused cells. Such studies may also suggest which of the T cell subsets, which act as effectors in the different in vitro and in vivo reactions, should be used for in vivo therapy under given conditions. Parenthetically, although it is critical to obtain from the basic cellular immunologist direction for attempts to use T cells for cancer therapy, in vivo therapy models conversely provide a unique opportunity for investigators who have been studying T cells and T cell clones for their activity in vitro to determine, document, confirm, or establish that in vitro results reflect some function or activity in vivo.

Allogeneic T cells have also been used for therapy, but in far fewer tumor models and with far less success (11,12). The principal tumor targets for adoptive allogeneic therapy against advanced tumor are listed in Table 4 (12). Allogeneic lymphocyte transfer for therapy

TABLE 4. <u>Models of effective allogeneic adoptive therapy</u>

$$
\left.\begin{array}{l}
\text{Moloney} \\
\text{Gross} \\
\text{L1210}
\end{array}\right\} \quad \text{Leukemia}
$$

$$
\left.\begin{array}{l}
\text{Moloney} \\
\text{Rat MC}
\end{array}\right\} \quad \text{Sarcoma}
$$

poses at least 3 additional issues not posed by syngeneic adoptive therapy: a) the rejection of donor cells by the host; b) the induction of graft-vs.-host (GVH) disease; c) the occurrence of the graft-vs.-tumor reaction. If donor cells must remain in the host for any length of time in order to affect tumor kill or eradication -- an assumption supported by several studies (11) -- then rapid donor graft rejection must be avoided. This implies a need for a dose of chemotherapy and/or radiation which will be sufficiently immunosuppressive to prevent or delay the rejection of donor cells and which will concurrently decrease the tumor load and potentially decrease host suppressive factors. However, the persistence of allogeneic T cells for any length of time can lead to a GVH reaction and GVH disease, as documented in animal models and in man. GVH disease -- which is often fatal -- is difficult to prevent and extraordinarily difficult to control or eradicate once it is established (12).

However, the GVH reaction is a double-edged sword. Although its deleterious effects on normal host tissue represent a major impediment to therapy, it also exerts a significant effect against tumors in some animal models (11). Most importantly, there is now strong circumstantial evidence for an anti-leukemic effect of GVH disease in man, from data obtained by the Seattle Bone Marrow Transplant Team (22,23). Patients with acute leukemia were treated with anti-leukemic therapy in the form of supralethal doses of cyclophosphamide and total body irradiation plus bone marrow from HLA-identical siblings or from a genetically identical twin. The patients receiving non-twin marrow also received small doses of the immunosuppressive chemotherapeutic agent methotrexate prophylactically for potential GVH disease for about 3 months after marrow transplantation. Despite the excellent matching and despite the methotrexate, however, a high incidence of acute GVH disease was observed. The GVH disease was of variable severity, i.e., no disease, mild disease involving only skin, or more severe disease involving skin, liver, and gastrointestinal tract.

A statistical analysis was performed (22) on the causes of death of the marrow transplant recipients, in an attempt to determine any association between acute GVH disease and post-transplant recurrence of leukemia. The results, in Figure 1, show that the probability of leukemic recurrence was significantly lower for patients who received allogeneic marrow and developed significant GVH disease than for patients who received allogeneic marrow and exhibited none or very mild GVH disease or for patients who received syngeneic marrow and, therefore, had no GVH disease.

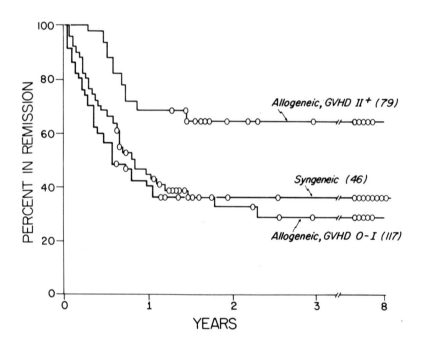

FIG. 1. Kaplan-Meier product limit estimate of the probability of remaining in complete remission from acute leukemia as a function of time after marrow transplantation. Forty-six patients received marrow from genetically identical twins, and 196 from HLA-identical siblings. 0-I = none or very mild GVHD; II$^+$ = severe GVHD; 0 = patient still alive in remission.

More recently, a similar analysis was performed with chronic GVH disease (23) -- a syndrome which occurs later and has different clinical manifestations with many autoimmune problems. The results show that the probability of remaining in remission after marrow transplantation was highest for those patients who had both acute and chronic GVH disease and lowest for allogeneic marrow recipients who had no GVH disease (23).

This striking association between GVH disease and decreased probability of leukemic relapse represents a major clinical example of an anti-tumor effect by adoptively transferred cells. The challenge remains to determine how to impart to this type of reaction a greater anti-tumor specificity as compared to anti-host reactivity and to identify the kind of cells and conditions necessary for optimal therapeutic results.

In conclusion, much has been learned in animals about T cell subsets and their ability to kill tumor cells in vitro and, under special conditions, to be therapeutic in vivo. Human T cells subsets are also being identified and can be rendered cytotoxic to tumor cells in vitro. Although the therapeutic effect of such cells has not yet been demonstrated in man, the graft-vs.-leukemia effect reported in man may represent such an effect. In toto, recent developments in cellular and tumor immunology instill optimism regarding the potential of T cells in cancer therapy. This workshop is expected to validate such optimism.

REFERENCES

1. Berendt, M.J., North, R.J. (1980): J. Exp. Med. 151:59.
2. Borberg, H., Oettgen, H.F., Choudry, K. and Beathie, E.J. (1972): Int. J. Cancer 10:539.
3. Cheever, M.A., Kempf, R.A., Fefer, A. (1977): J. Immunol. 119:714.
4. Cheever, M.A., Greenberg, P.D., Fefer, A. (1978): J. Immunol. 121:2220.
5. Cheever, M.A., Greenberg, P.D., Fefer, A. (1980): J. Immunol. 125:711.
6. Cheever, M.A., Greenberg, P.D., Fefer, A. (1981): Ca. Res. 41:2658.
7. Cheever, M.A., Greenberg, P.D., Fefer, A. (1981): J. Immunol. 126:1318.
8. Fefer, A. (1969): Ca. Res. 29:2177.
9. Fefer, A. (1974): In: Handbook of Experimental Pharmacology, edited by Sartorelli, A.C., and Johns, D.G., pp. 528-554. Springer Verlag, New York.
10. Fefer, A., Einstein, A.B., Cheever, M.A. and Berenson, J.R. (1976): Ann. N.Y. Acad. Sci. 276:573.
11. Fefer, A., Einstein, A.B., Cheever, M.A. (1976): Ann. N.Y. Acad. Sci. 277:492.
12. Fefer, A., Cheever, M.A. and Greenberg, P.D. (in press): In: Immunological Aspects of Cancer Therapeutics, edited by Mihich, E. John Wiley & Sons, Inc., New York.
13. Fernandez-Cruz, E., Halliburton, B., Feldman, J.D. (1979): J. Immunol. 123:1772.
14. Fernandez-Cruz, E., Woda, B.A., Feldman, J.D. (1980): J. Exp. Med. 152:823.
15. Gillis, S., Smith, K.A. (1977): Nature 268:154.
16. Greenberg, P.D., Cheever, M., Fefer, A. (1979): J. Immunol. 123:515.

17. Kedar, E., Weiss, D.W. (1980): In: Immunogenicity, edited by
     Borek, R.
18. Mills, G.B., Carlson, G., Paetkau, V. (1980): J. Immunol. 125:1904.
19. Rosenberg, S.A., Terry, W.D. (1977): Adv. Ca. Res. 25:323;347;366.
20. Smith, H.G., Harmel, R.P., Hanna, MG., Zwilling, B.S., Zbar, B.S.,
     Rapp, H.J. (1977): J. Natl. Ca. Inst. 58:1315.
21. von Boehmer, H., Haas, W., Pohlit, H., Hengartner, H., Nabholz, M.
     (1980): Springer Semin. Immunopathol. 3:23.
22. Weiden, P.L., Flournoy, N., Thomas, E.D., Prentice, R., Fefer, A.,
     Buckner, C.D., Storb, R. (1979): N. Engl. J. Med. 300:1068.
23. Weiden, P.L., Sullivan, K.M., Flournoy, N., Storb, R., Thomas, E.D.
     (1981): N. Engl. J. Med. 304:1529.

The Potential Role of T Cells in Cancer Therapy,
edited by A. Fefer and A. Goldstein,
Raven Press, New York © 1982.

Allosensitization to Obtain Anti-Tumor Immunity

Fritz H. Bach, Benny Leshem, Oded J. Kuperman, Hartwig Bunzendahl,
Barbara J. Alter, and Joyce M. Zarling

*Mayo Memorial Building, Immunobiology Research Center, University of Minnesota at Minneapolis,
Minneapolis, Minnesota 55455*

The concept of utilizing a "pool" of allogeneic cells from 10–20 unrelated, randomly chosen individuals as a sensitizing stimulus in mixed leukocyte culture (MLC) to obtain anti-tumor cytotoxic cells was based on a number of considerations (4). First, we had demonstrated in man that stimulation with such a pool resulted in proliferative responses that were as strong or stronger than stimulation with cells of any single individual included within that pool (19). Second, sensitization with a pool resulted in priming of lymphocytes such that virtually any unrelated restimulating cell, whether included in the pool or not, would elicit a highly significant accelerated, secondary-type proliferative response (a primed lymphocyte typing (PLT) response) (20). Third, sensitization with a pool led to lysis of essentially any unrelated target cell, once again whether that unrelated target cell was from an individual who had donated to the pool or not (14). It thus seemed that the pool included, either by direct representation or based on cross-reactivity, essentially all of the L-Determinant (LD) antigens which stimulate the majority of the proliferative response in an MLC or a PLT test as well as most or all of the C-Determinant (CD) antigens, which serve as targets for cytotoxic T lymphocytes (Tc).

Based on these findings, it seemed possible that pool sensitization would also sensitize those Tc that might be reactive to a syngeneic or autologous abnormal cell (saac), such as a tumor cell. As reviewed very briefly below, allosensitization by the pool or by cells of single allogeneic donors has been an effective means of generating anti-saac immunity in certain systems (17,18,21,22,26). In mouse, our studies have utilized primarily the RBL-5 tumor from BL/6 mice as the saac target; in man we have utilized both cells of Epstein-Barr (EB) virus transformed autologous lymphoblastoid cell lines (LCLs) as well as leukemia target cells.

An important issue to be addressed concerned the means by which allosensitization leads to anti-saac effector cells. One possibility is that lymphocytes manifesting anti-saac immunity are activated polyclonally in some manner by growth factors elaborated in MLC (7,8,10,11,12,15,16) (perhaps based on their previously having been sensitized to antigens cross-reactive with saac antigens thus possibly rendering them more susceptible to reactivation with T cell growth factor (TCGF) (interleukin-2)). Alternatively, allosensitization may lead to the generation of cytotoxic cells capable of lysing both the allosensitizing target and the saac target. Our findings, which are summarized below, demonstrate, at the clonal level, that the cells that become cytotoxic to saac following allosensitization are, for the most part, ones that also lyse the sensitizing allogeneic normal target. Since these results were obtained with Tc populations at the clonal level, the most reasonable conclusion is that it is sharing or cross-reactivity between alloantigens and saac antigens which forms the basis of the overall response.

Since anti-tumor cytotoxic lymphoid cells can include both Tc and natural killer (NK) cells, the question is raised whether cells generated following allosensitization, which are capable of lysing a saac target, are of the Tc or NK variety. Results reviewed below demonstrate that whereas NK-like cells are generated in an MLC that are capable of lysing NK-sensitive targets, the majority of anti-saac immunity, present at the height of sensitization in MLC against targets such as the RBL-5 mouse leukemia cells or LCLs, is mediated by Tc.

CHARACTERIZATION OF EFFECTOR CELLS

In mouse, sensitization with cells of certain single allogeneic strains leads to generation of anti-saac immunity (6,17,18). We have sensitized BL/6 cells in MLC with cells of B10.G, for instance, and tested, at 16 hours and at 5 days following sensitization, for the development of cytotoxicity on a number of targets including RBL-5 (a BL/6, Rauscher virus induced leukemia). The results presented in Table 1 demonstrate that high level cytotoxicity is present after 16 hours; these cytotoxic cells are not removed by treatment with anti-Thy-1 serum and complement (C) suggesting that they may be NK-like cells. At 16 hours, of course, there is no detectable cytotoxicity present against the allosensitizing target.

TABLE 1.   Effect of anti-Thy-1 treatment on BL/6 pool-sensitized cells cytotoxic for syngeneic tumors

	Targets	
Treatment	LR-6 melanoma[a]	RBL-5 leukemia[b]
None	18.3 ± 4.6	12.1 ± 3.2
Anti-Thy-1 + C	17.7 ± 5.8	1.1 ± 3.3
C	17.5 ± 7.1	15.8 ± 2.3

[a] ^{3}H-proline assay - 16 hrs after allostimulation

[b] ^{51}Cr release assay - 5 days after allosensitization

(Adapted from Paciucci et al., J. Immunol. 124:370-375, 1980. Copyright Williams and Wilkins Press.)

When evaluated at 5 days, cytotoxic activity against both the allosensitizing target and RBL-5 is, to a very large extent, sensitive to treatment with anti-Thy-1 serum plus C suggesting that

these cytotoxic cells are of the Tc class. Since Thy-1 has been
shown to be present on NK cells, we have also performed studies in
which the effector cytotoxic cells were treated with anti-Lyt-2 serum
plus C immediately prior to their being tested for cytotoxic activity;
the results obtained with day 5 sensitized cells confirm the interpretation above of studies with anti-Thy-1.

Similar results have been obtained in experiments in which Balb/c
cells sensitized to allogeneic normal cells lyse syngeneic Simian
virus 40 transferred solid tumor cells. Lysis is mediated nearly
exclusively by Thy.1+ cells (18) which are also Ly2+ (Hurrell, S.,
Zarling, J.M., and Bach, F.H. in preparation).

We have performed similar studies in humans aimed at determining
whether lysis of autologous EB virus transformed LCLs by pool-stimulated cells is mediated by Tc or NK-like cells, both of which are
generated in MLC. Differentiation of Tc from NK and NK-like cells
was based on findings by one of us (JMZ) and collaborators (25) that
these cells can be distinguished by virtue of reactivity with monoclonal antibodies directed against human mononuclear cell populations.
Whereas treatment of allosensitized cells with monoclonal antibodies
OKT3 or OKT8 and C ablated cytotoxicity against allogeneic normal
cells, these antibodies did not reduce the ability of either fresh
lymphocytes, polyinosinic:polycytidylic acid-activated lymphocytes or
pool-sensitized lymphocytes to lyse HLA-negative, NK-sensitive K562
cells. Thus, Tc can be distinguished from fresh and activated NK
cells as well as NK-like cells generated in MLC by anti-T cell
antibodies OKT3 or OKT8. Treatment of fresh or activated NK cells
with OKM1 and C does eliminate most NK cell activity; however, this
antibody is non-reactive with MLC generated NK-like cells (25).
Experiments were subsequently conducted to determine whether pool-
sensitized cells which lyse autologous LCLs would be mediated by
effectors which are phenotypically Tc or NK-like cells (23). Results
of one of six similar experiments shown in Table 2 indicate the
treatment of pool-stimulated cells was OKT3 or OKT8 and C virtually
eliminated cytotoxicity against autologous LCL cells in that the
total lytic units (LU) recovered following treatment of 1 x 107
effector cells with control ascites and C was 108 whereas less than
5 LU were recovered following treatment with either OKT3 or OKT8.
Similarly, treatment with OKT3 or OKT8 eliminated cytotoxicity
against allogeneic normal cells but this treatment had no effect on
NK-like cells lytic for K562 target cells. We have recently demonstrated that lysis of autologous and allogeneic EB virus transformed
LCLs by effector cells generated by stimulation with autologous LCLs
is mediated by Tc whereas lysis of EBV-negative, NK-sensitive leukemia
cells including K562, MOLT-4 and HSB-2 is mediated by cells which are
phenotypically NK-like cells (24).

From the results discussed above, it appears therefore that although
NK-like cells are generated in MLC, that lysis of syngeneic leukemia
and sarcoma cells by allo-stimulated mouse cells and lysis of EB
virus transformed LCLs by pool-stimulated human cells is mediated
primarily or exclusively by Tc. Studies discussed below were designed
to determine whether lysis of syngeneic or autologous abnormal cells
by allo-sensitized cells is mediated by Tc directed against antigens
shared with those expressed on the allogeneic stimulating cells.

TABLE 2. Differential effects of treatment of pool-sensitized human
cells with monoclonal anti-T cell antibodies on lysis of
allogeneic normal cells, autologous LCLs and K562 cells[a]

Treatment of pool-stimulated effector cells	Target Cells					
	Allogeneic normal cells		Autologous LCLs		K562	
	$LU/10^6$	total LU	$LU/10^6$	total LU	$LU/10^6$	total LU
Control + C	18	139	14	108	6	44
OKT8 + C	<1	<5	<1	<5	9	45
OKT3 + C	<1	<3	<1	<3	17	45

[a]Lymphocytes from a normal individual were stimulated with
pooled allogeneic normal cells for 7 days. The effector
cells were harvested and treated with control ascites,
monoclonal antibodies OKT8 or OKT3 and complement (C) as
previously detailed (25). Dead cells were removed by
ficoll-hypaque centrifugation and the live cells were
tested for their ability to lyse the target cells in a
6 hr ^{51}Cr release assay at several effector:target cell
ratios. One lytic unit (LU) was defined as the number
of effector cells required to mediate 25% specific ^{51}Cr
release from 8×10^3 target cells. The total LU recovered
was calculated by: $LU/10^6$ effector cells x number of
viable effector cells recovered. The number of cells
recovered after treating 1×10^7 cells was OKT3, OKT8 or
control ascites and C were 2.7, 5.1 or 7.7×10^6,
respectively. (Modified from Zarling et al., J. Immunol.
126:375-378, 1981. Copyright Williams and Wilkins
Press.)

Limiting Dilution Studies and Derivation of Cloned Cytotoxic Cells

We have previously demonstrated that growth of bulk populations
of allosensitized cells in TCGF-containing medium allows the very
marked expansion (by a factor of 1×10^6 to 1×10^7) of the cells
active against saac accompanied by a somewhat increased (2-3 fold)
specific activity of anti-saac killing based on a per effector cell
basis; no significant lysis of autologous normal cells was noted
(22). We have recently used the limiting dilution approach to
develop clones of cytotoxic cells following allosensitization that
are active against the saac target (Leshem, B., Kuperman, O.J., and
Bach, F.H., in preparation; Bunzendahl, H., and Bach, F.H., in
preparation) for at least two reasons. First, we wanted to ask
whether those cytotoxic cells active against saac were the ones that
also lysed the sensitizing allogeneic target, which would suggest
that anti-saac killing was based on sharing or cross-reactivity of
determinants on the allogeneic and saac targets and second, to the
extent that cells generated in bulk culture in the presence of
TCGF-containing medium could be used in adoptive immunotherapy, the
clonal approach would seem to minimize the possibility of reactions
mediated against cells other than the autologous tumor.

We have analyzed allosensitized cytotoxic cells that are also
active against the saac target (RBL-5 in mouse and the autologous

LCL in man) in an attempt to evaluate the basis of anti-saac lysis following allosensitization. Our findings in mouse are presented in Table 3.

BL/6 mice were sensitized to one of several allogeneic strains that led to anti-RBL-5 cytotoxicity; in the example shown in Table 3, B10.G sensitizing cells were used. Following 5 days of bulk sensitization, limiting dilution studies were done in which the cells were plated in microtitre wells at an average of 5 cells per well in the presence of secondary MLC supernatant and B10.G x-irradiated feeder cells (12). Subsequently, those cloids (a cell population,

TABLE 3.   Cytotoxicity to the allo-sensitizing strain B10.G
and the syngeneic tumor, RBL-5[a]

| | Cytotoxicity against | |
Cloid no.	B10.G	RBL-5
43-A6	70.9	20.0
43-A8	81.1	39.2
43-A9	12.6	0.7
43-B1	70.4	64.8
43-B10	34.7	1.7
43-C3	44.0	7.9
43-C5	39.4	63.7
43-D5	-8.4	7.8
43-D10	15.1	0
43-E2	23.4	-1.1
43-E9	18.4	-1.1
43-F8	22.9	19.8
43-G9	27.3	-1.2
43-H1	15.1	0
43-H11	62.0	46.8

[a]BL/6 spleen cells were sensitized, for 5 days, in bulk culture with irradiated B10.G spleen cells and then plated, at 5 cells per well, in lda conditions. Eight days later, each individual well was tested for cytotoxicity against FBS induced blasts of B10.G and against RBL-5. Cytotoxically positive wells were defined as those wells whose cytotoxicity exceeded minimal positive (i.e. mean + 3 S.D. of 24 spontaneous release wells). Minimal positive for B10.G was 12.3% and for RBL-5, 3.4%. Of 96 wells plated, 31 (32%) had growing cells; out of those, 7 wells (22.5%) showed cytotoxicity against B10.G only, 23 wells (74.2%) showed cytotoxicity against both RBL-5 and B10.G and only 1 well (3.2%) showed cytotoxicity against RBL-5 only. Data from 15 wells are shown in the table.

in these studies, derived from 5 or fewer antigen stimulated blasts where the probability of clonality is less than 95%) that were active against RBL-5 were tested against the sensitizing allogeneic target, in this case B10.G. Since in the great majority of all instances tested (more than 90%) the cells of cloids that lysed RBL-5 (on the basis of which the cloid was selected) also lysed B10.G, and on the basis of subcloning data to be published elsewhere

(Leshem et al., in preparation), we tentatively conclude that the basis of anti-saac cytotoxicity following allosensitization is primarily either true sharing (as is suggested by the alien histo-compatibility antigen model (2,5,13)) or cross-reactivity between alloantigenic determinants and saac determinants recognized in the syngeneic combination. In fact, in the few cloids that lysed RBL-5 targets and not the sensitizing allogeneic target, the level of anti-RBL-5 cytotoxicity was very low; sub-cloning of those cloids will be necessary to examine this question further. That the saac determinant recognized following allosensitization may well be the tumor-associated target, i.e. the determinant recognized when BL/6 mice are sensitized to RBL-5 directly, is evidenced by the following. We have cloned cells following in vivo sensitization of BL/6 with RBL-5 and tested them on allogeneic targets. Preliminary results indicate that following in vivo sensitization with RBL-5, some clones also lyse certain allogeneic targets (data not shown).

Frequency Estimates of Anti-allogeneic and Anti-saac Cytotoxic Cells

As shown in Figure 1, the limiting dilution analysis of the frequency of Tc against the sensitizing allogeneic target cells and against RBL-5 following 5 days of bulk allosensitization gives the following results. The frequency of anti-allogeneic cytotoxic cells is 1/11.1; as expected with increased numbers of responding cells per well the percentage of anti-allogeneic positive cytotoxic wells increases to 100% when the responding cell number per well is between 20 and 50 in this experiment. Further, as expected, with still higher numbers (up to 50,000 responding cells/well in one experiment) of responding cells, the percentage of wells cytotoxic to the sensi-tizing allogeneic target remains at 100%. In contrast, although tested from the same wells, the patterns of percent positive wells against RBL-5 and syngeneic, in vivo, fetal bovine serum-induced BL/6 blast targets showed a markedly different pattern. Initially, at relatively low responding cell numbers, i.e. less than 50/well for RBL-5 and less than 100 for BL/6, the percentage of positive wells against both of these targets gave a highly significant fit to the Poisson statistic allowing estimates of the precursor Tc frequency to be made for each of these two targets. However, as the responding cell number per well was increased still further (in 7 different experiments at numbers between 50 and 1000 responding cells per well) the percentage of positive anti-RBL-5 and positive anti-BL/6 blast cytotoxic wells began to decrease and, by 5000 cells per well in this experiment (with a range of 2000-5000 cells per well in different experiments) essentially no wells positive in cytotoxicity against RBL-5 or BL/6 blasts were found. We refer to this phenomenon as "suppression" of the response, even though the mechanism is not understood and we have not, to date, identified suppressor cells as being responsible or even present at various numbers of responding cells per well.

In man, it is possible to sensitize to a pool of as few as three individuals or, utilizing the limiting dilution approach from bulk culture to obtain clones or cloids, even to cells of single individuals, and in relatively high frequency obtain cytotoxic cells to the autologous LCL. Thus, bulk sensitization is carried out for four days, blasts from the allosensitized culture (utilizing either

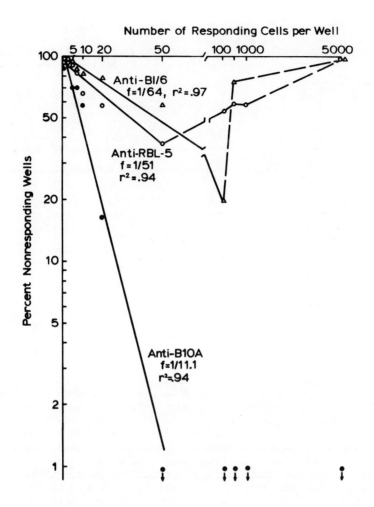

Legend to Figure 1

Spleen cells from BL/6 mice were sensitized, in bulk culture, for 5 days with irradiated B10.A spleen cells in DMEM medium (supplemented with 2% fetal bovine serum (FBS)) and then plated, in 1da conditions (MEM medium, 10% FBS and 30% 2° MLC supernatant (12)) at the number of responding cells per well as indicated and 1 x 10^{6} irradiated B10.A spleen cells per well. After 8 days, aliquots from each individual well were tested, in ^{51}Cr release assay, against B10.A targets (●), RBL-5 (o) and BL/6 FBS blasts (△). Frequency analysis was made by linear regression using the points that gave r^{2}>.90. Dashed lines connect points which were not used in frequency analysis.

a pool of three cells or single allogeneic cells) are isolated on a
unit gravity gradient and plated in microtitre wells in the presence
of TCGF-containing medium and allogeneic feeder cells. Cloids or
clones are derived under these conditions that show the patterns of
lysis seen in Table 4.

TABLE 4. Lysis of autologous LCL by allosensitized Tc cloids[a]

Clone	Autologous cell		Sensitizing Allogeneic cell		3rd Party Allogeneic	
	LCL	NP[b]	LCL	NP	LCL	NP
a	−	−	+	+	−	−
b	+	−	+	+	−	−
c	+	−	+	+	+	−
d	+	−	−	−	+/−	−

[a]Seeded at 1 cell/5 wells; p for clonality 0.9.
[b]Normal, fresh peripheral blood lymphocytes.

   In the experiment from which the cloids were derived which showed
the prototype results illustrated for clones a, b, c and d in Table 4,
responding cells were sensitized with a single allogeneic cell and
subsequently tested on the LCL and normal peripheral lymphocytes
autologous with the cloned cells, on the LCL and normal peripheral
blood lymphocytes of the allosensitizing cell donor and third party
allogeneic targets. The four patterns of reactivity demonstrated
were all seen. First, as illustrated by clone "a", some clones were
lytic neither to the autologous LCL nor to the autologous normal
cells but were lytic to the allosensitizing cell used as a target.
These clones showed the expected specificity following allosensitization in that they did not kill at least certain third party
allogeneic targets. Second, cloids were derived which did lyse the
autologous LCL but not the autologous normal peripheral blood
lymphocytes. These cloids also lysed the target cells of the
allosensitizing cell donor but frequently not third party normal
cells. Some of these cloids did lyse third party LCLs (cloid c)
while others did not (cloid b). Some cloids (e.g. d) filled the
autologous LCL but not the sensitizing allogeneic target. The basis
for lysis of third party LCLs is not understood in terms of antigens
that may be recognized by the cloid or clone.
   Based on our previous findings (see Table 2 and (23)) that pool-
sensitized cells lytic for autologous LCLs are OKT8+, a surprising
observation has been that the cytotoxic clones active against both
the autologous LCL and the sensitizing allogeneic target carry the
OKT3+, OKT4+, OKT8− phenotype as analyzed by a FACS. In 8/12 clones
examined that are positive for OKT4, there is no evidence for the
presence of the OKT8 antigen; in the other 4 clones examined, the
OKT4 antigen is very significantly present and there is a very slight
indication of a low level of OKT8 as shown in Figure 2.

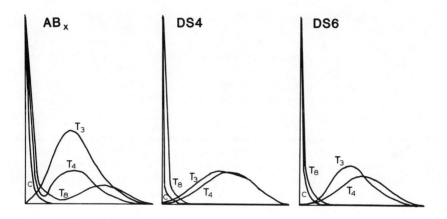

Legend to Figure 2

Results are from fluorescent activated cell sorting analysis of cells that have been grown for 6 days in a mixed leukocyte culture, AB_x, followed by 4 days cultivation in TCGF, and two cytotoxic clones (DS4 and DS6) derived following allosensitization with cells of a single individual. The clones represent examples in which very low level T8 expression was present in addition to high level expression of both T3 and T4.

SOME COMMENTS

The results presented above would appear to provide answers to at least two questions that have previously remained unresolved in this literature. First, the cytotoxic cells active against a saac target following allosensitization, at least for the systems and conditions examined, appear to be predominently cells that are phenotypically Tc rather than NK-like cells. Second, Tc active against the saac target frequently also recognize determinants on the allosensitizing cell; that is, there appears to be sharing or cross-reactivity between the allosensitizing cell and the saac target although exceptions exist. Obviously, experiments such as these cannot provide critical data to help in the resolution of whether this represents alien histocompatibility antigen expression or cross-reactivity (2).

The V-shaped pattern of reactivity to RBL-5 following allosensitization as analyzed by limiting dilution (see Figure 1) is perhaps most easily explained by hypothesizing the presence of suppressor cells which preferentially, or differentially, suppress those cytotoxic cells active against both the allosensitizing target and RBL-5 as opposed to those that lyse the allogeneic target only. We have,

however, no direct evidence that suppressive mechanisms are involved
in this reaction; other possibilities must be considered. Moreover,
whatever the mechanism that leads to a "return" to 100% non-responding
wells following the demonstration of an initial positive reaction
with a given frequency against RBL-5, does not lead to elimination of
anti-RBL-5 cytotoxic precursors. This is evidenced by our finding
(Leshem et al., in preparation) that if the cells are taken from
those wells that were plated at a number where 100% of the anti-
allogeneic wells are positive in cytotoxicity whereas 100% of the
anti-RBL-5 wells are again negative in cytotoxicity (e.g. at 5000
cells/well in the experiment pictured in Figure 1) and re-evaluated
in limiting dilution assay (lda), one obtains a frequency of anti-
RBL-5 cytotoxic precursors not very significantly different from that
initially demonstrated. In those experiments in which, in bulk
culture, no anti-saac effectors are detected following allosensitization, it may well be that a mechanism similar to that responsible
for the V-shaped curve (which has also been noted in other systems
(9)) may also be responsible.

Most of the studies done to date in which cells have been sensitized in vitro have tested populations for activity immediately after
the 5-7 day in vitro sensitization, either as a "primary" in vitro
response or following in vivo sensitization. Much of the emphasis,
since the initial description of TCGF activity and its ability to
maintain the long-term growth of T cell subpopulations, has been on
the expansion of specific cytotoxic, or other, T lymphocytes since
such cells maintain antigen-specificity and functional reactivity.
However, whether such cells will home properly and function in vivo
in an appropriate manner is largely unanswered.

There are observations which are consistant with the hypothesis
that the cell surface phenotype of T lymphocytes may change during
cultivation in TCGF-containing medium although at present the data
are not available to differentiate between such a mechanism and
growth in TCGF of a relatively small sub-population of cells. Thus,
one interpretation of the OKT4+, OKT8- phenotype of the cytotoxic
cloids discussed above is that these cells initially had a different
OKT phenotype but that with their continued growth in TCGF they
changed to the OKT4+, OKT8- cell surface expression. Experiments are
currently underway to evaluate the precursor phenotype of these
cells. Similarly, the Ly-5 antigenic system, which, in mouse, shows
molecular weight polymorphism (1) that may correlate with functional
subtypes of T lymphocytes, may well be influenced by culture in
secondary MLC supernatant. High molecular weight markers are present
on cytotoxic T lymphocytes that have been cloned in secondary supernatant (molecular weight forms above 200,000), yet there is a relative
lack of expression of these forms in cell populations prior to cultivation in secondary supernatant even though one out of every four T
lymphocytes, as a minimum estimate, is a cytotoxic cell. Given the
possibility of such changes, homing and function following growth in
TCGF may present a problem which needs careful and extensive testing.

Lastly, we, as well as other laboratories interested in generating
anti-syngeneic or autolgous tumor immunity following allosensitization, have emphasized studies of cytotoxic T cells. A question of
great import is to what extent helper cells as well as cytotoxic

cells, analogous to in vitro collaboration between such cells (3), may be functional in anti-tumor immunity, makes critical investigations concerning the generation and need for specificity of helper cells in the systems in which, to date, cytotoxic cell investigations have predominated.

ACKNOWLEDGEMENTS

We thank Lynn Guy for extremely able technical assistance and Jayne Ritter for editorial work. This work was supported by grants CA 27826, CA 26738, AI 18326, AI/GM 17687 and March of Dimes 6-255. JMZ is a Scholar of the Leukemia Society of America. HB is supported by a research training grant of the Deutsche Forschungsgemeinschaft. This is paper number 273 from the Immunobiology Research Center, University of Minnesota, Minneapolis.

REFERENCES

1. Bach, F.H., Alter, B.J., Widmer, M.B., Segall, M., and Dunlap, B. (1981): Immunol. Rev., 54:5-26.
2. Bach, F.H., and Bortin, M.M. Second International Symposium on Alloimmunization. The Biological and Clinical Significance of Alien Histocompatibility Antigens on Cancer Cells. In press.
3. Bach, F.H., Bach, M.L., and Sondel, P.M. (1976): Nature, 59:273-281.
4. Bach, M.L., Bach, F.H., and Zarling, J.M. (1978): Lancet, 1:20-22.
5. Bortin, M.M. and Truitt, R.L. (eds.) (1980): Alien Histocompatibility Antigens in Cancer. Grune and Stratton, New York.
6. Bortin, M.M., Truitt, R.L., Rimm, A.A., and Bach, F.H. (1979): Nature, 281:490-491.
7. Gillis, S., and Smith, K.A. (1977): Nature, 268:154-156.
8. Gillis, S., and Smith, K.A. (1977): J. Exp. Med., 146:468-482.
9. Goronzy, J., Schaefer, U., Eichmann, K., and Simon, M.M. (1980): J. Exp. Med., 153:857-870.
10. Inouye, H., Hank, J.A., Alter, B.J., and Bach, F.H. (1980): Scand. J. Immunol., 12:149-154.
11. Janis, M., and Bach, F.H. (1970): Nature, 225:238-239.
12. MacDonald, H.R., Cerottini, J-C., Ryser, J-E., Maryanski, J.L., Taswell, C., Widmer, M.B., and Brunner, K.T. (1980): Immunol. Rev., 51:93-123.
13. Martin, W.I., Esber, E., Cotton, W.G., and Rice, J.M. (1973): Br. J. Cancer, 28:48-61.
14. Martinis, J., and Bach, F.H. (1978): Transplantation, 25:39-41.
15. Morgan, D.A., Ruscetti, F.W., and Gallo, R.C. (1976): Science, 193:1007-1008.
16. Oppenheim, J.J., and Rosenstreich, D.L. editors. (1976): Mitogens in Immunobiology. Academic Press, Inc.
17. Paciucci, P.A., Macphail, S., Bach, F.H., and Zarling, J.M. (1980): J. Immunol., 125:36-39.
18. Paciucci, P.A., Macphail, S., Zarling, J.M., and Bach, F.H. (1980): J. Immunol., 124:370-375.

19. Segall, M., and Bach, F.H. (1976): Transplantation, 22:79-85.
20. Sondel, P.M., Sheehy, M.J., Bach, M.L., and Bach, F.H. In: Histocompatibility Testing 1975, edited by F. Kissmeyer-Nielsen, Munksgaard, Copenhagen, p. 581.
21. Zarling, J.M., and Bach, F.H. (1978): J. Exp. Med., 147:1334-1340.
22. Zarling, J.M., and Bach, F.H. (1979): Nature, 280:685-688.
23. Zarling, J.M., Bach, F.H., and Kung, P.C. (1981): J. Immunol., 126:375-378.
24. Zarling, J.M., Dierckins, M.S., Sevenich, E.A., and Clouse, K.A. Submitted for publication.
25. Zarling, J.M., and Kung, P.C. (1980): Nature, 288:394-396.
26. Zarling, J.M., Robins, H.I., Raich, P.C., Bach, F.H., and Bach, M.L. (1978): Nature, 274:269-271.

AUDIENCE DISCUSSION

Dr. Rosenberg: After you showed that allosensitization would generate cells lytic for the syngeneic tumor, we repeated those experiments and got the same results, plus some perplexing results. Allosensitization in the mouse generates cytotoxic cells that are lytic for syngeneic tumor when one uses a tissue culture target as you did. However, we never found lysis of fresh solid tumor cells as targets following allosensitization. In addition, normal fibroblast lines were lysed as well as the tumor tissue culture lines. Therefore, we don't know what the target antigen is, and whether it bears any importance to what would be tumor-related in vivo.

Dr. Bach: First, we cannot know whether the antigens being recognised will have import to reactions in vivo. We must be certain that cytotoxic cells play a role in immunotherapy in vivo. Some of the results I presented concerned the relationship between the alloantigens that are recognized as sensitizing determinants and the antigens subsequently recognized on the syngeneic tumors in both mouse and man. Second, I have a concern about what can be used as a "normal" autologous or syngeneic target. Utilizing fibroblasts, for instance, may well present those cells in a way that new antigenic determinants are exposed as compared with those that are on the surface of the cells from which the fibroblasts are derived as those cells exist in vivo. Third, I worry about studies that utilize cultured target cells. With regard to RBL-5, we have also performed some of these studies on RBL-5 immediately following its growth in vivo.

Dr. Fathman: I was intrigued by your V-shaped precursor frequency curve for cytolysis when you were sensitizing with BL6 strain and getting cross-reactive killing on the target RBL5 or ultimately syngeneic blasts. It's reminiscent of work from Hammerling's lab in which they've been able to show with similar CTL precursor estimates for allogeneic killing, that there is a dose-dependent appearance of cells which look at different targets on the same cells, that is on the H2K or D molecules for mouse allokilling. They can show this by using monoclonal antibodies directed at what they call clusters of antigens on these molecules. There is a time- or dose-dependent appearance of one low frequency effector which is then negated by the appearance of the second less frequent cell. Each of them look at a different target, so that you might be looking at different targets and the appearance of the second cell in Hammerling's system negates the cytolysis you saw with the first for reasons not known. It could be suppression since you're actually looking at three separate targets, all on B10A, with one of them shared on RBL5. Perhaps you're looking at the dose-dependence of suppression or the immunodominance of the effector.

Dr. Bach: All the possibilities you raise are reasonable. In regards to the interpretation of the V-shaped curve, although the presence of suppressors is an attractive hypothesis, there could be other mechanisms not involving suppressor cells. I want to stress that we test allo- and RBL5- and BL6-target killing all from the same well and obtain the patterns shown. To that extent there is a slight difference from the findings you described from Hammerling's laboratory.

Dr. Bonavida: Does a polyclonal activation take place during the allo-sensitization? What indication do you have that specific anti-tumor response is generated following allosensitization and challenge with syngeneic tumors?

Dr. Bach: Based on data of Glasebrook and Fitch, we would not expect the cytotoxic clones derived to respond to antigens that they can recognize directly. To that extent it would be very difficult to do the type of selection you propose since activation must be by presumed IL 2 which, in turn, must be produced by an alloactivated helper cell.

Dr. Bonavida: Following the original allosensitization, can you stimulate with syngeneic tumors and generate specific anti-tumor cytotoxic clones?

Dr. Bach: One could select the anti-tumor cytotoxic cells in the bulk culture by your enrichment procedure. Several years ago we attempted similar experiments in the allogeneic system and were able to enrich to some extent. Presumably if helpers stimulated in the bulk culture and the target antigen for the cytotoxic cells were there as well, then those cytotoxic clones should be selectively activated to expand.

The Potential Role of T Cells in Cancer Therapy,
edited by A. Fefer and A. Goldstein,
Raven Press, New York © 1982.

Alloimmunization of H-2-Compatible Donors for Adoptive Immunotherapy of Leukemia: Role of H-2, Mls, and Non-H-2 Antigens

Robert L. Truitt, Chiu-Yang Shih, *Alfred A. Rimm,
**Laurence D. Tempelis, and Mortimer M. Bortin

*May and Sigmund Winter Research Laboratory, Mount Sinai Medical Center, Milwaukee, Wisconsin
53201; *The Section of Biostatistics, The Medical College of Wisconsin, Milwaukee, Wisconsin 53226;
**Hematology/Oncology Section, Department of Medicine, University of Wisconsin Medical School,
Milwaukee, Wisconsin 53201*

A graft-vs-leukemia (GVL) reaction recently has been reported to occur in man following transplantation of HLA-compatible allogeneic bone marrow (18,27,28); however, this beneficial GVL effect was detected only in the presence of concurrent graft-vs-host (GVH) disease of moderate to severe intensity. Recurrent leukemia was a major complication if GVH disease was absent or mild (18,27,28). In view of these findings, it has been proposed that the transplant strategy be modified so as to increase the incidence of acute and chronic GVH disease in patients who are at high-risk of leukemia recurrence (27,28). Obviously, this is a dangerous course to pursue because of the potentially lethal consequences of GVH disease and its complications.

Using the T cell acute lymphoblastic leukemia of AKR (H-2^k, Mls^a) mice (AKR-L), we have investigated different approaches to the treatment of leukemia by allogeneic bone marrow transplantation. We demonstrated that although a GVH reaction always occurred coincident with a GVL reaction,

Supported by grants CA 18440, CA 20484, and CA 26245 from the National Cancer Institute, USDHHS, and grants from the Briggs and Stratton Corporation Foundation, the Henry W. Bull Foundation, the Elizabeth Elser Doolittle Trusts, the Evan and Marion Helfaer Foundation, the Kearney & Trecker Foundation, and the Pollybill Foundation.

RLT is a scholar of the Leukemia Society of America, Inc.

the two were clearly separable reactions (4,6,14). In particular, lymphoid cells from H-2-compatible (H-2^k) donors had no antileukemic reactivity, irrespective of the level of their GVH reactivity, unless the donors were pre-sensitized to the leukemia. As a consequence of presen-sitization the donors often acquired an unacceptable in-crease in GVH reactivity (6,14).

We recently reported that alloimmunization of H-2-compatible donors with lymphoid cells from a variety of individual or pooled allogeneic mouse strains induced sig-nificant and adoptively transferable reactivity against AKR-L (7). In most instances the level of GVL reactivity was comparable to that observed after specific tumor-immunization. Of particular relevance to clinical marrow transplantation was the finding that alloimmunization of H-2-compatible donors did not augment their GVH reactivity as measured in nonleukemic AKR mice (7,8,24,25).

The mechanism by which alloimmunization induced GVL reactivity in H-2-compatible donor mice is not known. We considered the possibility that lymphocyte activation via an H-2 or Mls-activated "allogeneic effect" might explain generation of GVL reactivity in our system. Products of the H-2 complex are known to activate strong helper T cell activity (allohelp) which can influence the magnitude of cellular immune responses through an allogeneic effect (1,10,12). Furthermore, Mls-locus products can substitute for differences in the H-2 complex in the induction of an allogeneic effect (20,22). Reported here are the results of experiments which suggest that the induction of GVL reacti-vity in the H-2-compatible donor mice was not due exclu-sively to activation of lymphocytes as a result of disparity between the donor and the alloimmunizing strain at either the H-2 complex or the Mls-locus. However, Mls-locus products may influence the strength of GVL reactivity in some donor-immunogen combinations. The possibility that other non-H-2, non-Mls alloantigenic differences between the donor and alloimmunizing strain are important for induction of GVL reactivity is discussed.

MATERIALS AND METHODS

Spleens from AKR mice bearing advanced, spontaneous leukemia (5) were the source of leukemia cells in the studies described. A fresh pool of 10-15 AKR-L spleens was used in each experiment to reduce variability in the growth pattern of AKR-L cells taken from individual mice. B10.K mice were generously provided by Dr. Donald Shreffler, St. Louis, MO, and Dl.LP mice were a gift from Dr. Gustavo Cudkowicz, Buffalo, NY. All other mice were purchased from The Jackson Laboratory, Bar Harbor, Maine.

GVL reactivity of cells from alloimmunized donors were evaluated in vivo using a bioassay that has been described in detail (3). Briefly, on day 0, 10^5 viable AKR-L cells were inoculated i.v. into lethally irradiated (8 Gy total body gamma radiation) 8-12 week old AKR "primary" hosts. One day later, as the sole antileukemic treatment, immuno-competent cells (2 x 10^7 spleen or 10^7 bone marrow plus 10^7 lymph node) from alloimmunized donors were transplanted into the AKR primary hosts. The GVL reaction was allowed to proceed for six days. To determine whether any viable leukemia cells remained, all spleen cells from each AKR primary host were transferred i.p. to an individual 8-9 week old AKR "secondary" recipient on day 7. GVL reactivity of the test cells is expressed as the proportion of leukemia-free AKR primary hosts as reflected by 90-day survival of the AKR secondary recipients. Using this protocol all but two of 508 historical and concomitant untreated control animals (i.e., mice given no cells on day 1) and all but one of 193 control animals given cells from unprimed H-2-compatible donors had leukemia as manifested by death of the AKR secondary recipients by day 53 (7,8,24-26). The theoretical and experimental bases for this bioassay and the rationale for use of the spleen as the most sensitive bio-assay organ were reported previously (3). Use of this bio-assay allowed GVL reactivity to be measured independent of radiation injury, failure to obtain engraftment, GVH disease, infections, etc. For this report we have arbitrar-ily divided the GVL reactivity of cells from alloimmunized donors into two categories; moderate to strong GVL reactiv-ity as evidenced by >54% survival of the AKR secondary at 90 days and weak or absent GVL reactivity as evidenced by survival of <34%.

For alloimmunization, H-2-compatible donors were given 2-6 weekly i.p. injections of 10^7 mixed spleen and thymus cells from various allogeneic strains of mice. Spleen cells or bone marrow plus lymph node cells from alloimmunized donors were transplanted one week after the last immuniza-tion.

RESULTS

Shown in Tables 1A and 1B are the results of several series of experiments testing the GVL reactivity of cells from H-2^k donors alloimmunized with lymphoid cells from individual allogeneic strains. The donor-immunogen combin-ations differed at H-2, Mls, both H-2 and Mls or neither H-2 nor Mls. The Mls phenotypes were based on those re-ported in the literature. In addition, we have tentatively accepted the contention of Molnar-Kimber and Sprent (19) that Mls^d and Mls^a are identical; thus, CBA/J is listed as Mls^a rather than Mls^d.

Role of H-2: Induction of GVL reactivity against AKR-L by in vivo alloimmunization of H-2^k donor mice was not

Table 1A: Effect of Mls-identity or disparity on induction of adoptively transferable reactivity against AKR (H-2^k, Mls^a) leukemia
in H-2^k donor mice alloimmunized with H-2-disparate lymphoid cells.

Group	H-2^k Donor (Mls)[*]		Alloimmunized with (H-2, Mls)[†]		GVL Reactivity[#] N Leukemia-Free at 90 Days/ N AKR Mice Tested (%)

H-2 Disparate, Mls-Disparate Combinations:

1	CBA/J	(a)[φ]	C57BL/10	(b,b)	29/35	(83)
2	CBA/J	(a)	BALB/c	(d,b)	22/29	(76)
3	CBA/J	(a)	A.CA	(f,c)	12/12	(100)
4	CBA/J	(a)	B10.P	(p,b)	10/12	(83)
5	CBA/J	(a)	SJL	(s,c)	46/74	(62)
6	CBA/J	(a)	B10.G	(q,b)	8/10	(80)
7	CBA/J	(a)	B10.D2	(d,b)	11/13	(85)
8	B10.BR	(b)	DBA/2	(d,a)	1/12	(8)

H-2 Disparate, Mls-Identical Combinations:

9	B10.BR	(b)	C57BL/10	(b,b)	1/12	(8)
10	B10.BR	(b)	BALB/c	(d,b)	0/20	(0)
11	B10.BR	(b)	B10.M	(f,b)	1/12	(8)
12	B10.BR	(b)	B10.P	(p,b)	0/11	(0)
13	C3H/He	(c)	SJL	(s,c)	2/9	(22)
14	CBA/J	(a)	DBA/1	(q,a)	8/42	(19)
15	CBA/J	(a)	DBA/2	(d,a)	4/13	(31)
16	CBA/J	(a)	D1.LP	(b,a)	3/14	(21)
17	CBA/H-T6	(b)	C57BL/10	(b,b)	4/7	(57)
18	CBA/H-T6	(b)	BALB/c	(d,b)	8/8	(100)

[*]Donor of 2 x 10^7 spleen or 10^7 bone marrow plus 10^7 lymph node cells.

[†]Donor mice were alloimmunized with 2-6 weekly i.p. injections of
10^7 spleen-thymus cells from the strains indicated.

[#]One week after the final immunization GVL reactivity of donor cells
was measured in vivo using the GVL bioassay described in the text.
All deaths were due to leukemia.

[φ]CBA/J is listed as Mls^a based on report of Molnar-Kimber and
Sprent (19).

consistently associated with either identity or disparity
between the donor and immunogen at H-2 (Tables 1A and 1B).
Alloimmunization of CBA/J mice with some H-2-disparate cells
resulted in moderate to strong levels of antileukemic reactivity (Groups 1-5); whereas, alloimmunization of B10.BR or
C3H/He mice with the same H-2-disparate haplotypes (Groups
9-13) did not. Other H-2-disparate cells failed to induce
significant GVL reactivity in either B10.BR or CBA/J mice
(Groups 8,14-16). Of particular note was the observation

that alloimmunization with cells expressing the H-2 haplotypes q,d and b induced strong GVL reactivity in CBA/J
donors when associated with B10 or BALB/c background (Groups
1,2,6,7) but weak reactivity when associated with a DBA
background (Groups 14-16). GVL reactivity was induced in a
variety of $H-2^k$ donor strains by alloimmunization with some,
but not all, H-2-identical strains (cf. Groups 19-24, 27-30,
with Groups 25,26,31-33). These data strongly indicate that
induction of significant GVL reactivity was not due exclusively to alloactivation by H-2 complex differences between
the donor and alloimmunizing strain.

Role of Mls: Generation of GVL reactivity following
alloimmunization might be due to lymphocyte activation as a
consequence of non-H-2 antigenic differences. The Mls-locus
is one of the better known lymphocyte activating determinants outside the H-2 complex (11). Therefore, we examined
the data in Tables 1A and 1B for an association between Mls-
disparity and induction of GVL reactivity. There were several Mls-identical and H-2-disparate (Groups 17,18) or H-2-
identical (Groups 27-30) donor-immunogen combinations in
which moderate to strong GVL reactivity was observed.
Overall, however, a significantly higher (P <0.01) proportion of the Mls-disparate donor-immunogen combinations (13
out of 16 combinations) resulted in moderate to strong GVL
reactivity (Groups 1-8, 19-26) as compared to Mls-identical
donor-immunogen combinations (6 out of 17 tested) (Groups 9-
18, 27-33). The association between Mls-disparity and
moderate to strong GVL reactivity was most obvious when $H-2-$
disparate strains were used for alloimmunization of the $H-2^k$
donor mice (Groups 1-8, Table 1A).

Role of Non-H-2, Non-Mls Antigens: Inasmuch as GVL reactivity was induced in donor mice when the alloimmunizing
strain was H-2 and Mls-identical (Groups 27-30) the question
arises as to whether non-H-2, non-Mls antigenic differences
between the $H-2^k$ donor and the alloimmunizing strains were
responsible for induction of GVL reactivity. Moderate to
strong GVL reactivity was generated in several $H-2^k$ donor
strains following alloimmunization with lymphoid cells which
carried the B10-background (Groups 1,4,6,7,17,21,22,27,30).
On the other hand, immunization of B10.BR or B10.K mice with
cells from C57BL/10 or B10 congenic strains consistently
failed to generate GVL reactivity (Groups 9,11,12,32,33).
These data do not conflict with an interpretation that
induction of GVL reactivity might be due to specific immunization of the $H-2^k$ donors with non-H-2 antigens shared by
the alloimmunizing strain and the AKR-L targets. Failure to
see significant GVL reactivity after alloimmunization with
tissue from mice of the DBA strains (Groups 8, 14-16) could
be due to the lack of cross-reactive antigens. Further
studies are necessary to evaluate the importance of non-H-2,
non-Mls antigens in either immunization against specific
antigens or via an allogeneic effect.

Table 1B: Effect of Mls-identity or disparity on induction of adoptively transferable reactivity against AKR ($H-2^k$, Mls^a) leukemia in $H-2^k$ donor mice alloimmunized with H-2-identical lymphoid cells.

Group	$H-2^k$ Donor (Mls)*		Alloimmunized with (H-2, Mls)[†]		GVL Reactivity[#] N Leukemia-Free at 90 Days/ N AKR Mice Tested (%)
	H-2 Identical, Mls-Disparate Combinations:				
19	CBA/J	(a)[Φ]	C3H/He	(k,c)	62/81 (77)
20	B10.BR	(b)	C3H/He	(k,c)	11/11 (100)
21	CBA/J	(a)	B10.BR	(k,b)	89/93 (96)
22	C3H/He	(c)	B10.BR	(k,b)	10/11 (91)
23	B10.BR	(b)	CBA/J	(k,a)	9/9 (100)
24	C3H/He	(c)	CBA/J	(k,a)	6/11 (55)
25	C3H/He	(c)	BRVR	(k,a)	2/10 (20)
26	B10.BR	(b)	BRVR	(k,a)	1/11 (9)
	H-2-Identical, Mls-Identical Combinations:				
27	CBA/H-T6	(b)	B10.K	(k,b)	9/9 (100)
28	B10.K	(b)	CBA/H-T6	(k,b)	5/8 (63)
29	CBA/J	(a)	BRVR	(k,a)	6/10 (60)
30	CBA/H-T6	(b)	B10.BR	(k,b)	6/11 (55)
31	B10.BR	(b)	CBA/H-T6	(k,b)	3/9 (33)
32	B10.K	(b)	B10.BR	(k,b)	1/9 (11)
33	B10.BR	(b)	B10.K	(k,b)	0/9 (0)

*, †, #, Φ See Footnotes to Table 1A.

DISCUSSION

As originally described by Katz et al. (12,13) the term allogeneic effect referred to amplification of immune responses in animals undergoing a transient GVH reaction. Subsequent studies led to a broader interpretation of the term to encompass augmentation of both T and B cell responses in various systems of alloactivation (1,10,20,22). Our interest in the allogeneic effect began with a desire to find the mechanism by which alloimmunization with cells from a variety of individual or pooled H-2-incompatible strains induced reactivity against AKR-L in mice that were allogeneic, but H-2-compatible with AKR (7).

The data reported here clearly indicate that induction of GVL reactivity in $H-2^k$ donor mice was not the result of an allogeneic effect due exclusively to incompatibility between the donor and immunogen at H-2. Likewise, on the basis of the data presented, we cannot state that induction of GVL

reactivity was due solely to alloactivation as a consequence
of incompatibility at Mls. This is consistent with our
previous observation that alloimmunization with cells from
F_1 hybrid mice ($H-2^k$ donor strain crossed with an H-2-
compatible or H-2-incompatible strain) induced GVL reactivity despite their inability to mount a transient GVH
reaction or "classical" allogeneic effect (24,26).

It is conceivable that while an allogeneic effect may not
be the mechanism responsible for induction of GVL reactivity, it influences the reaction in some donor-immunogen
combinations. Alloactivation with Mls-disparate cells has
been reported to have both positive (9,17) and negative
(15,16) effects on T cell responses. In our studies,
Mls-disparity showed a significant association with induction of moderate to strong GVL reactivity; whereas, Mls-
identity was associated with weak or absent GVL reactivity.
The lack of Mls-congenic strains hampers a thorough analysis
of the role of Mls activation.

We have been unable consistently to detect in vitro a
significant population of cytotoxic lymphocytes in the alloimmunized $H-2^k$ donors prior to transplant into the leukemic
AKR hosts (unpublished). This argues against antigen-specific immunization. A donor T cell is involved since treatment of the alloimmunized donor spleen cells with theta-
specific antiserum prior to transplant abolished the GVL
reactivity (24). Conceivably, leukemia-specific killer
cells may be generated after adoptive transfer of the alloimmunized $H-2^k$ donor cells into the leukemic AKR primary
host. The size and therapeutic effectiveness of this cytotoxic response may be influenced by the amount of allohelp
induced during alloimmunization. This in turn may be regulated by immune response genes of the $H-2^k$ donor and influenced by the alloantigenic differences (such as Mls or non-
H-2, non-Mls products) between the $H-2^k$ donor and the immunizing strain. Recently, we have been able to detect
leukemia-specific cytotoxic lymphocytes in the spleens and
lymph nodes of lethally irradiated leukemic AKR mice five to
seven days after transplant. We are in the process of
characterizing the antigenic phenotypes and target specificities of these cells. At present, we cannot completely
exclude the possibility that radio-resistant cells in the
AKR primary host may be recruited by the alloactivated donor
cells and participate in the antileukemic reaction.

Several laboratories have reported the induction of
antitumor reactivity following alloactivation in vitro and
alloimmunization in vivo (2,7,21,23,29,30). Tumors which
are susceptible to alloactivated killing by autologous or
allogeneic lymphocytes include both human and animal, solid
and disseminated tumors. The potential for using T cell
subpopulations that are alloimmunized in vivo or alloactivated in vitro for the adoptive immunotherapy of cancer

justifies a thorough analysis of animal models which can contribute to our understanding and awareness of the reactions and pitfalls involved. For leukemic patients who are candidates for bone marrow transplantation and who are at high-risk of relapse post-transplant, transplantation of cells with GVL reactivity and without GVH reactivity may help overcome the problem of recurrent leukmia without exposing these patients to the risks associated with GVH disease (7,8,18,24).

REFERENCES

1. Altman, A. and Katz, D.H. (1980): Immunol. Rev., 51: 3-34.
2. Bear, R.H., Roholt, O.A., and Pressman, D. (1980): Transplant. Proc., 12: 150-151.
3. Bortin, M.M., Rimm, A.A., and Saltzstein, E.C. (1973): Science, 179: 811-813.
4. Bortin, M.M., Rimm, A.A., Saltzstein, E.C., and Rodey, G.E. (1973): Transplantation, 16: 182-188.
5. Bortin, M.M. and Truitt, R.L. (1977): Biomedicine, 26: 309-311.
6. Bortin, M.M., Truitt, R.L., and Rimm, A.A. (1978): In: The Handbook of Cancer Immunology: Immunotherapy, (Vol. 5), edited by H. Waters, pp. 239-246. Garland STPM Press, New York.
7. Bortin, M.M., Truitt, R.L., Rimm, A.A., and Bach, F.H. (1979): Nature, 281: 490-491.
8. Bortin, M.M., Truitt, R.L., Shih, C-Y., and Rimm, A.A. (1981): In: Graft-versus-Leukemia in Man and Animal Models, edited by J.P. OKunewick and R.F. Meredith, pp. 139-156. CRC Press, Boca Raton, Florida.
9. Butler, L.D. and Battisto, J.R. (1979): J. Immunol., 122: 1578-1581.
10. Delovitch, T.L., Watson, J., Battistella, R., Harris, J.F., Shaw, J. and Paetkau, V. (1981): J. Exp. Med., 153: 107-128.
11. Festenstein, H. (1973): Transplant. Rev., 15: 62-88.
12. Katz, D.H. (1972): Transplant. Rev., 12: 141-179.
13. Katz, D.H., Paul, W.E., Goidl, E.A., and Benacerraf, B. (1971): J. Exp. Med., 133: 169-186.
14. LeFeber, W.P., Truitt, R.L., Rose, W.C., and Bortin, M.M. (1977): In: Experimental Hematology Today, edited by S.J. Baum and G.D. Ledney, pp. 403-429. Springer-Verlag, New York.
15. Lilliehook, B., Blomgren, H., Jacobsson, H., and Andersson, B. (1977): Cell. Immunol., 29: 223-231.
16. Matossian-Rogers, A. and Festenstein, H. (1977): Transplantation, 23: 316-321.
17. Matter, A. (1978): Cell. Immunol., 37: 107-117.
18. McIntyre, R. and Gale, R.P. (1981): In: Graft-versus-Leukemia in Man and Animal Models, edited by J.P. OKunewick and R.F. Meredith, pp. 1-10. CRC Press, Boca Raton, Florida.
19. Molnar-Kimber, K.L. and Sprent, J. (1981): Transplantation, 31: 376-378.

20. Panfili, P.R. and Dutton, R.W. (1978) J. Immunol. , 120: 1897-1901.
21. Parmiani, G. and Sensi, M.L. (1981): Transplant. Proc., in press.
22. Rollinghoff, M. and Wagner, H. (1975): J. Immunol., 114: 1329-1332.
23. Strausser, J.L., Mazumder, A., Grimm, E.A., Lotze, M.T., and Rosenberg, S.A. (1981): J. Immunol., 127: 266-271.
24. Truitt, R.L. and Bortin, M.M. (1981): In: Organ Transplantation: Present Status, Future Goals, edited by S. Slavin, in press. Elsevier/North Holland, Amsterdam.
25. Truitt, R.L., Bortin, M.M., and Rimm, A.A. (1980): Transplant. Proc., 12: 143-146.
26. Truitt, R.L., Shih, C-Y., Rimm, A.A., Tempelis, L.D., and Bortin, M.M. (1981): Transplant. Proc., in press.
27. Weiden, P.L., Flournoy, N., Sanders, J.E., Sullivan, K.M., and Thomas, E.D. (1981): Transplant. Proc., 15: 248-251.
28. Weiden, P.L., Sullivan, K.M., Flournoy, N., Storb, R., and Thomas, E.D. (1981): N. Engl. J. Med., 1529-1533.
29. Zarling, J.M. and Bach, F.H. (1978): J. Exp. Med., 147: 1334-1340.
30. Zarling, J.M., Robins, H.I., Raith, P.C., Bach, F.H., and Bach, M.L. (1978): Nature, 274: 269-270.

AUDIENCE DISCUSSION

Dr. Bach: You showed one Mls heterozygote involving the Mls^a haplotype and that one also did not give you a GVL. Have you tested others? Does the Mls^a in some way suppress the ability to induce a GVL reaction?

Dr. Truitt: No, we plan to do so by using (B10xDBA/1)F$_1$ hybrid. Allo-immunization of the H-2^k donor with such a hybrid should tell us whether or not the Mls^a is actually regulating the ability to respond.

Dr. Bach: Did you look at lytic units/culture/10^6 cells?

Dr. Truitt: These experiments have just been done within the last month and their design was based on Shendel's pre-emption experiment. We were trying to determine if there was a pre-emption type of situation. We couldn't find that, but in the course of those studies, we found this apparent suppression. The in vitro experiments I presented are not the best way to look at whether Mls^a is involved in suppressing the GVH response in our system. The limiting dilution cytotoxicity assays will be better. There we can quantify in vitro the number of cytotoxic cells generated in vivo.

Dr. Fathman: I am worried about the choice of two strains which have very similar background. What about the reciprocal experiment -- if you prime with DBA/1 or DBA/2 and then work with your BRVR or whatever you Mls^a mouse was -- will you see the same type of suppression, or is that something that is on the DBA/1 or DBA/2 background which has nothing to do with Mls at all?

Dr. Truitt: We are concerned that both the strains were of DBA background. We recently obtained BRVR mice which are H-2^k and supposedly Mls^a. We are now testing them. Our donor has to be H-2^k because we want a histocompatible situation. There are very few strains which are

$H-2^k$ and of the various Mls types which fit into this situation. We're testing BRVR both as the donor and as the immunizing strain. Unfortunately, there are no Mls-congenic strains available.

Dr. Rosenberg: Are the cells that are lytic the transferred cells or are host cells that withstood 800 R?

Dr. Truitt: We suspect they are the donor cells, because when we use CBA as the donor, they will kill AKR targets, but not CBA targets. We have not done Thy 1.1, 1.2 specificities to confirm that it is the donor cell. For example, spleen cells from nu/nu mice do not work in the GVL bioassay. We've never been able to induce the AKR to react against the respondent.

Dr. Rosenberg: If you do the bioassay with transferred tissues other than spleen, do you get the same answer?

Dr. Truitt: Yes. You do not have to bioassay the spleen. You can use the lymph nodes.

Dr. Mitchell: In transfer experiments, the simplest cell to demonstrate seems to be the helper T cell. That is, your may have situations in which you generate direct killer cells but when you do a transfer experiment, because of the recruitment by these inducer cells, their effect is much more amplified and you are more likely to spot them than cells that require a high ratio in order to effect their killing. I was wondering whether this is an element here.

Dr. Truitt: Yes, it's entirely possible.

Dr. Cheever: Is it possible that your original observation reflected the fact that you had a very sensitive anti-leukemic assay but a very insensitive graft-vs.-host assay?

Dr. Truitt: We have confirmed the GVH results in both adult mortality and Simonsen spleen weight-gain assays and are currently using popliteal lymph node assays. All three assays gave us the same results, that is, there was no significant augmentation of GVH reactivity after alloimmunization. The Simonsen assay, which is more sensitive, does indicate that there was a slight increase in GVH reactivity following alloimmunization, but the level was not lethal with CBA donors.

Dr. Cheever: Was it due to the same amplifer cell you hypothesized?

Dr. Truitt: We're trying to determine that.

Dr. Greenberg: In terms of the apparent suppression induced by sensitization to the Mls locus on allogeneic cells, isn't there evidence that Mls is recognized in an Ia-restricted fashion? Wouldn't that make interpretation difficult?

Dr. Truitt: Why would that make it difficult?

Dr. Greenberg: The suppression is presumably generated by priming to Mls in the context of allo-Ia on the sensitizing cell. After transferring these primed cells into an AKR mouse which expresses the Mls determinant in the context of a different H-2, why would the suppression be induced and/or expressed?

Dr. Truitt: One possibility is, as Bevan has shown with minor antigens such as H-Y, that in vivo the restriction occurs at the induction level with the H-2 of the strain being sensitized. That is, if you alloimmunize with B10 cells, which are Mls^b and $H-2^b$, the restriction occurs in vivo with $H-2^k$ and Mls^b, not $H-2^b$ and Mls^b. So it's entirely possible that H-2 restriction does occur in vivo, but the H-2 restriction is at the level of the antigen presenting cell in the animal being stiumulated.

The Potential Role of T Cells in Cancer Therapy,
edited by A. Fefer and A. Goldstein,
Raven Press, New York © 1982.

Prerequisites for Successful Adoptive Immunotherapy: Nature of Effector Cells and Role of H-2 Restriction

P. D. Greenberg, M. A. Cheever, and A. Fefer

*Division of Oncology, BB1015 Health Sciences RK-25, University of Washington,
Seattle, Washington 98195*

In vitro cytotoxicity studies have readily demonstrated that tumor
cells can be lysed by syngeneic cytotoxic T lymphocytes immune to tumor-
associated antigens. Similarly, in vivo studies of tumor protection and
tumor neutralization have demonstrated that transplanted tumor cells can
be prevented from growing in syngeneic hosts by immune T cells adoptively
transferred shortly before, with, or shortly after the inoculation of
tumor. However, attempts at immunotherapy after such antigenic tumors
have become established in the host have generally revealed that therapy
with adoptively transferred lymphocytes alone is ineffective in eradicating tumor (25). The limited ability of adoptive immunotherapy to eradicate established tumors presumably reflects negative consequences of a
growing tumor, such as a large tumor burden and induction of suppressor
cells or suppressor factors in the host (2,11). Thus, in addition to
providing or promoting immune effector cells, successful immunotherapeutic approaches have generally required that the underlying host-tumor
relationship be modified prior to adoptive transfer (2,8,10).

The Adoptive Chemoimmunotherapy (ACIT) Model

Several immunotherapy models have been developed in our laboratory in
which established disseminated syngeneic leukemias can be eradicated by
a combination of noncurative, nonlethal chemotherapy with cyclophosphamide followed by adoptively transferred immune cells (8). In these
adoptive chemoimmunotherapy models, mice are inoculated with syngeneic
leukemia intraperitoneally on day 0 (Fig. 1). Five days later, tumor
growth and dissemination can be readily demonstrated by bioassay of
peripheral blood or spleen for tumor cells (16). Mice receiving no
therapy on day 5 will shortly develop ascites, splenomegaly and lympha-
denopathy and die within 1-2 weeks. Treatment on day 5 with immune
cells alone has no apparent in vivo anti-tumor effect. Chemotherapy on
day 5 with cyclophosphamide, which has a direct tumoricidal effect (16),
prolongs survival for 2-3 weeks, but cures no mice. By contrast, therapy
on day 5 with cyclophosphamide followed in 6 hours by immune cells can
eradicate tumor and cure mice.

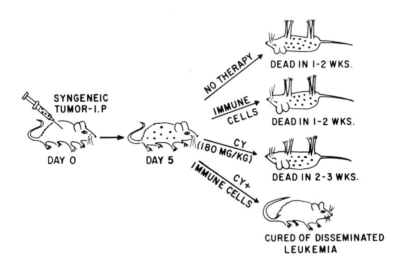

FIG. 1. Adoptive chemoimmunotherapy (ACIT). Mice are inoculated with syngeneic tumor i.p. Five days later, after tumor has disseminated to blood and spleen, mice bearing potentially lethal tumor can be cured by a combination of cydophosphamide (CY) and adoptively transferred syngeneic immune cells.

The efficacy of such ACIT in the treatment of C57BL/6 mice bearing disseminated FBL-3, a syngeneic Friend virus-induced leukemia is depicted in survival curves in Figure 2. C57BL/6 mice inoculated with 5×10^6 FBL on day 0 and left untreated all died by day 19. Therapy on day 5 with 180 mg/kg cyclophosphamide (CY) alone prolonged survival but cured no mice, whereas therapy on day 5 with CY plus 2×10^7 immune spleen cells, obtained from C57BL/6 mice which had been immunized in vivo with 3 biweekly inoculations of irradiated FBL, cured 24 of 25 mice. Several important characteristics of the immune effector population have been previously reported. Firstly, immune cells exhibit a dose-response curve in tumor therapy, in that decreasing numbers of immune cells have progressively smaller effects on prolonging survival and curing mice (4,5). Secondly, therapeutic efficacy requires specifically immune syngeneic cells. Thus, in ACIT of two non-crossreactive C57BL/6 tumors, FBL-3, a virus-induced erythroleukemia, and EL-4(G-), a chemically-induced T cell lymphoma, immune cells are effective only in therapy of the tumor to which they have been sensitized (5). Thirdly, immune

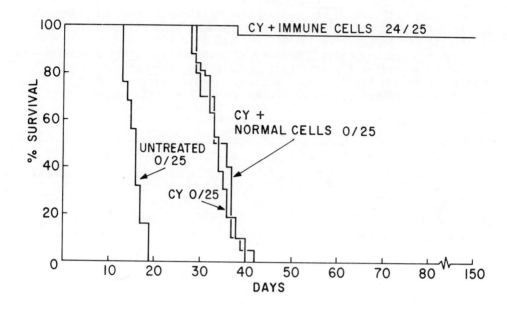

FIG. 2. Efficacy of ACIT of disseminated FBL-3. C57BL/6 mice were inoculated on day 0 with 5×10^6 FBL. On day 5, mice remained untreated,
were treated with only i.p. CY (180 mg/kg), or were treated i.p. with CY
plus either 2×10^7 normal C57BL/6 spleen cells or spleen cells immune to
FBL-3. Fractions represent mice surviving per total mice in group.

cells must be capable of proliferating in the host after adoptive transfer, in that irradiation prior to transfer abolishes the therapeutic
effects (8).
     We have examined the mechanisms by which adoptively transferred T
cells mediate tumor destruction in vivo and the factors which can promote or interfere with the in vivo therapeutic efficacy of immune cells.
Simplistically, tumor eradication following chemoimmunotherapy could
reflect destruction of a large fraction of the tumor by drug followed by
rapid killing of the residual tumor cells by infused cytotoxic donor
cells. However, this explanation of immune cell function does not
coincide with the experimental data. Immune cells obtained from donors
at a time point when no direct cytotoxicity can be demonstrated are
effective in ACIT; and, although a subpopulation of such non-cytolytic
immune cells may become cytotoxic upon reexposure to tumor in the host,
the capacity of immune cells to generate cytolytic reactivity, as
reflected by assaying in vitro tumor lysis following secondary in vitro
sensitization of in vivo primed cells, does not correlate with the

in vivo efficacy of the immune cells (6). Moreover, the cytolytic
activity of CTL contained in a population of immune effector cells
generated by secondary in vitro sensitization is not diminished by
X-irradiation with 1000 R, if measured immediately in a 4-hour CRA
(1,15), but such irradiation renders the immune population unable to
proliferate and ineffective in ACIT (Figure 3). Adoptive transfer of
$5x10^6$ immune effector cells generated by secondary in vitro sensitization, which were directly cytotoxic to tumor in vitro at the time of
adoptive transfer, significantly prolonged median survival of the
treated mice. However, irradiation with 1000 R eliminated the

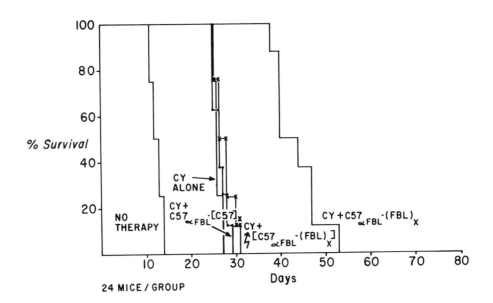

FIG. 3. Effect of irradiation on efficacy of immune cells in ACIT.
C57BL/6 mice inoculated with $5x10^6$ FBL on day 0 received either no
therapy or treatment on day 5 with CY alone, CY plus $5x10^6$ C57BL/6
spleen cells which had been primed to FBL in vivo and secondarily sensitized in vitro by 5 day co-culture with irradiated FBL ($C57_{\alpha FBL} \cdot (FBL)_x$),
CY plus in vivo primed C57BL/6 spleen cells which had been co-cultured
with irradiated syngeneic spleen cells as a control for secondary
in vitro sensitization ($C57_{\alpha FBL} \cdot (C57)_x$), or CY plus in vivo primed
C57BL/6 spleen cells which had been secondarily sensitized in vitro but
which were irradiated with 1000 R immediately prior to adoptive transfer
($\xi[C57_{\alpha FBL} \cdot (FBL)_x]$).

therapeutic potential of these immune cells, although the capacity to mediate direct in vitro tumor lysis was unaffected. These studies have served to highlight that the requirements and mechanisms operative in vivo during eradication of established tumors are not adequately or completely reflected by a 4-hour assay of in vitro cytolytic function. Subsequent studies, to be described in more detail, have identified several principles of immunotherapy which in part explain these disparities.

Requirement for a Prolonged Anti-tumor Response In Vivo

The time course of tumor elimination following curative ACIT has been examined by bioassaying the peripheral blood and spleen of curatively treated mice for the presence of tumor cells at varied intervals following therapy. Suprisingly, these studies demonstrated that curative treatment with ACIT did not reflect rapid elimination of all leukemia, but rather viable proliferating tumor cells were detectable for several weeks following therapy before being completely eliminated (16). We hypothesized that if ultimate tumor rejection is immunologically mediated, then immunosuppression of mice long after potentially curative ACIT should result in progressive tumor growth. To test this, rabbit anti-thymocyte serum, ATS, was utilized as an immunosuppressant in vivo. Prior to these in vivo therapy experiments, we confirmed, by in vitro assays, that a single inoculation of 0.04 ml of ATS into FBL-primed mice partially depleted the spleen of tumor-specific memory cells (16). The effect of ATS, given 10-14 days after adoptively transferred cells, on the outcome of ACIT was examined (Fig. 4). Therapy on day 5 with cyclophosphamide plus 10^7 immune spleen cells cured 80% of the mice. However, when such mice treated on day 5 with CY plus immune cells also received a single intraperitoneal injection of 0.04 ml of ATS on days 15, 17, or 19, a significantly increased rate of tumor recurrence and mortality was observed, with 50% of mice dying from progressive tumor. The fact that reduction in survival was only partial following ATS immunosuppression could result from incomplete removal of primed effector cells and/or participation of an additional mechanism in the eventual tumor rejection. However, the data do imply that immune cells are required to participate in tumor elimination for a period exceeding 2 weeks following adoptive transfer.

Suppression of the Efficacy of Immune Cells in ACIT by Suppressor Cells

Since ACIT requires that immune cells proliferate in the host and mediate an anti-tumor effect over a prolonged time period, the therapeutic efficacy of such immune cells might be susceptible to immunoregulation in the host. Therefore, we generated suppressor cells, demonstrated that such cells could suppress the immune response to syngeneic tumor, and examined whether these suppressor cells could interfere with immunotherapy (15). Culture-induced suppressor cells were utilized, since these T suppressor cells, which are nonspecifically induced during in vitro culture in heterologous serum, are easily generated, non-specifically suppress immune responses, and might be of importance when attempting to generate effector cells by in vitro sensitization (9,15,20).

Prior to testing in vivo, we first demonstrated that culture-induced suppressor cells could abrogate secondary in vitro sensitization of

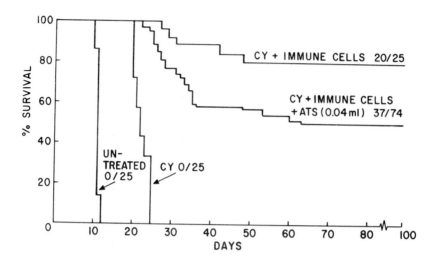

FIG. 4. Effect of in vivo immunosuppression with ATS on the outcome of ACIT. C57BL/6 mice were inoculated with 5×10^6 FBL-3 on day 0 and treated on day 5 with CY plus 10^7 immune cells. Mice receiving CY plus immune cells were either observed for development of lethal tumor, or given a single inoculation of 0.04 ml ATS i.p. between days 15 to 19. Fractions represent mice surviving per total mice in group.

spleen cells immune to FBL-tumor. Sensitization was examined in mixed leukocyte tumor culture and suppression assessed with mixing experiments (Table I). Fresh unprimed C57 spleen cells failed to generate a primary cytotoxic response. Culture-induced suppressor cells, denoted $(C57)_{CULT}$, were induced by culturing C57 spleen cells for 5 days in 5% FCS. Reculture of these cells with FBL similarly failed to generate a primary response. C57 spleen cells obtained from mice primed in vivo with irradiated FBL, denoted $C57_{\alpha FBL}$, and cultured with FBL generated a secondary response. Addition of previously cultured C57 cells at the initiation of sensitization culture suppressed the secondary response. Appropriate controls confirmed that this suppression did not merely reflect alteration of responder to stimulator ratio, dilution of effector cells, or toxicity to responder cells (15). Moreover, this suppression occurred at the level of sensitization since, in data not shown, mixing $(C57)_{CULT}$ with cytotoxic effector cells immediately prior to testing in the 4-hour CRA did not inhibit cytotoxicity (15). Thus,

Table I. Suppression of <u>in vitro</u> sensitization to syngeneic tumor[a]

CTL-Generation Culture[b]			% Specific Lysis[c]	
Responder	Stimulator	Test Population	40:1	20:1
C57	$(FBL)_x$		6	3
	$(FBL)_x$	$[C57]_{cult}$	7	3
C57	$(C57)_x$		7	4
$C57_{FBL}$	$(FBL)_x$		26	15
$C57_{FBL}$	$(C57)_x$		5	3
$C57_{FBL}$	$(FBL)_x$	$[C57]_{cult}$	9	5
$C57_{FBL}$	$(FBL)_x$	C57	27	16
$C57_{FBL}$	$(FBL)_x$	$C57_{FBL}$	34	20

[a]The data represent the means of 4 experiments.
[b]All cells were added at the initiation of 5-day culture. Cell groups are represented as C57, fresh normal C57BL/6 spleen cells; $C57_{FBL}$, fresh cells from C57BL/6 mice previously primed <u>in vivo</u> to FBL; $(FBL)_x$, FBL-3 tumor cells X-irradiated with 10,000 R; $(C57)_x$, C57BL/6 spleen cells X-irradiated with 10,000 R; $[C57]_{cult}$, normal spleen cells previously cultured for 5 days in 5% FCS.
[c]Cytotoxicity to RBL-5 was measured in a 4-hr CRA at the designated effector to target ratio.

these suppressor cells were capable of inhibiting the generation of cytotoxic cells from primed precursors, but did not affect the expression of already differentiated cytotoxic cells. Further studies have shown that the culture-induced suppressor is a T cell which is radiation-sensitive and adheres to nylon wool columns (15).

The effect of these suppressor cells on the efficiacy of immune cells in ACIT was assessed, C57BL/6 mice were inoculated with FBL on day 0 (Fig. 5). Therapy on day 5 with CY + 10^7 fresh <u>in vivo</u> primed cells cured approximately 50% of mice. However, when mice received on day 5, in addition to CY and immune cells, 5×10^6 culture-induced suppressor cells, the efficacy of therapy was significantly diminished. $(C57)_{CULT}$, when inoculated into mice treated with CY alone, had no demonstrable <u>in vivo</u> efficacy or toxicity. Thus, analogous to the suppression of <u>in vitro</u> secondary sensitization, suppressor cells can interfere with the <u>in vivo</u> anti-tumor response of transferred tumor-primed cells.

The effector population used in the above experiments, fresh spleen cells obtained from mice primed <u>in vivo</u> to FBL, is not directly cytotoxic to tumor as measured in a 4-hour CRA. Therefore, we examined whether ACIT with effector cells generated by secondary <u>in vitro</u> sensitization to FBL, which renders <u>in vivo</u> primed cells more effective in ACIT and cytotoxic <u>in vitro</u> (4), would also be affected by inoculation of suppressor cells. Therapy of disseminated FBL on day 5 with CY plus 5×10^6 immune cells generated by secondary <u>in vitro</u> sensitization significantly prolonged survival (Fig. 6). However, when mice received on day 5, in

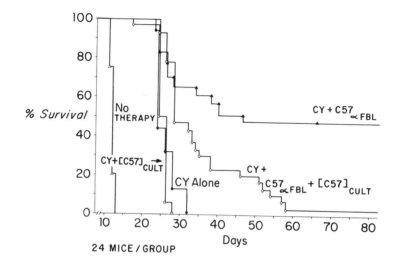

FIG. 5. Effect of culture-induced suppressor cells on ACIT of FBL with in vivo primed cells. C57BL/6 mice inoculated with 5×10^6 FBL on day 0 received either no therapy (△-△); treatment on day 5 with only CY (◆—◆CY alone); or treatment with CY plus 10^7 fresh in vivo tumor-primed cells (▲-▲ CY + C57$_{\alpha FBL}$), CY plus 5×10^6 normal cells cultured for 5 days (□—□ CY + [C57]$_{cult}$), or CY plus both 10^7 fresh tumor-primed cells and 5×10^6 cultured cells (◇—◇ CY + C57$_{\alpha FBL}$ + [C57]$_{cult}$).

addition to CY plus immune cells, an equal number of cultured C57 spleen cells by separate injection, the in vivo efficacy was significantly diminished. Thus, although culture-induced suppressor cells do not interfere with the cytolytic activity of already differentiated cytotoxic cells, these suppressor cells can interfere with the in vivo anti-tumor effect of an immune effector population containing directly cytotoxic cells.

Phenotype of Effector Cells in ACIT

The previous studies demonstrated that cells other than cytotoxic cells may influence the outcome of ACIT. Therefore, we attempted to characterize the functional T cells subsets, as determined by Lyt antigen expression, which are operative in tumor therapy (18). In general,

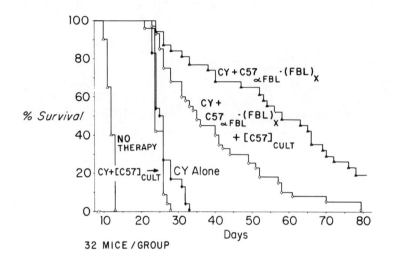

FIG. 6. Effect of culture-induced suppressor cells on ACIT of FBL with in vitro secondarily sensitized cells. C57BL/6 mice inoculated i.p. with 5×10^6 FBL on day 0 received either no therapy ($\triangle$-$\triangle$), treatment on day 5 with only CY ($\blacklozenge$-$\blacklozenge$ CY alone), or CY plus 5×10^6 normal cells cultured for 5 days ($\square$-$\square$ CY + $[C57]_{cult}$), CY plus 5×10^6 primed cells secondarily sensitized in vitro ($\blacktriangle$-$\blacktriangle$ CY + $C57_{\alpha FBL}$-$(FBL)_x$), or CY plus both 5×10^6 secondarily sensitized cells and 5×10^6 cultured normal cells ($\diamond$-$\diamond$ CY + $C57_{\alpha FBL}$ $(FBL)_x$ + $[C57]_{cult}$).

T cells can be operationally separated into Lyt 1^+2^- cells containing the helper, amplifier, and DTH effector cells, Lyt 1^-2^+ cells containing cytotoxic and suppressor cells, and an Lyt 1^+2^+ compartment containing precursors for the other T cell subsets as well as a portion of cytotoxic and suppressor cells (3,22). The T cell subsets analyzed in ACIT were defined operationally by susceptibility to lysis by monoclonal antibody to Lyt antigens. Since the source and titer of antibody and complement can influence the separation of subsets, we examined the ability of our reagents to lyse T cells of well-described phenotype. Both αLyt 1 and αLyt 2 plus complement lysed greater than 80% of fresh thymocytes, which are predominantly Lyt 1^+2^+. To analyze the phenotypes of CTL to allo-antigens and syngeneic tumors, cells from (BALB/c x C57BL/6)F_1 mice, denoted CBF, were utilized, since these mice permit maximal flexibility for future planned ACIT studies on effector cell specificity with regard to tumor and H-2 antigens. Culture of CBF spleen cells in MLC with allogeneic B10.G($H-2^q$) stimulators induced CTL which specifically recognized B10.G blast targets rather than FBL, the C57BL/6 parental strain tumor (Table II). Treatment of alloreactive effector cells immediately prior to testing in a 4-hour CRA with αThy 1.2 and complement eliminated all cytotoxicity. The majority of cytotoxic reactivity was similarly eliminated by treatment of effector cells with αLyt 2 and C, whereas depletion of Lyt 1[+] cells had only a minimal effect on cytotoxicity. Thus, as defined functionally, alloreactive CTL were predominantly of

Table II. Phenotypes of CBF_1 Cytotoxic Cells

Cytotoxicity Generation Culture[a]		Treatment[b] of Effector Cells	% Specific Lysis[c]	
Responder	Stimulator		B10.G ($H-2^q$)	FBL ($H-2^b$)
I. Allogeneic Response				
CBF	-	None	0	0
CBF	$(B10.G)_x$	None	33	2
CBF	$(B10.G)_x$	C only	31	
CBF	$(B10.G)_x$	αThy 1.2 + C	0	
CBF	$(B10.G)_x$	αLyt 1 + C	25	
CBF	$(B10.G)_x$	αLyt 2 + C	9	
II. Syngeneic anti-Tumor Response				
CBF	-	None		2
CBF	$(FBL)_x$	None		5
$CBF_{\alpha FBL}$	Not Cultured	None		0
$CBF_{\alpha FBL}$	-	None	0	3
$CBF_{\alpha FBL}$	$(FBL)_x$	None	1	53
$CBF_{\alpha FBL}$	$(FBL)_x$	C only		50
$CBF_{\alpha FBL}$	$(FBL)_x$	αThy 1.2 + C		5
$CBF_{\alpha FBL}$	$(FBL)_x$	αLyt 1 + C		27
$CBF_{\alpha FBL}$	$(FBL)_x$	αLyt 2 + C		11

[a] 60×10^6 responder cells derived from normal unprimed CBF_1 mice (CBF) or mice primed and boosted *in vivo* with irradiated FBL ($CBF_{\alpha FBL}$) were cultured with 15×10^6 irradiated allogeneic B10.G spleen cells or 3×10^6 irradiated FBL tumor cells.

[b] After 5 day culture, the potential effector cells were harvested. Prior to testing for cytotoxicity, specific cell subpopulations were depleted by incubating these cells with the denoted monoclonal antibody and C.

[c] Cytotoxicity of potential effector populations was measured in a 4-hr CRA with labeled Con A-induced B10.G spleen cell blast targets or FBL tumor cells at an effector:target ratio of 20:1. The results are the mean cytotoxicities of 4 experiments.

the Lyt 1^-2^+ phenotype. The phenotype of CTL for syngeneic tumor was similarly assessed (Table II). CBF_1 cells obtained from normal nonimmune mice did not become significantly cytotoxic after primary in vitro sensitization to FBL. Fresh, non-cultured tumor-primed spleen cells, obtained from mice which had been immunized twice in vivo with FBL, were not directly cytotoxic to tumor, but specific cytotoxic reactivity was readily detectable following 5 day in vitro sensitization of these in vivo primed cells. Treatment of the effector cells with either αThy 1.2 or αLyt 2 and C eliminated most cytotoxicity, whereas approximately 50% remained after depletion of Lyt 1^+ cells. Thus, as defined functionally, the CTL to syngeneic FBL tumor were most likely of two phenotypes, Lyt 1^-2^+ and Lyt 1^+2^+. The demonstration in our studies that Lyt 1^+2^+ cells represent a significant fraction of CTL to syngeneic tumor, but only a minor fraction of alloreactive CTL, is similar to that

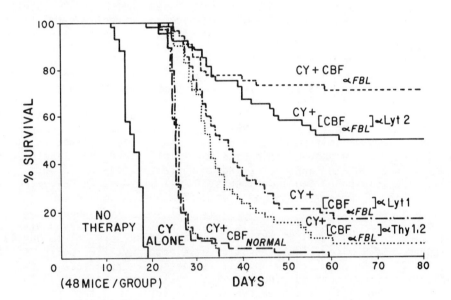

FIG. 7. In vivo efficacy of T cell subpopulations in chemoimmunotherapy of FBL. CBF_1 mice were inoculated with 5×10^6 FBL i.p. on day 0, and left untreated (——— NO THERAPY), treated on day 5 with cyclophosphamide (—··— CY ALONE), or treated with CY plus 5×10^6 CBF_1 donor cells obtained either from normal non-immune CBF_1 mice (— — CBF_{NORMAL}) or mice that had been primed and boosted in vivo with irradiated FBL. Donor immune spleen cells were used either unseparated (— — — $CBF_{\alpha FBL}$) or after depletion of subpopulations by in vitro incubation prior to adoptive transfer with complement and antibody to Thy 1.2 (······[$CBF_{\alpha FBL}$]αThy 1.2), Lyt 1 (—·—[$CBF_{\alpha FBL}$]αLyt 1), or Lyt 2 (———[$CBF_{\alpha FBL}$]αLyt 2).

reported with most conventional alloantisera (14,24,26).

The efficacy of adoptive immunotherapy with these T lymphocyte sub-populations was examined (Fig. 7). The ACIT model in CBF_1 mice is the same as in C57BL/6 mice. CBF_1 mice were inoculated ip with $5x10^6$ FBL-3 on day 0. Mice receiving no therapy died by day 19, and therapy on day 5 with cyclophosphamide alone or CY plus normal, non-immune CBF_1 spleen cells prolonged median survival time to day 26. Immune spleen cells, obtained from mice primed and boosted in vivo with FBL, were used either directly or after depletion of populations with lytic monoclonal Ab and C. Therapy with CY plus cells immune to FBL prolonged survival and cured 70% of mice. Depletion of T cells from the immune population by in vitro treatment with αThy 1.2 and C prior to adoptive transfer abrogated most of the therapeutic effect. Immune cells depleted of Lyt 1^+ cells (i.e., which contain only Lyt 1^-2^+ T cells) were ineffective in therapy, similar to immune cells depleted of all T cells. By contrast, immune cells depleted of Lyt 2^+ cells (i.e., which contain only Lyt 1^+2^- T cells) retained most of the therapeutic potential of the initial unseparated population. It should be emphasized that Lyt 1^+2^- T cells are not cytolytic and are not capable of becoming directly cytolytic to tumor. Therefore, the in vivo anti-tumor effect must be mediated either by cooperation with another cell type or secretion of a cell product.

Preliminary experiments have been performed using T cells subsets positively selected on the FACS. Unfortunately, since the cell yield obtained from sorting is low, only a small number of mice receiving a low dose of potential effector cells have been studied -- thus only limited conclusions can be drawn. However, the results are consistant with the studies analyzing negatively selected populations. Prior to sorting, spleen cells from CBF_1 mice immunized in vivo 3 times to FBL were passed over nylon wool to enrich for T cells, and then labeled with fluorescein-conjugated anti-Lyt 2 and/or rhodamine-conjugated anti-Lyt 1. The results of two experiments of ACIT of FBL-3 in CBF_1 mice are shown in Fig. 8. Treatment on day 5 with CY alone prolonged median survival to day 26. Therapy on day 5 with CY and $5x10^5$ nonadherent immune unselected CBF_1 spleen cells cured 5 of 9 mice. Therapy with CY plus $5x10^5$ selected Lyt 1^+2^- cells prolonged median survival to day 49 and cured 2 of 7 mice. Thus, positively selected Lyt 1^+2^- cells, similar to Lyt 1^+2^- cells obtained by negative selection, were effective in eradicating tumor in vivo. Therapy with equal numbers of Lyt 1^+2^+ cells, a subpopulation which was shown to be lytic in vitro, had an apparently smaller but detectable in vivo anti-tumor effect.

In these experiments positively selected Lyt 1^-2^+ cells were not examined since all T cells expressed at least some Lyt 1 antigen by this sensitive immunoflourescence technique. However, in a concurrent control group, therapy with Lyt 1^+2^- immune cells obtained by negative selection with Lyt 2 antibody and complement were again ineffective as an adjunct to CY.

The results of positive and negative selection studies demonstrate that the major effector population required for in vivo therapy has the Lyt 1^+2^- phenotype and is not cytolytic in vitro. The Lyt 1^+2^+ and Lyt 1^-2^+ T cell subsets, which are cytolytic in vitro, may provide slight additive effects but are not essential. The potential mechanisms by which Lyt 1^+2^- T cells can promote in vivo eradication of established FBL tumor must reflect one or several of the T effector functions characterized by this subset -- helper cells for antibody responses,

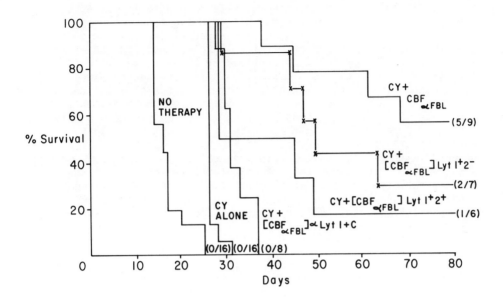

FIG. 8. In vivo efficacy of positively-selected T cell populations in ACIT of FBL. CBF₁ mice were inoculated with 5×10^6 FBL on day 0, and left untreated (No therapy), treated on day 5 with cyclophosphamide (CY alone), or treated with CY plus 5×10^5 CBF₁ donor cells obtained from mice that had been immunized three time in vivo with irradiated FBL. Donor immune cells were passed over nylon wool columns, and the non-adherent cells were used either unseparated ([CBF$_{\alpha FBL}$]), after depletion of Lyt 1⁺ cells by in vitro incubation with αLyt 1 and complement ([CBF$_{\alpha FBL}$]αLyt 1 + C), or after positive selection on the FACS. Prior to sorting on the FACS, immune cells were incubated with fluoresceinated-αLyt 2 antibody and rhodaminated-Rabbit-anti-arsanilate plus arsanilated-αLyt 1 antibody. Cells were then selected for bright luminescence in the rhodamine and negative luminescence in the fluorescein channel ([CBF$_{\alpha FBL}$]Lyt 1⁺2⁻) or brightness in both channels ([CBF$_{\alpha FBL}$]Lyt 1⁺2⁺). Cells not bright for Lyt 1 (rhodamine) were rejected. Fractions represent the number of mice surviving/group from 2 experiments.

initiators of DTH responses, and amplifiers of CTL responses. A critical requirement for in vivo amplification of an effector cell population would be consistant with our previous studies in the ACIT model, which have demonstrated the necessity for proliferation and a prolonged anti-tumor effect in vivo.

The potential of Lyt 1⁺2⁻ T cells to amplify the generation of CTL in vivo was indirectly assessed using techniques for in vitro

generation of CTL (Table III). The cytotoxicity generated to alloantigens and syngeneic tumor in standard MLC and MLTC using unseparated
responder CBF_1 spleen cells was compared to the cytotoxicity generated
in cultures using CBF_1 responder cells depleted of Lyt 1^+ cells prior to
in vitro sensitization and to the cytotoxicity generated in cultures
with such Lyt 1^+ cell-depleted cultures but to which a supernatant
containing IL2, a T cell growth factor, was added at the initiation of
culture. This factor, produced by Lyt 1^+2^- T cells, has been shown to
reconstitute the amplifier function provided by Lyt 1^+2^- cells in the
generation of cytotoxic responses (19,30). Unfractionated responder
spleen cells generated significant alloreactive cytotoxicity following
stimulation by $H-2^k$ AKR cells (Table III). Responder cells depleted of
Lyt 1^+ cells prior to in vitro sensitization failed to generate a cytotoxic response. However, when cultures with Lyt 1^+ depleted responder
cells were supplemented with IL2, most of the specific cytotoxic reactivity detected with unfractionated responder cells was restored. These
results suggest that IL2 adequately reconstituted the amplifier function
eliminated by depletion of the Lyt 1^+ population. The small diminution
of cytotoxicity could reflect elimination of a minor fraction of CTL
precursors expressing Lyt 1 antigen, since alloreactive CTL were previously shown to contain predominantly cells of the Lyt 1^-2^+ phenotype
with a small subpopulation of Lyt 1^+2^+ cells.
     The cytotoxic response to syngeneic tumor was similarly assessed. No
cytotoxicity was generated by primary in vitro sensitization, including
those cell cultures which had been depleted of Lyt 1^+ cells and supplemented with IL2. Since responder cells in this situation contain
only Lyt 1^-2^+ cells, this is consistant with a relative absence of
Lyt 1^-2^+ CTL precursors to syngeneic tumor in unprimed populations.
In vitro sensitization of CBF_1 cells previously immunized in vivo to FBL
induced a strong cytotoxic response to the syngeneic tumor target.
Depletion of Lyt 1^+ cells prior to in vitro culture prevented the
generation of a significant cytotoxic response, and addition of IL2 to
these cultures permitted only partial restoration of cytotoxicity. The
low level of cytotoxicity generated in the presence of IL2 was specific
for the tumor target. The ability of IL2 to only restore a fraction of
the cytotoxic potential of unseparated cells is consistent with our
previous results demonstrating that, unlike alloreactive CTL, a significant fraction of CTL and/or CTL presursors to syngeneic tumors are
eliminated by αLyt 1 and complement. However, despite this limitation
which resulted in the generation of only low levels of cytotoxicity, the
results suggest that Lyt 1^+ cells, or a product derived from these
cells, can augment the in vitro generation of cytotoxic responses to
syngeneic tumor. Perhaps more importantly, depletion of Lyt 1^+ cells
prevented the generation of significant cytotoxicity. Since our studies
in ACIT demonstrated that Lyt 1^+2^- cells are critical for therapeutic
efficacy in immunotherapy, these Lyt 1^+2^- cells may similarly be required
in vivo to permit sufficient expansion and expression of cytotoxic cells
to mediate a significant anti-tumor effect. Of particular note, if
Lyt 1^+2^- cells, which are devoid of CTL and CTL precursors do in fact
function in vivo by amplifying CTL induction, then adoptively transferred cells must be capable of inducing the host to make a positive
contribution to the outcome of therapy by providing the necessary CTL
precursors.
     These studies have confirmed that the mechanisms operative in vivo
which determine if an immune population can effect tumor eradication are

Table III. CTL Responses in Lyt 1$^+$-Depleted Populations

Cytotoxicity Generation Culture[a]			Addition[b] to Culture	% Specific Lysis[c]	
Responder	Pre-culture Treatment	Stimulator		AKR (H-2^k)	FBL (H-2^b)
I. Allogeneic Response					
CBF	None	-		0	0
CBF	None	(AKR)$_x$		25	0
CBF	αLyt 1 + C	-		0	
CBF	αLyt 1 + C	(AKR)$_x$		1	
CBF	αLyt 1 + C	-	IL2	2	0
CBF	αLyt 1 + C	(AKR)$_x$	IL2	20	1
II. Syngeneic Anti-tumor Response					
CBF	None	-		0	0
CBF	None	(FBL)$_x$		0	0
CBF	αLyt 1 + C	-			0
CBF	αLyt 1 + C	(FBL)$_x$			0
CBF	αLyt 1 + C	-	IL2	2	1
CBF	αLyt 1 + C	(FBL)$_x$	IL2	2	0
CBF$_{αFBL}$	None	-		0	0
CBF$_{αFBL}$	None	(FBL)$_x$		0	27
CBF$_{αFBL}$	αLyt 1 + C	-			0
CBF$_{αFBL}$	αLyt 1 + C	(FBL)$_x$			2
CBF$_{αFBL}$	αLyt 1 + C	-	IL2	1	0
CBF$_{αFBL}$	αLyt 1 + C	(FBL)$_x$	IL2	0	9

[a]Responder cells, derived from normal unprimed CBF$_1$ mice (CBF) or mice primed and boosted <u>in vivo</u> with irradiated FBL (CBF$_{αFBL}$), were either used directly without pretreatment, or were depleted of Lyt 1$^+$ cells by incubation with αLyt 1 and C prior to <u>in vitro</u> sensitization. These cells were washed and then placed into culture with irradiated allogeneic AKR spleen cells or irradiated FBL at Responder:Stimulator ratios of 4:1 and 20:1 respectively.

[b]Partially purified supernatants containing IL2 were added to the designated responder-stimulator combinations at the initiation of 5 day culture at a final dilution of 1:10.

[c]After 5 day culture, effector cells were harvested and washed. Cytotoxicity was measured in a 4-hr CRA with labeled Con A-induced AKR spleen cell blast targets or FBL tumor cells at an E:T ratio of 20:1.

distinct from and more complex than the requirements that can be derived by studying in vitro tumor lysis by effector populations in short term cytotoxicity assays. However, these studies do not imply that CTL can have no in vivo function, or that insights learned from analyzing in vitro cytotoxicity are unimportant in therapy.

H-2 Restriction of ACIT

One fundamental immunologic principle which has evolved largely from analysis of in vitro cytotoxicity assays is that of H-2 restriction of lymphocyte-tumor interactions. According to the rules of H-2 restriction, T cells are sensitized to tumor antigens in association with the major histocompatability antigens expressed on the tumor cells, and subsequently will lyse in vitro only tumor targets which express both the tumor and H-2 antigens of the sensitizing tumor cell (31). However, prolongation of in vitro assays to permit 12 to 20 hours for lysis has revealed apparent antigen-specific non-restricted lysis of tumor targets (i.e. targets sharing the tumor-associated antigen but disparate at H-2), as well as a requirement for a T amplifier cell for maximal expression of cytotoxicity (12,21,23,27,28,29). In many respects, these long-term assays appeared more analagous to the conditions operative during in vivo therapy than short-term cytotoxicity assays. Therefore, we examined whether H-2 restriction of lymphocyte-tumor interactions is important in vivo for eradication of established tumors.

To test the in vivo role of H-2 restriction, ACIT of tumors which differ at H-2 but which share tumor-associated antigens and are not

Table IV. H-2 Restricted Lysis of FMR Tumors By CBF Cells[a]

Mixed Leukocyte Tumor Culture[b]		% Specific Lysis[c]			
		RBL ($H-2^b$)		LSTRA ($H-2^d$)	
Responder	Stimulator	20:1	5:1	20:1	5:1
$CBF_{\alpha msv}$	$(FBL)_x$	61	27	7	2
$CBF_{\alpha msv}$	$(LSTRA)_x$	5	3	52	25
$CBF_{\alpha msv}$	-	3	1	2	1
CBF	$(FBL)_x$	8	3	13	3
CBF	$(LSTRA)_x$	2	1	23	14
CBF	-	1	1	8	3

[a]The data represent the means of 4 experiments.

[b]60×10^6 responder CBF_1 spleen cells derived from MSV-primed mice ($CBF_{\alpha msv}$) or normal unprimed mice (CBF) were cultured without stimulation, with 3×10^6 irradiated FBL, or with 1.5×10^6 irradiated LSTRA.

[c]After 5-day culture, the nylon wool nonadherent cells were tested in a 4-hr CRA for cytotoxicity to the $H-2^b$ and $H-2^d$ FMR tumor targets at effector to target ratios of 20:1 and 5:1. RBL-5, a Rauscher virus-induced leukemia of C57BL/6 origin was used as the $H-2^b$ target since it releases less chromium spontaneously and is more sensitive to lysis than is FBL-3.

allogeneic to the host or donor was studied. The tumors used, FBL-3 and
RBL5 of C57BL/6 origin and LSTRA of BALB/c origin, were induced respectively by Friend, Rauscher and Moloney viruses, and express FMR
tumor-associated antigens which cross-react with each other and other
FMR tumors (7, 13). CBF_1 mice bearing a disseminated parental strain
FMR tumor served as the host for ACIT. To obtain effector cells, donor
CBF_1 mice were inoculated with Moloney sarcoma virus, which induces a
spontaneously regressing tumor that cross-reacts with transplantable FMR
tumors. The MSV-primed CBF_1 spleen cells were secondarily sensitized
in vitro for 5 days with parental strain FMR tumors, enriched for
T cells by passage over nylon wool, and then tested in ACIT and for
in vitro cytolytic activity in a 4-hour CRA. MSV-primed cells secondarily sensitized with FBL, the $H-2^b$ tumor, preferentially lysed the
$H-2^b$ FMR tumor target (Table IV). Primed cells sensitized with LSTRA

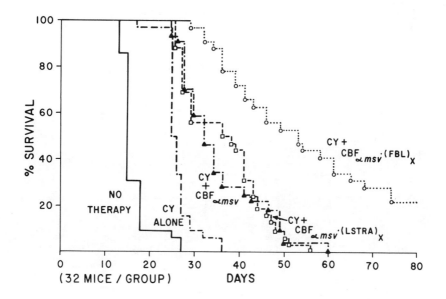

FIG. 9. H-2 restricted efficacy of immune cells in ACIT of FBL-3. CBF_1
mice were inoculated with 5×10^6 FBL i.p. on day 0, and left untreated
(———, no therapy), treated on day 5 with CY (—·—, CY alone) or
treated with CY plus 1×10^7 immune cells. Donor cells were MSV-primed
CBF_1 spleen cells that had been cultured for 5 days without stimulation
(▲--▲, $CBF_{\alpha msv}$ cultured), or secondarily sensitized in vitro to FBL
(o····o, $CBF_{\alpha msv}$ $(FBL)_x$) or to LSTRA (□---□, $CBF_{\alpha msv}·(LSTRA)_x$), and
passaged over nylon wool before adoptive transfer.

preferentially lysed the $H-2^d$ tumor target. MSV-primed cells cultured without a stimulator cell were only minimally cytotoxic to either target. Normal unprimed CBF_1 cells were significantly less cytotoxic then MSV-primed cells following <u>in vitro</u> sensitization. Therefore, MSV primed CBF_1 mice to FMR tumors of both parental strains, but secondary <u>in vitro</u> sensitization induced CTL with lytic activity restricted to target cells sharing FMR and H-2 antigens with the stimulating tumor cells.

These secondarily sensitized CBF_1 cells were tested in ACIT of disseminated tumors in CBF_1 hosts (Fig. 9). Therapy of FBL on day 5 with cyclophosphamide alone prolonged median survival to day 25. Therapy on day 5 with CY plus 10^7 MSV-primed CBF_1 spleen cells further prolonged median survival to day 32. Therapy with spleen cells secondarily sensitized <u>in vitro</u> to LSTRA was no more effective than with the MSV-primed cells cultured without stimulation. However, therapy with CY plus cells secondarily sensitized to FBL significantly extended median survival to day 53. Thus, secondary <u>in vitro</u> sensitization with FBL but not LSTRA rendered MSV-primed cells more effective in chemoimmunotherapy of FBL.

Reciprocal experiments for ACIT of disseminated LSTRA in CBF_1 mice

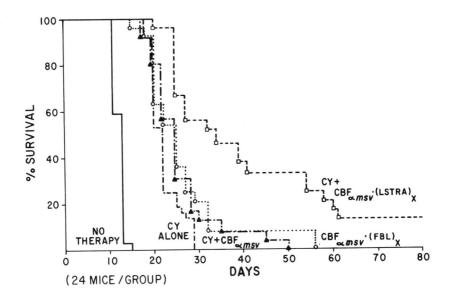

FIG. 10. H-2 restricted efficacy of immune cells in ACIT of LSTRA. CBF_1 mice were inoculated with 2×10^5 LSTRA i.p. on day 0 and left untreated (——, no therapy), treated on day 5 with CY (—·—, CY alone) or with CY plus 1×10^7 immune cells. Immune CBF_1 donor cells were derived from the same groups of nylon wool nonadherent cells used in Table I and Figure 1.

revealed analagous results (Fig. 10). Day 5 therapy with CY alone
prolonged median survial to day 22. Therapy on day 5 with CY plus MSV-
primed cells cultured without stimulation or secondarily sensitized to
FBL were no more effective than CY alone. Therapy with CY plus primed
cells secondarily sensitized to LSTRA was significantly more effective
than all other treatment groups. Thus, eradication of established
tumors by adoptively transferred lymphocytes results from H-2 restricted
lymphocyte-tumor interactions.

Conclusions

In summary, we have examined some of the principles underlying
successful immunotherapy of established tumors. Several conclusions can
be drawn:
1) Tumor therapy is mediated by specifically immune H-2 restricted
T lymphocytes.
2) Tumor eradication requires a prolonged in vivo anti-tumor response.
3) As a result of this requirement for a prolonged response, the
immune effector cells are susceptible to positive and negative influences
during an extended time period.
4) Successful therapy is mediated in large part by adoptive transfer
of non-cytolytic Lyt 1^+2^- T cells. The mechanism by which these T cells
mediate tumor destruction in vivo has not yet been fully elucidated, but
it presumably requires induction or amplification of another effector
cell.

Acknowledgments

The authors wish to thank M. Bolton, S. Emery, and B. Keniston for
expert technical assistance; and J. Hoak and M. Lund for preparation of
the manuscript.

REFERENCES

1. Anderson, R.E. and Warner, N.L. (1976): Adv. in Immunology,
   26:216.
2. Berendt, M.J. and North, R.J. (1980): J. Exp. Med., 151:69.
3. Cantor, H. and Boyse, E. (1977): Contemp. Top. Immunobiol., 7:47.
4. Cheever, M.A., Greenberg, P.D. and Fefer, A. (1978): J. Immunol.,
   121:220.
5. Cheever, M.A., Greenberg, P.D. and Fefer, A. (1980): J. Immunol.,
   125:711.
6. Cheever, M.A., Greenberg, P.D., and Fefer, A. (1981): JNCI,
   67:169.
7. Fefer, A., McCoy, J.L., and Glynn, J.P. (1967): Cancer Res.,
   27:962.
8. Fefer, A., Einstein, A.B., Cheever, M.A., and Berenson, J.R. (1976):
   Ann. N.Y. Acad. Sci., 276:573.
9. Ferguson, R.M., Anderson, S.M., and Simmons, R.L. (1978):
   Transplantation, 26:331.
10. Fernandez-Cruz, E., Woda, B.A., and Feldman, J.D. (1980): J. Exp.
    Med., 152:823.
11. Fujimoto, S., Greene, M.I., and Sehon, A.H. (1976): J. Immunol.,
    116:791.
12. Gomard, E., Duprez, V., Henin, Y., and Levy, J.P. (1976): Nature,
    260:707.

13. Gomard, E. Levy, J.P., Plata, F., Henin, Y., Duprez, V., Bismuth, A., and Reme, T. (1978): Eur. J. Immunol., 8:228.
14. Green, W.R., Nowinski, R.C., and Henney, C.S. (1979): J. Exp. Med, 150:51.
15. Greenberg, P.D., Cheever, M.A., and Fefer, A. (1979): J. Immunol., 123:515.
16. Greenberg, P.D., Cheever, M.A., and Fefer, A. (1980): Cancer Res., 40:4428.
17. Greenberg, P.D., Cheever, M.A. and Fefer, A. (1981): J. Immunol., 126:2100.
18. Greenberg, P.D., Cheever, M.A., and Fefer, A. (1981): J. Exp. Med., 154:952.
19. Henney, C.S., Okada, M., and Gillis, S. (1980): Behring Inst. Mitt., 67:26.
20. Hodes, R.J. and Hathcock, K.S. (1976): J. Immunol., 116:167.
21. Holden, H.T. and Herberman, R.B. (1977): Nature, 268:250.
22. McKenzie, I.F.C. and Potter, T. (1979): Adv. Immunol. 27:179.
23. Plata, F., Jongeneel, V., Cerottini, J.-C., and Brunner, K.T. (1976): Eur. J. Immunol., 6:823.
24. Roehm, N.W., Alter, B.J., and Bach, F.H. (1981): J. Immunol., 126:353.
25. Rosenberg, S.A. and Terry, W.D. (1977): Adv. in Cancer Res., 25:323.
26. Shiku, H., Takahashi, T., Bean, M.A., Old, L.J., and Oettgen, H.F. (1976): J. Exp. Med., 144:1116.
27. Stutman, O. and Shen, F-W. (1978): Nature, 276:181.
28. Stutman, O., Shen, F-W, and Boyse, E.A. (1977): Proc. Natl. Acad. Sci. 74:5667.
29. Ting, C-C and Law, L.W. (1977): J. Immunol., 118:1259.
30. Wagner, H., Hardt, C., Heeg, K., Pfizenmaier, K., Solbach, W., Bartlett, R., Stockinger, H., and Röllinghoff, M. (1980): Immunolog. Rev., 51:215.
31. Zinkernagel, R.M. and Doherty, P.C. (1979): Adv. Immunol., 27:51.

AUDIENCE DISCUSSION

Dr. Altman: In the experiments on the effect of culture-induced suppressor cells on tumor immunity, it is possible that these nonspecifically activated cells are mediating suppression by competing with tumor specific CTL precursors for T cell helper factors rather than by a direct suppressive effect. Have you attempted to overcome this nonspecific suppression by supplementing with exogenous IL 2?

Dr. Greenberg: That is an interesting hypothesis. However, although it might be possible to override nonspecific suppression in vitro by providing excess nonspecific help with IL 2, I'm not sure this would elucidate the mechanism by which suppression is mediated either in vitro or in vivo.

Dr. Altman: In the immunotherapy experiments, it is possible that the Lyt 1⁺2⁻ cells are more effective in vivo because they have a more prolonged life span than the Lyt 1⁻2⁺ CTL, which may be terminally differentiated. Can you make the Lyt 1⁻2⁺ CTL more effective in therapy if you inject them several times over an extended time period rather than only once?

Dr. Greenberg: The question of whether or not adoptively transferred CTL can mediate an antitumor effect against established tumors is critical to resolve. The experiments you mentioned have already been planned. The problem may be related to survival of the transferred cells. Studies from Cantor's laboratory have shown that Lyt 1^+2^+ precursors and CTL have a longer lifespan than Lyt 1^-2^+ cells, and, in the positive selection experiments we performed, a significant antitumor effect was noted with positively selected doubly-positive cells.

Dr. Bach: With regard to the studies examining the activity of Lyt 1 and Lyt 2 cells, after treatment of unfractionated cells with αLyt 2 serum, the remaining cells retained a small amount of residual cytotoxicity to your tumor target. Although you seem to be stressing that the Lyt 1^+2^- population is working by a noncytotoxic mechanism, there is an alternative explanation. Several laboratories have demonstrated that cells cytotoxic to Class II antigens may be of the Lyt 1^+2^- phenotype. Similarly, we have demonstrated that CTL to human Ia antigens are of the OKT 4^+8^- phenotype. Since you have residual cytolytic activity after depletion of Lyt 2^+ cells, is it possible that the _in vivo_ activity results from Lyt 1^+2^- cells lytic for Class II antigens?

Dr. Greenberg: Although that is possible, it should be noted that we are clearly enriching for a therapeutic effect by selecting Lyt 1^+2^- cells. It would be surprising if _in vivo_ efficacy is mediated by a small fraction of the CTL, which exhibit _in vitro_ activity for a small repertoire of the antigens on the tumor cells. However, we need to examine positively selected Lyt 1^+2^- T cells for residual cytotoxicity and the specificity of such cytotoxicity.

Dr. Ihle: Your H-2 restriction studies primarily rely on the use of RBL and LSTRA. Since the predominant target antigens for cytotoxicity would normally be the viral antigens, it should be noted that the products of Rauscher and Moloney viruses vary considerably, as reflected by sequence analysis. Have you taken the viruses and put them in different cells to make sure that the restrictions still exist at that level?

Dr. Greenberg: No. However, we have shown that _in vivo_ priming of CBF_1 mice with any one of these FMR parental tumors results in cross-priming to the other FMR tumors. Thus, there is little question that they express crossreactive FMR antigens and should thus be reasonable tumors for H-2 restriction analysis.

[Unidentified]: Although the Lyt 1^+2^- T cells may be functioning in therapy by amplifying CTL, is it not also possible that these cells are augmenting the reactivity of non T cells such as natural killer cells or macrophages by production of lymphokines such as interferon or MAF?

Dr. Greenberg: The precise mechanisms by which Lyt 1^+2^- cells promote tumor eradication are not yet defined. McKenzie showed that rejection of skin allografts is mediated by a DTH mechanism rather than CTL, and potentially, tumor eradication may be mediated by similar mechanisms.

Dr. North: In your models, it would seem likely that the effect of cyclophosphamide is not just reduction of the number of tumor cells, but that it also modifies host suppressor cells which interfere with immunotherapy.

Dr. Greenberg: We have done bioassay experiments which have demonstrated that cyclophosphamide clearly has a significant direct antitumor effect, but we have not yet sufficiently analyzed what effect it has on underlying host tumor immunity. However, experiments are planned using positively-selected T cells from tumor-bearing and cyclophosphamide-treated tumor-bearing mice to analyze this question.

The Potential Role of T Cells in Cancer Therapy,
edited by A. Fefer and A. Goldstein,
Raven Press, New York © 1982.

Immunotherapy of Progressive Tumors with T Cell Subsets

E. Fernandez-Cruz and J. D. Feldman

Department of Immunopathology, Scripps Clinic and Research Foundation, La Jolla, California 92037

In this presentation we shall describe some of the recent data we have obtained studying the cellular mechanisms involved in the immune response to two syngeneic tumors in a rat model system. We shall discuss data related to the generation of anti-tumor effector cells in vitro and to the analysis and phenotypic characterization of the effector cell populations. We shall also present results on the successful elimination of established tumors in vivo by treatment with T cell subsets.

MATERIALS AND METHODS

First, we will describe the tumors we have used in our system. One of the sarcomas is a Moloney sarcoma tumor (MST) induced in a neonatal BN rat by inoculation of Moloney sarcoma virus from a mouse spleen. This tumor expresses, on its surface, virus, the viral antigens gp 70 and p30 and the histocompatibility antigens of the BN rat. A dose of 5×10^4 tumor cells inoculated subcutaneously into a BN adult rat is fatal in 30-40 days (4). The other tumor is a sarcoma induced in a BN rat by injection of methylcholanthrene (BC5). BC5 tumor cells express tumor associated-antigens and RT1 BN histocompatibility antigens. Murine leukemia virus or rat virus antigens are not detectable on its surface. 1×10^5 BC5 cells inoculated subcutaneously into a BN rat is lethal within 50 days.

The effector cells are generated in vitro in a mixed lymphocyte-tumor culture (MLTC) over a period of seven days (1). We remove spleens from donor animals that have been immunized with the MST or BC5. For controls spleens are removed from donor rats that have been inoculated with an irrelevant tumor, or removed from normal unmanipulated rats. The spleen cells are then incubated in the MLTC with the original immunogen (tumor) treated with mitomycin-C (1×10^7 tumor cells with 100 µg Mit.C/ml). After 7 days MLTC cells are harvested, analyzed for surface markers, and transferred intravenously to a recipient animal.

The in vivo assay animal is a BN rat 3-4 months old, 150-170 gm, either x-rayed with 400R or unmanipulated, bearing at the time of the treatment a subcutaneous inoculum of BC5 or MST, approximately 1 cm in diameter by day 6, with an established blood supply.

RESULTS

In the viral induced MST system 5×10^7 immune spleen cells, cultured <u>in vitro</u> in an MLTC, and transferred intravenously into a recipient bearing an established MST tumor, 1 cm in diameter, eliminates
the tumor within 35 days. Adoptive transfer successfully eliminates MST
in x-rayed and normal recipients (1).

Figure 1 illustrates that relatively large established MST can be
eliminated in test rats. We allowed the MST to grow for 12 days, to
2.5-3 cm in diameter, or 18-20 days, to 4-6 cm in diameter, about 4-6
gm. The 12-day growth curve shows that 3×10^8 immune spleen cells of
a 7-day MLTC were necessary to eliminate a 3 cm tumor, over a period
of 60 days; the 18-day growth curve shows that 1.5×10^9 immune spleen
cells, given in 4 infusions, were needed to eliminate a 6 cm in diameter
tumor over a period of 100 days. Both curves reveal that despite infusion of a large number of effector cells, a period of time is required before regression is recognizable and that the larger the tumor
load at the time of the treatment the greater the number of effector
cells that were required to eliminate the tumor. Controls show linear
growth of MST with death of the recipients within 30 days.

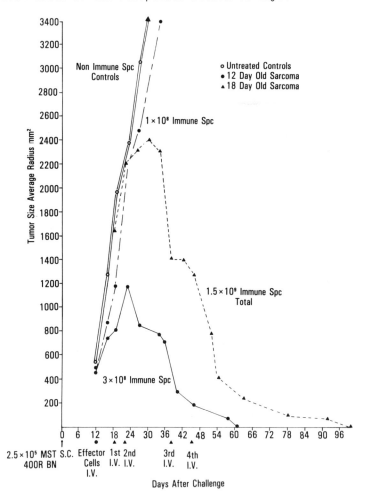

FIG. 1.

Figure 2 presents one of the rats with an 18-day tumor: A) at the start of the treatment and; B) after treatment wit- 1.5 x 10^9 immune spleen cells, 100 days later. We have followed a number of treated animals for longer than two years and have observed no recurrence.

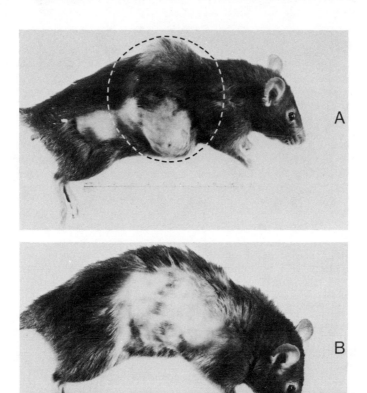

FIG. 2. Photograph showing: (A) an assay rat bearing a lethal sub-cutaneous MST-1 sarcoma, 6 cm in diameter, on day 27 after tumor inoc-ulation. The test rat was treated with repeated intravenous infusions of effector spleen cells (total = 1.5 x 10^9), beginning on day 18 after inoculation of tumor; (B) elimination of the tumor 98 days after tumor inoculation and 80 days after infusion of effector cells. Reprinted from Fernandez-Cruz et al, (2), 1980. The Rockefeller University Press.

FIG. 1. Elimination of malignant sarcomas, 2.5-7 cm in diameter, by in-fusion of effector immune spleen cells. Assay rats bearing a 12-day old sarcoma (o) were treated with a single infusion of effector cells and assay rats bearing an 18-day old malignancy were treated with repeated infusions (▲) of effector cells. Data are pooled from three separate experiments. Each point of the experimental groups represents the mean of 6 assay rats and each point of the control curves is the mean of 15 control assay rats (o). Reprinted from Fernandez-Cruz, et al., (2), 1980. The Rockefeller University Press.

Phenotypic markers of the effector cells generated in the MLTC were studied (2). We used three monoclonal anti-rat T cell antibodies, W3/13, W3/25 and OX8, to identify T cells (W3/13) and T cell subsets (the helper-W3/25 and the cytotoxic/suppressor OX8) (5); a monoclonal anti-rat Ia antibody to detect Ia antigens; and F(ab')$_2$ fragments of a polyvalent goat antibody to the rat immunoglobulins to detect surface immunoglobulins.

Table I shows the composition of effector cells in MLTC derived from spleens of normal donors, spleens of rats that have a progressive tumor, and spleens from immune animals that have rejected tumor. Most importantly, at the end of 7 days only in MLTC with immune spleen cells was there an increase in the number of T cells. 55% of the cells were T cells by W3/13 marker and 50% by W3/25 marker. The yield at the end of 7 days of culture was 40-50% of the original number of spleen cells. 70% of the elements in MLTC were blast cells and 60% of those blasts displayed Ia antigens. Interestingly, 55% of total T cells were blast cells and Ia+ (Table II). In addition, Ig+ cells were decreased to 25%, null cells were 18%, and tumor cells and macrophages were less than 1%. In all other MLTC, derived from control spleens, the composition of effector cells after 7 days in culture was not statistically significantly different from the composition of day 0 cultures (Tables I and II).

Table 1.　Surface Markers on Uncultured and Day 7 MLTC Cells[a]

Uncultured Spleen Cells (Day 0)	T (W3/13+) %	T (W3/25+) %	Ig+ %	T-Ig-[b] %
Normal Spleens	45 + 1 (4)[c]	38 + 1 (4)	48 + 2 (4)	7
Progressor Spleens	46 + 2 (4)	34 + 2 (4)	46 + 1 (4)	8
Regressor Spleens	46 + 1 (4)	38 + 1 (4)	45 + 1 (4)	9
Day 7 MLTC Cells				
Normal Spleens	39 + 3 (3)	35 + 3 (3)	31 + 2 (2)	30
Progressor Spleens	37 + 3 (3)	35 + 3 (3)	39 + 2 (2)	24
Regressor Spleens	57 + 3 (6)	50 + 3 (6)	24 + 6 (4)	19
P[d]	P = <0.02	P <0.02	P <0.02	

[a] 3×10^6 uncultured and day 7 MLTC spleen cells were stained with fluorescein labeled goat anti-rat-Ig (Fl-GARG), monoclonal mouse anti-W3/13 or anti-W3/25 followed by fluorescein labeled goat anti-mouse-IgG (Fl-GAMG). 1×10^5 viable cells were analyzed for fluroescence intensity in a FACS IV.

[b] Determined by substracting from 100% of the total number of T cells (W3/13+) and B cells (Ig+).

[c] Number of trials in parenthesis.

[d] P value was calculated by student's t-test and compared uncultured (day 0) regressor spleen cells and day 7 MLTC regressor spleen cells.

Table II. Surface Markers on Uncultured and Day 7 MLTC Cells

Uncultured Spleen Cells (Day 0)	Ia+ %	T (W3/13+) Ia+ %	T (W3/25+) Ia+ %
Normal Spleens	27 + 1 (12)	3 + 7 (7)	2 + 1 (7)
Progressor Spleens	28 + 1 (2)	4 + 1 (2)	4 + 1 (2)
Regressor Spleens	29 + 1 (2)	5 + (2)	4 + 1 (2)
Day 7 MLTC Cells			
Normal Spleens	18 (1)	1 (1)	2 (1)
Progressor Spleens	21 + 2 (2)	5 + (2)	4 + 2 (2)
Regressor Spleens	58 + 4 (5)	54 + 7 (4)	55 + 2 (2)
P	P < 0.01	P < 0.01	P < 0.01

For the determination of Ia+ cells and Ia+ T cells, 3 x 10⁶ cells were stained with monoclonal anti-W3/13 or anti-W3/25 and rhodamine labeled-GAMG followed by Fl-anti-Ia. The percentage of Ia+ lymphoid cells and Ia+ T cells was determined in the fluorescence microscope. Tables I and II are reprinted from Fernandez-Cruz, et al., (2), 1980. The Rockfeller University Press.

Figure 3 illustrates that most of the cells in an immune-MLTC are large blast elements (left panel). There are no tumor cells present and there are very few small lymphocytes. In control MLTC (right panel) there is a mixture of tumor cells and some small lymphocytes, but relatively few or no blast elements. The effector cells generated in control MLTC yielded 5-15% of the original number of spleen cells.

FIG. 3.

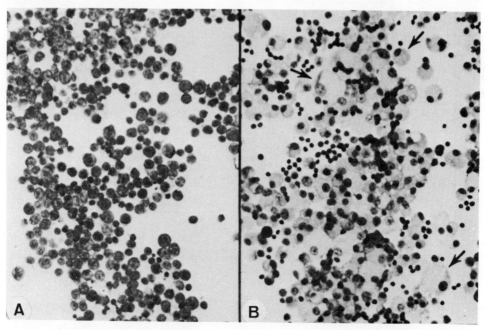

FIG. 3. (A) Photomicrograph of effector cells in 7-day MLTC containing immune spleen cells from donor with regressed tumor and MST-1mit.
Blast lymphocytes are numerous and tumor cells are rarely encountered.
Giemsa stain; cytocentrifuged preparation; X250. (B) Photomicrograph of
cells in 7-day MLTC controls. A mixture of tumor cells (arrows) and
small lymphocytes are seen. Reprinted from Fernandez-Cruz, et al., (2),
1980. The Rockefeller University Press.

We wanted to find out if the model we were working with had any
generality, or were we simply looking at an immune response peculiar to
viral-induced tumors. We decided to examine the chemically-induced
sarcoma BC5 (3). We used the same kind of protocol.
The generation of effector cells that operate in vivo in the BC5
system require stringent culture conditions, different from those used
in the viral MST system. Donor BN rats were immunized with repeated inoculations of mitomycin-treated BC5 and provided spleen cells that were
cultured with mitomycin-treated BC5 in MLTC. Immune spleen cells (Spl)
in a 7-day MLTC displayed a poor proliferative response in vitro and did
not affect tumor growth when infused into rats bearing BC5 (Fig. 4).
There was suppression of the generation of effector cells in vitro.

FIG. 4.

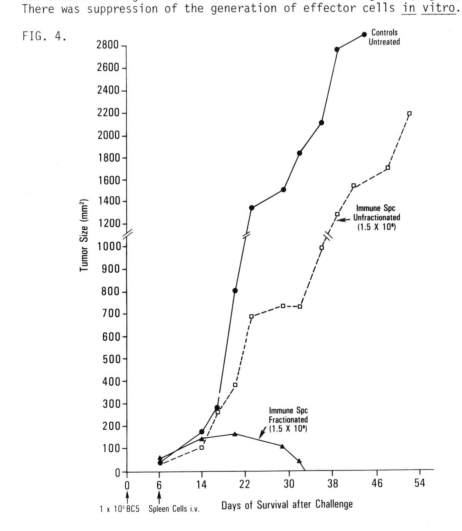

To overcome the suppression in this system, adherent spleen cells (macrophages) were depleted at the start of MLTC. Spleen cells were applied to nylon-wool packed syringes and the effluent spleen cells were further depleted of macrophages by plating on plastic culture dishes for 3-4 hours. The non-adherent population (fractionated Isp) represented 25% of the original spleen cell number and contained 0.3% of macrophages. In order to generate effector cells in vitro, normal macrophages were added back at the start of MLTC at a concentration of 0.5% of the cells in culture.

With these manipulations we found that an increased number of macrophages present in the spleens of donors immune to BC5 suppressed the generation of effector cells in MLTC. However, generation of effector cells in MLTC was dependent on low ratios of macrophages. In addition, on day 5 of MLTC, TCGF (supernatant of Con A stimulated rat splenocytes) was added at a concentration of 0.5 units/ml to expand the population of effector cells.

Figure 4 shows that 1.5×10^8 7-day MLTC cells treated as above, infused i.v. into BN rats bearing a BC5 tumor 0.5 - 1 cm in diameter, eliminated the tumor within 35 days. We learned also that an infusion of effector cells i.v. and a second intraperitoneal injection of effector cells and TCGF, accelerated significantly the elimination of BC5 tumors.

When spleen cell populations were depleted of macrophages and then given 0.5% normal macrophages, the cellular composition of 7-day MLTC-immune spleen cells was significantly different from unmanipulated spleen populations or the control spleen populations in MLTC. 65% of the cultured cells were T cells and 50-60% of the T cells were Ia+ blasts. Ig+ cells were decreased to 5% from 25% of the cultured cells and null cells were relatively increased to 25%. No viable tumor cells and less than 0.2% macrophages remained in culture. MLTC with control spleen cells or unmanipulated immune spleen cells showed no expansion of T cells, nor the development of blast cells, and tumor elements were numerous.

Next, we present data on the nature of the effector cell that eliminates tumors in vivo in both systems. We have separated in a FACS the cells of MLTC into W3/25+ and W3/25- fractions (2). Figure 5 shows an experiment in which rats, bearing MST 0.8 cm in diameter, were infused intravenously with 5×10^6 W3/25+ cells, with equal numbers of W3/25- cells, or with 1.5×10^7 unfractionated immune spleen cells of 7-day MLTC. The infusion of 5×10^6 W3/25+ cells eliminated the tumor in 15 days. The infusion of W3/25- population, containing OX8+ T cells, null cells, Ig+ cells and macrophages, was associated with tumor enhancement; and unsorted immune spleen cells, containing at least 5×10^6 W3/25+ cells, failed to eliminate tumor. These latter results indicated the presence of suppressor cells in the effector population.

FIG. 4. Elimination of BC5 in vivo by infusion of 1.5×10^8 fractionated cells of 7-day MLTC. With the same number of unfractionated cells of 7-day MLTC, the growth of BC5 was inhibited and rats only survived for 50 days. Untreated controls survived less than 40 days. Each point on the curves represents seven assay rats.

FIG. 5.

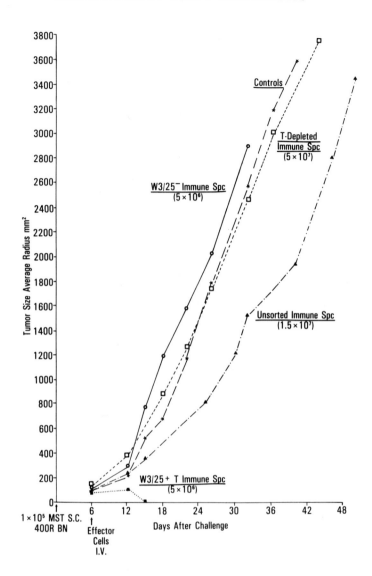

FIG. 5. Effect of W3/25+ and W3/25- effector immune spleen cells of 7-day MLTC on tumor growth in vivo. The unfractionated population contains a mixture of 5 x 10⁶ W3/25+ T cells and 5 x 10⁶ W3/25- cells. The elimination of the tumor was accomplished by the helper subset W3/25+ T cells. Each curve represents three different experiments with three assay rats per experiment. Reprinted from Fernandez-Cruz, et al., (2), 1980. The Rockefeller University Press.

We have performed similar experiments with W3/25+ and W3/25- fractions in the BC5 tumor model and we have been able to confirm that the effector cell that eliminates the tumor in vivo is a T lymphoblast with W3/25 antigen on its surface. 5 x 10⁷ W3/25+ cells eliminated a BC5 tumor within 3 weeks after the treatment. However, 1 x 10⁸ unsorted Isp -MLTC, which contains at least 5 x 10⁷ W3/25+ cells, failed to eliminate

the tumor (3). Unfortunately, these data are derived from 2 trials and
we will not present to you any representative figure.

     There is a disparity between what we find in the in vivo results as
compared to what we find in the in vitro cytotoxicity results. Figure
6-A shows that in the MST system, when fractionated effector cells are
incubated with ^{51}Cr-labeled MST, W3/25+ T cells are poorly cytotoxic.
However, the whole population (W3/25+ plus W3/25-) displayed significant
cytotoxicity. Figure 6-B also shows that in the BC5 tumor model the
whole effector cell populations, fractionated or unfractionated, displayed little cytotoxicity in vitro against ^{51}Cr-labeled target BC5;
W3/25+ T cells were also not cytotoxic. When we infuse W3/25+ cells into a test animal bearing MST or BC5, the tumor is eliminated.

FIG. 6.

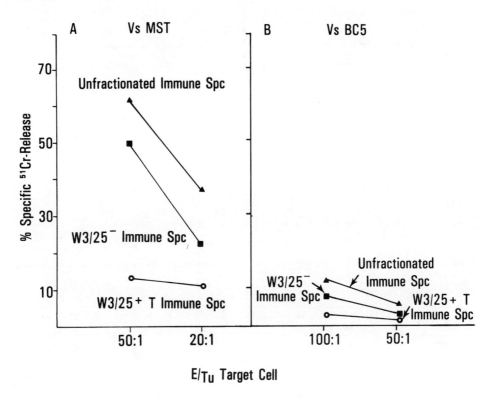

E/T$_u$ Target Cell

FIG. 6. In vitro cytotoxicity of W3/25+ and W3/25- immune spleen cells
and the unfractionated population from which these were derived, of 7-
day MST and BC5 MLTC's. Immune effector cells and control spleen cells
were tested in an 18h ^{51}Cr-release assay against MST and BC5. Each
point is the mean of three trials at E:T ratios of 20:1, 50:1, and 100:1
E/T, spleen (E): tumor cells (T). Reprinted from Fernandez-Cruz, et al,
(2), 1980. The Rockefeller University Press and unpublished observations.

The fact that: a) the W3/25 cell is poorly or not cytotoxic in vitro; b) carries on its surface the W3/25 antigen which identifies helper or amplifier cells in other systems; and c) there is a time lag between infusion of effector cells and noticeable regression of tumors, suggest to us that this cell may function as a helper cell in the tumor bearing host. Still, we cannot exclude that a small number of OX8+ cells (less than 10%) contained in the W3/25+ effector population may expand and contribute to the elimination of the tumor in vivo.

Figure 7 shows that cells of the MLTC are specific. Cells that have geen generated in MLTC with specificity for MST will not eliminate a BC5 tumor, nor will cells that have been prepared in MLTC specific for BC5 show any effect on growth of MST.

FIG. 7.

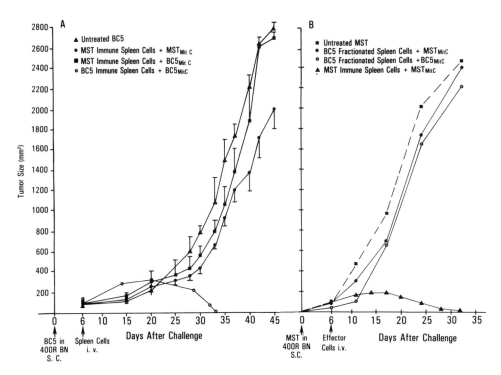

FIG. 7. Specificity in vivo of MST and BC5 effector immune lymphocytes, which do not eliminate challenge of BC5 or MST, respectively. Recipients were pre-irradiated (400R) and bore a 1 cm in diameter tumor. At 6 days postinoculum in each experiment, groups of 5 experimental and 5 controls were infused i.v. with: (A) effector MST immune cells incubated in MLTC with MST_{mit} or $BC5_{mit}$ and; (B) effector BC5 immune cells incubated in MLTC with $BC5_{mit}$ or MST_{mit}. Three experiments are shown. Reprinted from Fernandez-Cruz, et al., (1), 1979. The Williams and Wilkins Co., and unpublished observations.

Our observations in these two in vivo tumor models suggest that in the immunotherapy of established tumors it is important, first, to separate from the mixed effector cell population of MLTC the effector T cell subset from other cells with suppressor activity; second, provide to the tumor-bearing host sufficient numbers of the effector cells; third, in a tumor model resembling the BC5 chemically-induced tumor, it will be necessary to manipulate the cells of MLTC in vitro to overcome the suppression and to generate specific effector cells. Finally, the successful treatment of an expanding tumor with helper cells may indicate that this is a possible way to override the suppression induced by tumor in vivo, amplifying and recruiting the host's immune responses against the tumor.

REFERENCES

1. Fernandez-Cruz, E., Halliburton, B. and Feldman, J.D. (1979): J. Immunol., 123: 1772-1777.

2. Fernandez-Cruz, E., Woda, B.A. and Feldman, J.D. (1980): J. Exp. Med., 152: 823-841.

3. Fernandez-Cruz, E., Gilman, S. and Feldman, J.D. Manuscript in preparation.

4. Jones, J.M., Jensen, F., Veit, B.C. and Feldman, J.D. (1974): J. Natl. Cancer Inst., 52: 1771-1777.

5. Mason, D.W., Brideau, R.J., McMaster, W.R., Webb, M., White, R.A.H., and Williams, A.F. (1980): In: Monoclonal antibodies; hybridomas. A new dimension in biological analysis. Edited by R.H. Kennett, T.J. McKearn andK.B. Bechtol, p. 251. Plenum Press, New York.

AUDIENCE DISCUSSION

Dr. Bortin: You said that the expression of IA antigen on T cells might be important. Do you have any evidence whether IA is being expressed on the cells that are killing the tumor?

Dr. Fernandez-Cruz: I have no direct evidence for that. We consider IA an important marker to tell us that we are generating some T cells that probably will be effective in vivo.

Dr. Ihle: What degree of purity was the IL 2 that was used?

Dr. Fernandez-Cruz: We used a supernatant from Con A stimulated blood.

Dr. Kedar: Can you show any therapeutic effect if you try sensitizing lymphocytes from either unimmunized animals or from tumor-bearing animals?

Dr. Fernandez-Cruz: No. With cells from tumor-bearers you can get some effect against the chemical tumor. Uncultured cells or normal cells never work.

Dr. Greene: Do you have any evidence of suppressive molecules in this system?

Dr. Fernandez-Cruz: We have not looked.

The Potential Role of T Cells in Cancer Therapy,
edited by A. Fefer and A. Goldstein,
Raven Press, New York © 1982.

T Cell-Mediated Negative Regulation of Concomitant Antitumor Immunity as an Obstacle to Adoptive Immunotherapy of Established Tumors

Robert J. North, Earl S. Dye, and Charles D. Mills

The Trudeau Institute, Saranac Lake, New York 12983

HYPOTHESIS

A review of the literature reveals (13) that there are very few examples of the successful adoptive immunotherapy of established immunogenic tumors using cells or serum from tumor-immune donors. In those few cases where tumor regression was achieved by intravenous infusion of immune cells, very large numbers of lymphocytes from hyperimmunized donors had to be passively transferred, and the recipients' tumors needed to be below a certain critical size (4,14). The difficulty in demonstrating adoptive immunotherapy against established tumor contrasts with the relative ease at which immunity can be passively transferred against the growth of a tumor implant, particularly if the Winn assay is employed. It is apparent, therefore, that something happens during early growth of transplantable immunogenic tumors which results in the development of a mechanism that protects these tumors from the antitumor functions of intravenously infused tumor-sensitized lymphocytes. It seems highly likely, moreover, that this same mechanism protects these tumors from the immunotherapeutic effects of intralesional injection of immunoadjuvants, such as BCG and C. parvum, because this form of therapy also fails to cause the regression of tumors above a certain critical size (1).

In searching for an explanation for this apparent tumor-induced obstacle to adoptive and active immunotherapy of established tumors, it becomes important to consider what is known about the immunological events that are evoked in the syngeneic host by the emergence of its immunogenic tumor. The knowledge that immediately comes to mind is that the growth of an immunogenic tumor can evoke the generation of a paradoxical state of concomitant antitumor immunity that enables the host, in spite of the progressive growth of its primary tumor, to inhibit the growth of cells of the same tumor implanted at a distant site. Concomitant antitumor immunity is a well documented (16) though neglected phenomenon. There is evidence that it is T cell-mediated (12) and that it decays when the tumor grows beyond a certain size. We venture to suggest, moreover, that concomitant immunity is a consequence of the growth of all immunogenic tumors. Indeed, it seems highly possible that the first demonstration of tumor immunogenicity by Foley (7) and the demonstrations that followed may not have required ligation or excision of the primary tumor to reveal specific immunity to growth of a subsequent tumor implant. Instead, immunity may have been expressed against the implants, provided the implants were given before the primary tumors became too large.

On the basis of what is known about concomitant immunity in general,
we hypothesize that the emergence of any immunogenic will evoke, to a
greater or lesser degree, the generation of a state of concomitant immunity that will undergo progressive decay after the tumor grows beyond a
certain critical size. We further hypothesize that the decay of concomitant immunity is an active event that represents negative immunoregulation. Moreover, on the basis of what has been learned in this laboratory about concomitant immunity to the Meth A fibrosarcoma syngeneic in
BALB/c mice, and the P815 mastocytoma syngeneic in DBA/2 mice, we propose
that negative regulation of concomitant immunity is mediated by a population of suppressor T cells which is generated in response to progressive tumor growth. If this is so, then it follows that any attempt to
cause the regression of an established tumor, either by active, or by
adoptive immunotherapy represents an attempt to superimpose an immune
response on an already ongoing concomitant immune response that may be
undergoing positive or negative regulation depending on the size of the
tumor. Therefore, if immunotherapy is commenced too late, it will be
subjected to the same T cell-mediated mechanism that functions to negatively regulate concomitant immunity. It is predicted that this will
prove to be the major barrier to active and adoptive immunotherapy of
established immunogenic tumors. This, of course, would represent a
difficult situation, because it would mean that the only tumors which
should be susceptible to immunotherapy are the ones that evoke the generation of a state of T cell-mediated immunoregulation that acts to block
immunotherapy.

EVIDENCE FOR THE GENERATION OF A T CELL-MEDIATED MECHANISM OF IMMUNOSUPPRESSION IN TUMOR-BEARING MICE

That growth of the Meth A fibrosarcoma syngeneic in BALB/c mice results
in the generation of a state of concomitant immunity that undergoes decay
was first suggested by the results of a study of endotoxin-induced regression of established tumors. It was shown (2) that the Meth A fibrosarcoma is susceptible to endotoxin-induced regression for only a brief
period of its growth which corresponds to the time of peak concomitant
immunity in the host. After this time, the tumor suddenly becomes refractory to the effects of endotoxin, and this is associated with the
onset and progressive decay of concomitant immunity. This suggests that
the decay of concomitant immunity is in some way related to the development of the refractoriness of the tumor to endotoxin immunotherapy. It
was reasoned, that if concomitant immunity decays because it is negatively regulated by a mechanism of T cell-mediated immunosuppression, then,
this mechanism of immunosuppression should block attempts to adoptively
immunize against an established Meth A tumor with sensitized T cells.
This proposition was tested by determining whether intravenous infusion
of sensitized T cells from tumor-immune donors would cause the regression of tumors in recipients that were incapable of generating concomitant immunity. This involved infusing tumor-sensitized T cells into
tumor-bearing recipients that had been made T cell deficient by thymectomy and gamma irradiation, and protected with bone marrow (TXB mice).
The donors of immune spleen cells were immunized by causing their 6 day
Meth A tumors to completely regress 3 weeks earlier by intravenous
injection of endotoxin (3), or by treating the tumors with C. parvum (6).

It was found that, whereas intravenous infusion of one spleen equivalent of immune cells (1.5×10^8) had no effect on 4 day Meth A tumors growing in normal recipients, the same number of immune spleen cells caused complete and permanent regression of the same sized tumors growing in TXB mice that were incapable of generating concomitant immunity. Moreover, because regression did not commence until 6 days after giving immune spleen cells, the tumors had time to grow to a large size before they underwent immunologically-mediated regression. The immune spleen cells were T cells, as evidenced by the finding that their capacity to passively transfer immunity was totally ablated by treatment with anti-Thy-1.2 antibody plus complement. These results can be interpreted as showing that immune T cells failed to cause the regression of tumors in normal mice because of a tumor-induced, T cell-dependent mechanism that functioned to block the antitumor function of the infused T cells. Direct evidence for the existence of this tumor-induced mechanism of immunosuppression in normal tumor-bearing mice was supplied by the results of an experiment that attempted to block adoptive T cell-mediated regression of tumors in TXB mice by prior intravenous infusion of splenic cells from normal mice bearing 10-12 day Meth A tumors. It was found that prior infusion of Thy-1.2 positive spleen cells from mice bearing 12 day Meth A tumors completely inhibited the capacity of passively transferred immune spleens to cause the regression of tumors in TXB recipients. In contrast, normal spleen cells were without suppressive effect. On the basis of these and other results, we hypothesized (3) that progressive growth of immunogenic tumors results in the generation of a state of T cell-mediated immunosuppression that functions to negatively regulate concomitant antitumor immunity. The generation of this state of T cell-mediated immunosuppression not only serves to explain the central paradox of progressive growth of immunogenic tumors in their immunocompetent hosts (3), but also represents an explanation for the refractoriness of established tumors to adoptive immunotherapy.

Our confidence in the validity of these conclusions was reinforced by the results of similar more recent studies with the P815 mastocytoma. The results we obtained with this tumor were identical to those obtained with the Meth A fibrosarcoma (5). In the case of the P815 mastocytoma, concomitant immunity was measured as the generation in the node draining the tumor of the T cells that were cytolytic for ^{51}Cr-labelled P815 tumor cells in vitro. It can be seen in Fig. 1 that the cytolytic response to this tumor was relatively modest and that it peaked on about day 10 of tumor growth and then progressively decayed. It was next shown that it is possible to cause the regression of P815 tumors growing in TXB mice, but not in normal mice, by the intravenous infusion of splenic T cells from immune donors that had regressed their tumors 3 weeks earlier in response to intralesional therapy with C. parvum. This was followed by the demonstration that adoptive T cell-mediated regression of this tumor in TXB recipients could be inhibited by prior intravenous infusion of splenic T cells from mice bearing established 10-12 day P815 tumors, i.e. with T cells harvested during the decay of concomitant immunity. There can be little doubt, therefore, that the P815 mastocytoma also evokes the generation of a T cell-mediated mechanism of immunosuppression that inhibits the antitumor function of passively transferred, sensitized T cells (Fig. 2). The P815 tumor is more interesting than the Meth A fibrosarcoma, however, because it metastasizes to cause systemic disease. Indeed, additional experiments that involved excision of primary tumors after metastatic seeding, revealed (5) that micrometastases were

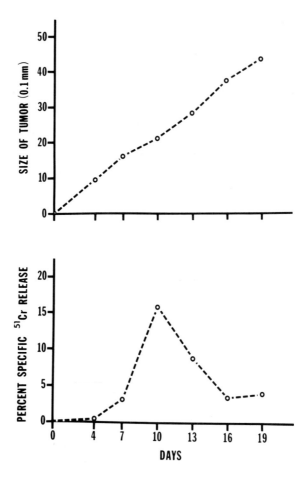

FIG. 1. Generation against time of cytolytic T cells
in the node draining a progressively growing intra-
footpad P815 tumor. Cytolytic activity is expressed
as the percent specific release of radiolabel from
^{51}Cr-labelled P815 cells in a 4 hour assay with a
50:1 effector to target ratio.

eliminated in TXB mice by passively transferred sensitized T cells. It
is important to point out in this connection, moreover, that TXB mice are
much more susceptible to metastatic spread of the P815 than are normal
mice. Indeed, we suggest that this is good evidence for hypothesizing
that concomitant immunity plays a useful role by functioning to successfully retard the spread of metastases during early growth of the primary
tumor.

More recent studies (to be published) have revealed that yet another
tumor, the L5178Y lymphoma gives identical results to the Meth A fibrosarcoma and P815 mastocytoma. More important,this tumor,because it is
syngeneic with the P815 mastocytoma gave us the opportunity to perform
reciprocal passive transfer experiments to determine whether the T cells
that mediate adoptive immunity and the T cells that suppress this immunity
are specific for the tumor that elicits their generation. It was found

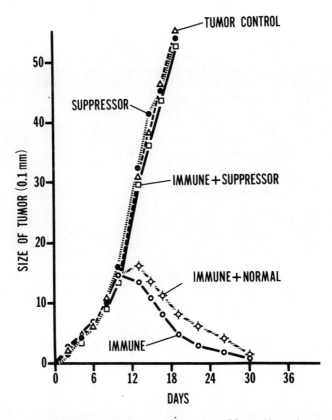

FIG. 2. Evidence that adoptive T cell-mediated regression of the P815 mastocytoma growing in TXB recipients, which results from intravenous infusion of immune spleen cells on day 4 of tumor growth, is inhibited by an infusion 4 hours earlier of spleen cells (suppressor) from tumor-bearing donors.

that T cells generated in response to the P815 mastocytoma cause adoptive T cell-mediated regression of the P815 in TXB recipients, but not the L5178Y lymphoma and vice versa. Likewise, suppressor T cells generated against the P815 mastocytoma only suppress adoptive T cell-mediated regression of the P815 mastocytoma in TXB recipients. These results will form the subject matter of a forthcoming publication.

FUNCTION OF SUPPRESSOR CELLS

The demonstration that growth of immunogenic tumors eventually results in the generation of a state of T cell-mediated immunosuppression was based on the use of an assay that employed TXB tumor-bearing recipients that are incapable of generating concomitant immunity. Thus, because of a deficiency of T cells, TXB mice are incapable of generating the suppressor T cells that inhibit the antitumor function of passively trans-ferred immune T cells. A conspicuous aspect of adoptive T cell-mediated regression of tumors in TXB recipients is that the onset of tumor regression does not begin until 6 days after the sensitized T cells are passively transferred (3,5). We believe that an understanding of the reason for this delay is important for an understanding of the mode of action of suppressor T cells. For example, there is enough evidence to propose that the delay is necessary because the tumor-sensitized T cells that are passively transferred do not themselves mediate tumor regression. Instead, it is first necessary for the infused T cell to replicate and expand to a number that is large enough to cause regression. It is important to realize, in this connection, that sensitized T cells are routinely harvested from immune donors 3 weeks after their tumors have been caused to regress by endotoxin (2) or C. parvum therapy (6). Consequently, these donors are in a state of immunological memory that is based on the possession of a population of sensitized memory T cells. Moreover, because memory T cells have no immediate capacity to destroy tumor cells, they must give rise to a population of effector T cells that are lytic for tumor cells before tumor regression begins. In other words, a secondary cytolytic T cell response of high enough magnitude must develop in response to the growing tumor in the adoptively immunized TXB recipient. This could explain why Ly1$^+$ T cells appear more effective than Ly2$^+$3$^+$ cytolytic T cells in passively transferring antitumor immunity to recipients that have had their tumor burdens reduced by cyclophosphamide, as shown by Dr. Greenberg at this meeting. This explanation is also in keeping with the results of recent experiments in this laboratory which show that the onset of tumor regression in TXB recipients which follows intravenous infusion of sensitized T cells is preceded by the generation of a substantial cytolytic T cell response in the node draining the tumor (Fig. 3). More important, this cytolytic T cell response is reduced by 70% in the nodes of adoptively immunized TXB recipients that are infused with suppressor T cells 24 hours before they are infused with immune T cells. It is apparent, therefore, that suppressor T cells function in this model to inhibit the replication of passively transferred, sensitized memory T cells, and thereby prevent the generation of a population of effector T cells that is large enough to cause tumor regression. Because it takes approximately 6 days for a large enough population of effector T cells to be generated in TXB tumor-bearing test recipients, it can be anticipated that suppressor T cells will suppress adoptive T cell-mediated tumor regression if they are given before, at the time of, or soon after infusing immune T cells. However, the level of suppression should decrease as the interval between the infusion of memory T cells and suppressor T cells is increased. This, in fact, was found to be the case (5). More recent work has shown, moreover, that infusing suppressor T cells at the time of onset of tumor regression has practically no effect on the regression process. This indicates again, that suppressor T cells function to inhibit the generation of effector T cells rather than to block the effector function of already generated cytolytic T cells.

CYCLOPHOSPHAMIDE-FACILITATED ADOPTIVE IMMUNOTHERAPY OF ESTABLISHED TUMORS AS EVIDENCE FOR TUMOR-INDUCED IMMUNOSUPPRESSION

There are a number of published reports which claim (9) that correctly timed treatment with cyclophosphamide favors the generation of cell-mediated immunity because this drug preferentially eliminates suppressor T cells or their precursors. In fact, there is direct evidence that suppressor T cells are cyclophosphamide sensitive in some

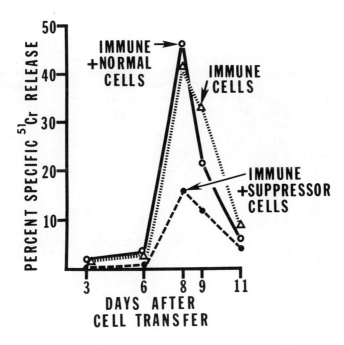

FIG. 3. Evidence that intravenous infusion of sensitized
T cells from immune donors into TXB recipient bearing 5 day
P815 tumors imparts to the recipients the capacity to
generate cytolytic T cells in the nodes draining the tumor.
Cytolytic activity was measured with a 4 hour ^{51}Cr-release
assay at an effector to target ratio of 50:1. The recipients' cytolytic response was substantially suppressed,
however, by prior infusion of splenic T cells from tumor-
bearing donors (suppressor cells). TXB tumor-bearing
controls were incapable of generating cytolytic T cells
(not shown).

experimental systems (8,10,15). These published results prompted the
design of recent experiments in this laboratory to determine whether
cyclophosphamide treatment augments the level of concomitant immunity in
tumor-bearing mice, and whether the augmented immunity is associated
with tumor regression. We failed to find a dose of cyclophosphamide that
would augment concomitant immunity. On the contrary, whereas small
doses of cyclophosphamide decreased the level of concomitant immunity,
larger doses (>150mg/kg) completely ablated the immunity, or prevented
its generation depending on the stage of tumor growth that the drug was
injected. It was reasoned, on the basis of these results, and on the
results and hypothesis presented in the foregoing discussion, that
cyclophosphamide-treated tumor-bearing recipients should be able to
substitute for TXB tumor-bearing recipients for demonstrating adoptive
immunotherapy of established tumors. It was predicted, that if
appropriately timed cyclophosphamide treatment prevents the generation
of concomitant immunity it will automatically prevent the generation of
suppressor T cells that function to negatively regulate concomitant
immunity. This possibility was tested in CB6F$_1$ mice bearing   4 day Meth

A tumors. The Meth A tumor was chosen for this study because, unlike the P815 mastocytoma and L5178Y lymphoma, it is only slightly susceptible to cyclophosphamide. Therefore, any tumor regression that resulted from giving immune T cells after treatment with cyclophosphamide could be attributed to the antitumor action of the immune cells, rather than to the direct cytotoxic action of cyclophosphamide. It was found (Fig. 4) that when mice bearing 5 day Meth A tumors were injected intravenously with cyclophosphamide (150mg/kg) 1 hour before infusing them intravenously with 1.5×10^8 spleen cells from tumor-immune donors, their tumors underwent complete and permanent regression after a delay of 6 days. In contrast, immune cells alone had no effect on tumor growth, and cyclo-

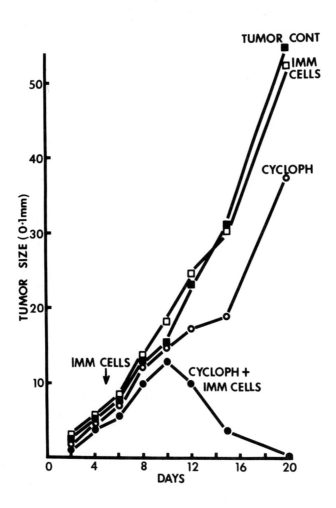

FIG. 4. Evidence for cyclophosphamide-facilitated adoptive immunotherapy. An intravenous injection of cyclophosphamide (150mg/kg) given to 5 day Meth A tumor bearers 1 hour before infusing them intravenously with 1.5×10^8 spleen cells from immune donors resulted in complete and permanent regression of the tumors. In contrast, cyclophosphamide or immune cells alone failed to cause regression.

phosphamide alone caused only a temporary reduction in the rate of tumor growth. It can be concluded, therefore, that cyclophosphamide treatment of tumor-bearing mice acts to prevent the development of a tumor-induced barrier that prevents intravenously infused immune T cells from realizing their antitumor function. It seems logical to suggest that this barrier consists of a cyclophosphamide-sensitive population of suppressor T cells that functions in the negative regulation of concomitant immunity. We have no evidence that cyclophosphamide selectively destroys suppressor T cells or their precursors. This would not be necessary for adoptive immunotherapy to succeed.

Similar results were obtained with recipient mice that had been given 800 rads of whole-body gamma irradiation 1 hour before implanting their test tumors. It can be seen in Fig. 4 that intravenous infusion of immune spleen cells into gamma-irradiated mice bearing 4 day Meth A tumors caused complete and permanent tumor regression after a delay of 6 days. In contrast, tumor regression failed to occur in mice that were not irradiated before tumor implantation. We interpret these results as showing that 800 rads of gamma-irradiation served to deplete the capacity of tumor-bearing mice to generate suppressor T cells within the time frame of the experiment.

SUMMARY AND CONCLUSION

Enough evidence was discussed in the foregoing sections to hypothesize that the emergence and growth of an immunogenic tumor in its immuno-competent syngeneic host evokes the generation of a state of T cell-mediated concomitant immunity that undergoes T cell-mediated negative regulation before a large enough number of effector T cells is produced to reject the tumor. The presence of a T cell-mediated mechanism of negative regulation in tumor-bearing mice was revealed in two ways. First, by showing that passively transferred tumor-sensitized T cells failed to cause the regression of established tumors in normal mice, but caused the complete and permanent regression of tumors growing in mice that had been made T cell-deficient by thymectomy and irradiation, and protected with bone marrow (TXB mice). Second, by showing that failure of passively transferred tumor-sensitized T cells to cause regression of tumors in normal mice was associated with the presence in these mice of splenic T cells that were capable, on passive transfer, of inhibiting adoptive T cell-mediated regression of tumors in TXB mice. This model is depicted in Fig. 5. It seems almost certain, therefore, that progressive growth of immunogenic tumors results in the generation of a T cell-mediated mechanism of immunosuppression that functions to down regulate concomitant immunity. It follows,therefore, that any attempt to cause the regression of an established immunogenic tumor by adoptive immunotherapy with tumor-sensitized T cells represent an attempt to superimpose an adoptive immune response on an already ongoing concomitant immune response that may be undergoing negative regulation. Consequently, passively transferred, sensitized T cells will be subjected to this T cell-mediated negative regulation if they are infused into mice with tumors above a certain critical size. It is suggested that this is the reason for the difficulty experienced in demonstrating adoptive immuno-therapy of established tumors. Furthermore, if the tumor-induced generation of suppressor T cells is the only mechanism responsible for the failure of passively transferred sensitized T cells to cause tumor regression, then, it should be possible for the sensitized T cells to

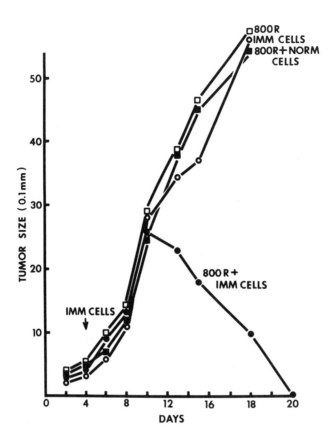

FIG. 5. Evidence for gamma irradiation-facilitated adoptive immunotherapy of established Meth A fibrosarcomas. Exposing mice to 800R of whole-body gamma-irradiation 1 hour before implanting them with Meth A cells enabled subsequently infused immune cells to cause complete regression of established tumors.

cause tumor regression, provided the tumor-bearer is treated in a way that results in a temporary depletion of suppressor T cells or their precursors. We propose that this is the reason why combination therapy with cyclophosphamide and tumor-sensitized T cells results in complete and permanent regression of the Meth A fibrosarcoma. This is not to say, however, that regression depended on the selective elimination of suppressor T cells. Based on the results with TXB mice, this would not be a requirement.

An understanding of the way that suppressor T cells inhibit the anti-tumor function of passively transferred immune cells requires a consideration of the events that must take place before adoptive immunotherapy is expressed. All of the adoptive immunity experiments on which the foregoing discussion was based were performed with the cells of tumor-immune donors, that more likely than not, possessed a state of immuno-logical memory at the time their immune spleen cells were harvested. In the case of experiments performed with the P815 mastocytoma, donor mice

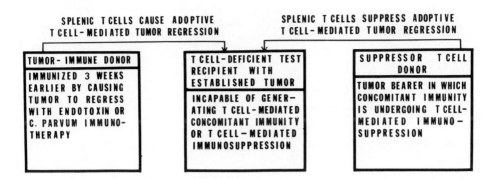

FIG. 6. Diagrammatic representation of the model used to reveal the presence of suppressor T cells in mice with established tumors.

were immunized by causing their tumors to regress 3 weeks earlier by C. parvum therapy. It was shown recently (11) that this is long past the time that cytolytic T cells have disappeared from the draining node and spleen. Therefore, adoptive immunotherapy of established tumors in TXB test recipients was not achieved by cytolytic T cells. Instead, the tumor-sensitized T cells that were passively transferred almost certainly were memory T cells that had to give rise to a secondary in vivo immune response to cause tumor regression. Hence the reason for the 6 day delay before the onset of tumor regression. It is apparent, therefore, that it is the generation of this secondary response in the TXB recipient that is inhibited by intravenously-infused suppressor T cells. Theoretically, it should be possible, therefore, to bypass the influence of suppressor cells by passively transferring cytolytic T cells, provided enough of them are infused and that they are physiologically capable of homing to target tumor tissue. It should be stressed, in this connection, that successful adoptive immunotherapy of tumors in TXB mice requires the use of highly immune donors with a substantial level of immunological memory. Needless to say, the passive transfer of a relatively large number of memory cells into a host with a relatively large progressive immunogenic tumor represents a situation that should be conducive to the generation of a large population of effector cells. Whether intravenously infused cytolytic $Ly2^+3^+$ T cells have the capacity to expand in vivo in response to antigen supplied by the growing tumor has yet to be determined.

SUPPORT

This work was supported by Grant CA-16642 and CA-27794 from the National Cancer Institute, Grant IM-266 from the American Cancer Society and Grant RR-05705 from the Division of Research Resources, National Institutes of Health.

REFERENCES

1. Bast, R.C., Bast, B.S., Rapp, H.J. (1976): Ann. N.Y. Acad. Sci., 277:60-85.
2. Berendt, M.J., North, R.J., and Kirstein, D.P. (1978): J. Exp. Med., 148:1560-1569.
3. Berendt, M.J., and North, R.J. (1980): J. Exp. Med., 151:69-80.
4. Borberg, H., Oettgen, H.F., Choudy, K., and Beattie, E. (1972): Int. J. Cancer, 10:539-547.
5. Dye, E.S., and North, R.J. (1981): J. Exp. Med., 154:(in press).
6. Dye, E.S., North, R.J., and Mills, C.D. (1981): J. Exp. Med., 154: (in press).
7. Foley, E.J. (1953): Cancer Res., 13:835-848.
8. Germain, R.N., and Benacerraf, B. (1978): J. Immunol., 121:608-612.
9. Goto, M., Misuoka, A., Sugiyama, M., and Kitano, M. (1981): J. Exp. Med., 154:204-209.
10. Green, M.I., Bach, B., and Benacerraf, B. (1979): J. Exp. Med., 149: 1069-1083.
11. Mills, C.D., North, R.J., and Dye, E.S. (1981): J. Exp. Med., 154: (in press).
12. North, R.J., and Kirstein, D.P. (1977): J. Exp. Med., 145:275-292.
13. Rosenberg, S.A., and Terry, W.D. (1977): In: Advances in Cancer Research, edited by G. Klein, and S. Weinhouse, pp. 323-394. Academic Press, New York.
14. Smith, H.G., Harmel, R.P., Hamm, M.G., Zwilling, B.S., Zbar, B., and Rapp, H.J. (1976): J. Natl. Cancer Inst., 58:1315-1322.
15. Sy, M-S., Miller, S.D., Moorhead, J.W., and Claman, H.N. (1979): J. Exp. Med., 149:1197-1207.
16. Vaage, J. (1971): Cancer Res., 31:1655-1662.

AUDIENCE DISCUSSION

Dr. Fernandez-Cruz: Have you tried to generate the specific effector cells by a secondary in vitro response?

Dr. North: Yes. Spleen cells from animals whose tumors regressed in response to C. parvum when exposed to Mitomycin C-treated tumor cells become cytolytic to P815. If you transfer 5 x 10^7 of these cells intravenously into TXB tumor-bearers, there is no tumor regression. If you leave these cells and allow the cytolytic response to decay, then you do cause tumor regression.

Dr. Fernandez-Cruz: Did you look at the effect of suppressor cells on the generation of the immune population in vitro?

Dr. North: No.

Dr. Mitchell: There is a theory that high doses of X-rays or cyclophosphamide clear out a lot of cells, making room for the cells you are infusing. Have you used any low dose cyclophosphamide or specific anti-suppressor cell monoclonal antibodies to specifically remove suppression and then transfer immunity?

Dr. North: I agree. There will be experiments with varying doses of cyclophosphamides to eliminate existing suppressors from tumor bearers. When we give 800 rads, we are certainly making room, but I don't know what the room theory really means. Certainly, 800 rads given early will destroy the precursors of suppressor cells, and 800 rads given later at the onset of the negative regulation will destroy mature suppressor cells.

Dr. Rapp: Have you ruled out the possiblity that your suppressor cell population contains one or more living tumor cells?

Dr. North: Tumor cells infused intravenously have no effect on our immune cells. But it is well to point out that in these T cell-deficient animals, by the time the tumor starts regressing after infusing immune cells, the animals already have metastases. The other reason why contaminating tumor cells in our spleen cells is unlikely to be involved is because the Meth A fibrosarcoma is notorious for not metastasizing. So with the Meth A and P815 you get exactly the same results. A 15-day spleen from the P815 tumor bearer does contain tumor cells. Another reason for believing that the suppressors are T cells is that they are Thy-1 positive in all systems studied.

Dr. Fathman: With low dose radiation, you should have removed the potential suppressor population. If so, you should have had a normal immune response which wasn't down regulated. You showed concomitant immunity after 500 rads but didn't get tumor regression, but got growth.

Dr. North: Right. That would depend on how fast the animal reconstitutes itself after 500 rads. I think the reason for lack of tumor regression is that there is not enough time for reconstitutuion to occur for the recipient animal to generate immunity. Other laboratories have shown that irradiation sometime before implanting a tumor yields a large percentage of subsequent regressions. I think it is the earlier reconstitution of effector elements before suppressor elements that results in regressions.

Dr. Bortin: What is the dose of cyclophosphamide used? What was the timing of the immune cells relative to surgery?

Dr. North: The immune cells were given 2 hours after surgery. The dose of cyclophosphamide was 150 mg/kg. Half that dose doesn't work.

Dr. Greenberg: Have you looked at the specificity of suppression? In particular, did spleen cells from mice bearing the L5178Y suppress the P815 response and vice versa?

Dr. North: The experiment was up to day 12 when I left. The evidence thus far shows that suppression is specific.

Dr. Douglas Green: With respect to the question of Dr. Mitchell, we have shown that doses of cyclophosphamide as little as 5-20 mg/kg are effective in a similar type of model. We have also shown that conventional alloantisera directed against IJ determinants is also effective, and it has now been shown by Dr. Wlatman that monoclonal anti-IJ antibodies can specifically inhibit tumor growth by in vivo depletion of suppressor T cells.

Dr. Oldham: Did you autopsy the animals which were "cured" at 60 days? Did they have any residual tumor cells? How late after tumor inoculation can you give 800 rads and immune cells and be effective?

Dr. North: On day 8 -- but not later -- combination therapy with 500 rads plus immune cells causes complete regression of very large tumors. We did no autopsies.

[Unidentified]: The P815 is known to produce soluble factors which can enhance tumor growth. Have you looked at extracts of the P815 in the light of inducer or suppressor population?

Dr. North: We haven't looked, but I would be suspicious of crude extracts in terms of enhancement of tumor growth.

Dr. Warner: I want to ask Dr. Greene a question in view of his comment. We are trying to manipulate the regulatory mechanism of immunity to tumor. This morning caution has been raised about the use of anti-IJ antibody to destroy suppressors. Is the monoclonal which inhibits suppressors distinct from the monoclonal anti-IJ which we heard earlier as negating the contra-suppressor, which would give you, in fact, the opposite response in therapy?

Dr. M. Greene: Right. This monoclonal removed suppressor factors in the tumor system. There has been at least one demonstration that administration of an anti-IJ antibody can lead to enhanced tumor growth. That might reflect the mechanism alluded to by Dr. Douglas Green.

Dr. Douglas Green: Monoclonal anti-IJs might also activate a suppressor system. We might see abrogation of suppressor either by destruction of the suppressor cell or by activation of a contra-suppressor. Maybe we destroy contra-suppressor or activate suppressor to get the enhanced tumor growth in these in vivo experiments. Merello and McDevitt showed that there was an Ly-1$^+$, IJ$^+$ cell that was required for immunity in that system, although the necessary experiments to show that this was actually the functional immunogenic cell was not done. Dr. North, when you inject tumor with C. parvum and take the cells from the animal at day 12, when you have cytolytic cells, will those cells transfer immunity to normal animals?

Dr. North: Yes, if you infuse enough of them.

Dr. Shu: In your adoptive transfer experiments, of the roughly 10^8 immune spleen cells transferred, there must be many T cells which are not committed to the tumor antigens. Do those T cells reconstitute the irradiated mice to a degree comparable to normal mice? How do you explain the difference in the adoptive transfer results?

Dr. North: I think it is a matter of timing. I think we do transfer the precursors of suppressor cells with immune cells, but the suppressors are dominant. If you do not put in suppressors until day 9, the tumor is already beginning to regress and you will not stop it with suppressors. This is probably because the destruction of tumor cells and regression as we measure them by increased thickness are dissociable. I think that most of the tumor cells are killed in a very short time; there is not enough time for suppressors to be generated from uncommitted T cells.

Dr. Shu: Have you tried to reconstitute the TXB and irradiated mice with normal spleen cells and then do the adoptive transfer studies?

Dr. North: No, that's part of the reconstitution work we will be doing soon with selected populations.

Dr. Rosenberg: You show no correlation between the in vitro cytotoxicity and the cells which were effective in your in vivo assay. Have you ever taken cells from the draining lymph node of a tumor-bearing animal on day 10, at a time when those draining lymph node cells are cytolytic in vitro, and tested whether they were capable of mediating an in vivo effect?

Dr. North: Yes, and they don't.

Dr. Bach: There is evidence that activated cytotoxic T lymphocytes are very hard to reactivate, at least in vitro. The comment you made earlier may be critically important: that you have to let those cells revert so they are reactivable before you use them. If you put them in at a time when they are very active in vitro, they are the worst cells to reactivate in vivo.

Dr. North: Our results suggest that is the case.

The Potential Role of T Cells in Cancer Therapy,
edited by A. Fefer and A. Goldstein,
Raven Press, New York © 1982.

Adoptive Immunity to a Syngeneic Guinea Pig Hepatoma: Characteristics of Effectors and Quantitative Analysis of Tumor Rejection

S. Shu, J. T. Hunter, H. J. Rapp, and L. S. Fonseca

*Laboratory of Immunobiology, National Cancer Institute, National Institutes of Health,
Bethesda, Maryland 20205*

The adoptive transfer of specifically sensitized lymphoid cells to naive animals has prevented the growth of inoculated tumors, caused regression of established local tumors and eradicated metastases (4,7, 14,17). The mechanism whereby the cellular immune system eliminates tumor in the recipient is not known. Direct killing of malignant cells by transferred immune lymphoid cells has been postulated and generally accepted as the counterpart of the in vivo mechanism of tumor eradication since several types of neoplastic cells were lysed upon contact with immune lymphocytes in vitro (3,5,10,13). However, parallel activities detected in cytotoxicity assay and adoptive transfer for a given lymphoid cell preparation could be due to functionally different subpopulations. In the first part of this presentation, I will summarize our experience in an effort to correlate in vitro findings of lymphoid-tumor cell interactions with adoptive immunity at effector cell level in a syngeneic guinea pig tumor model.

The line-10 hepatoma was originally induced in a male strain 2 guinea pig by feeding diethylnitrosamine. The tumor has been converted to the ascites form and is passed intraperitoneally in weanling strain 2 guinea pigs (6,11). Inoculation of 10^6 viable ascites line-10 cells intradermally (id) in the side of the guinea pig leads to progressive tumor growth, regional axillary lymph node metastases and death in 60 to 90 days (18). It has been reported by this laboratory that the line-10 tumor specific immunity could be adoptively transferred with mineral oil induced immune peritoneal exudate cells (17). In our studies, spleen cells from guinea pigs that had been immunized to line-10 or another antigenically distinct guinea pig hepatoma, line-1, served as effector cells for in vivo and in vitro assays. Routinely, adoptive transfer was carried out by intraveneous (iv) injection of spleen cell suspension and id inoculation of tumor cells. Table 1 summarizes the result of two experiments in which specificity of the adoptive immunity was studied. It is clear that the adoptive immunity to line-10 and line-1 hepatomas was tumor line specific; the growth of line-10 was inhibited in animals receiving line-10 immune but not in those receiving line-1 immune spleen cells whereas the growth of line-1 tumor was inhibited in animals receiving line-1 but not those receiving line-10 immune spleen cells.

LSF is a Guest Worker supported by CAPES-Brazil.

TABLE 1. Specificity of adoptive immunity to guinea pig hepatomas

| | Tumor incidence in guinea pigs challenged with | |
Source of spleen cells[a]	Line-10	Line-1
Medium control	12/12[b]	6/6
Normal	12/12	6/6
Line-10 immune	2/12	11/11
Line-1 immune	6/6	0/6

[a]Each guinea pig received 200 x 10^6 spleen cells iv and was challenged id on the same day with 10^6 ascites line-10 or 3 x 10^6 ascites line-1 cells.

[b]No. of animals with tumor/no. tested.(tumor growth was observed for 48 days).

Spleen cells capable of conveying adoptive antitumor immunity were tested in vitro for tumor cytotoxic activity. The cytotoxicity was measured by a 48-hour ^{3}H release assay as previously described (16). The ascites form of line-10 cells grew in suspension when cultured To use these cells as targets, they were converted to adherent mono- layers of epitheloid-type cells with the aid of fibronectin (8). Line-1 hepatoma cells grew as adherent monolayers without fibronectin. In several preliminary experiments we found that line-10 immune spleen cells consistently mediated line-10 cytotoxicity whereas normal spleen cells occasionally produced high levels of ^{3}H release from line-10 targets. The activity expressed by normal but not immune spleen cells, however, could be removed either by passing the spleen cells through nylon wool columns or by incubating the spleen cells on fibronectin coated plastic culture dishes.   The specificity of the in vitro cytotoxicity was then assessed in reciprocal protocols that included line-10 or line-1 cells and immune spleen cells to each tumor line. In seven similar experiments, three patterns of specificities were observed. They are representatively depicted in Fig. 1: A. Cross-reactivity was observed in four of the seven experiments. B. Partial cross-reactivity was observed in two experiments. C. Specific reactivity was observed in one experiment.

The apparent lack of tumor line specific reactivity in the majority of cytotoxicity assays does not exclude the possibility that cells immune to tumor specific rejection antigens that were detected by adoptive transfer were also participating in the destruction of tumor targets in vitro. The presence of tumor line specific reactivity in one of the seven experiments suggests that the tumor line specific cytotoxicity might frequently be masked by a high level of tumor specific but not tumor line specific activity. To investigate this possibility, we developed an absorption procedure to study the correlation between cells mediating in vitro cytotoxicity and cells conveying adoptive immunity. Cultured monolayers of line-10 and line-1 cells were used as specific immunoabsorbents. At approximately 50 percent confluence the absorbing monolayers cultured in 100 mm polystyrene tissue culture dishes were washed free of nonadherent tumor cells. Then, 100x to 150x 10^6 spleen cells in 10 ml of RPMI 1640 supplemented with 10 percent fetal bovine serum were dispensed into each dish. The dishes were incubated at 37°C for 3 hours on a stationary platform. After the

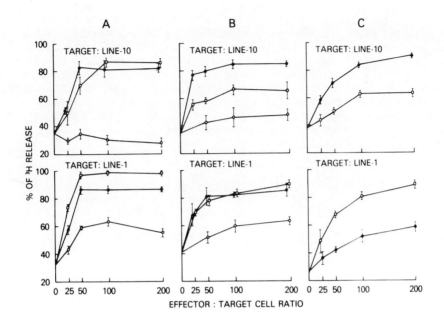

FIG. 1. Specificity studies on the in vitro cytotoxicity assay. Spleen cells from normal (o), line-10 immune (●) and line-1 immune (□) guinea pigs were tested for cytotoxic activities against line-10 or line-1 targets. Vertical brackets depict ± 1 S.D.

incubation, nonadherent spleen cells harvested by gentle swirling were dispensed into a culture dish containing a fresh monolayer of the same type of cells used in the first absorption. The nonadherent cells were assayed for their activity in the cytotoxicity assay and in adoptive transfer.

Fig. 2 affords an example of three experiments each indicating that the cytotoxic activity of line-10 immune spleen cells was abrogated after absorption with either line-10 or line-1 monolayers. Since both absorbing monolayers were capable of depleting cytotoxic effectors, we suspected that the absorption reflected nonimmunological adherence of cytotoxic spleen cells to cultured tumor cells. We, therefore, included a primary kidney fibroblast culture and a nontumorigenic embryonic fibroblast cell line (line 103), both were syngeneic to the strain 2 guinea pig, in our absorption protocol. In the experiment depicted in Fig. 3, we tested line-10 cytotoxicity mediated by line-10

or line-1 immune as well as normal spleen cells before and after two
3 hour incubations on various monolayers. It is apparent that the
in vitro cytotoxicity for line-10 cells mediated by immune spleen cells
was depleted after absorption with line-10 or line-1 monolayers but not
with monolayers of syngeneic kidney fibroblasts or the embryonic line
103. These findings suggest that the in vitro cytotoxicity detects or
is directed toward antigens or other cell properties common to both
line-10 and line-1 cells. The normal spleen cells used in this experiment mediated substantial line-10 cytotoxicity before absorption.
However, this activity was depleted after incubations on fibronectin
coated culture dishes and was characteristically different from that
produced by immune spleen cells.

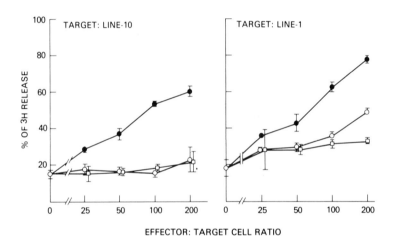

FIG. 2. Cytotoxicity on line-10 and line-1 targets mediated by unab-
sorbed (●), line-10 monolayer (o), or line-1 monolayer (□) absorbed
line-10 immune spleen cells. Vertical brackets depict ± 1 S.D. (Shu,
S. et al., Cancer Res., 1981, in press).

The possibility of separate lymphoid cell populations mediating in
vitro cytolysis and in vivo tumor specific rejection was evaluated by
studying tumor rejection activity of the absorbed line-10 immune spleen
cells. In two preliminary experiments we found that absorption of line-
10 immune spleen cells with monolayers of line-10 but not line-1 abrogated their ability to transfer systemic immunity agaisnt line-10 tumor

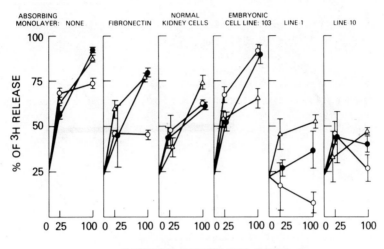

FIG. 3.   Specificity of line-10 cytotoxicity studied by absorption of
spleen cells on monolayers of various strain 2 guinea pig cells.   Spleen
cells were from normal (o), line-10 immune (●), or line-1 immune (△)
guinea pigs.   Vertical brackets depict ± 1 S.D. (Shu et al., Cancer
Res., 1981, in press).

challenge.   In an expanded protocol, besides line-10 and line-1 monolayers, we included monolayers of syngeneic kidney fibroblasts and line
103 embryonic cells as additional immunosorbent controls.   The result
of this experiment illustrated in Fig. 4 demonstrated that spleen cells
from line-10 immune guinea pigs lost their capacity to transfer specific
immunity after absorption on line-10 but not on other control monolayers.
Thus the tumor line specifc depletion, by absorption, of the capacity of
immune cells to transfer specific immunity is indicative of the in vitro
interaction involving tumor specific rejection antigen.   Comparison of
findings of in vitro cytotoxicity and adoptive immunity by absorption
studies indicates that spleen cells committed to tumor specific rejection
antigen react specifically in vitro with tumor targets.   However, this
interaction alone does not lead to the target cell destruction in vitro
even after 48 hour incubation.

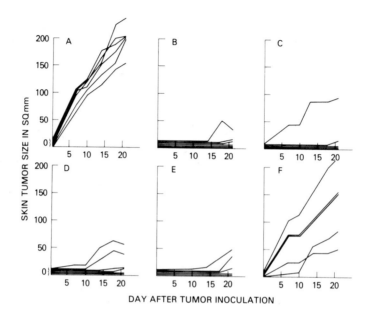

FIG. 4. Evidence of in vitro cell interaction involving tumor specific
rejection antigen revealed by abrogation of the adoptive immunity
after absorption of effectors with specific tumor targets. Normal guinea
pigs (A) and those receiving iv transfer of 100 x 10^6 line-10 immune
spleen cells (B), 100 x 10^6 immune cells absorbed twice with monolayers
of kidney fibroblasts (C), embryonic cell line, line 103 (D), line-1 (E),
or line-10 (F) were challenged id with 10^6 ascites line-10 cells. Each
line illustrates the growth of the tumor in an individual animal.

     Distinction between lymphoid cells mediating tumor specific rejection
and those effecting cytolysis in vitro was also evident in several
experimental tumor models (see chapters by P. D. Greenberg, E. Frenandez-
Cruz, and M. A. Cheever). In the light of these findings, adoptive
transfer may provide a more realistic approach than an in vitro cytotoxicity assay of undefined in vivo relevancy in the mechanistic study
of protective tumor immunity. Although the therapeutic efficiency of
adoptive immunity against tumors has been established since the
demonstration by Mitchison (9), the underlying mechanism of adoptive
antitumor immunity remains an enigma. In the second part of this

presentation, I will summarize recent experimental results in an effort
to elucidate some mechanistic aspects of adoptive antitumor immunity
by quantitative analyses. The relationship between iv transferred
immune spleen cells and id line-10 challenges was analyzed by a two-
dimensional titration (15).

Table 2 summarizes results of two experiments demonstrating that
tumor resistance increased as a function of increased numbers of
immune spleen cells. The data presented in Table 2 were based on

TABLE 2. Quantitative analysis of adoptive immunity to the line-10
hepatoma by a two-dimensional titration

| No. of immune spleen cells transferred[a] | Tumor incidence | | | | |
| | Line-10 challenge dose | | | | |
	10^3	10^4	10^5	10^6	10^7
0	2/6[b]	10/11	12/12	12/12	12/12
12.5×10^6		6/6			
25×10^6		1/10	9/11		
50×10^6		2/12	4/12	11/12	6/6
100×10^6		0/11	0/12	2/12	12/12
200×10^6				0/12	10/11
400×10^6					0/6

[a]Each guinea pig received immune spleen cells iv and was challenged
id on the same day.
[b]No. of animals with tumor/no. tested. (tumor growth was observed
for 38 days).

complete tumor suppression. Subsequently, quantitative tumor resistance
was estimated by comparison of the TD_{50} which was defined as tumor take
in 50 percent test animals and was calculated according to the Reed-
Muench formula (12). The TD_{50} values were then plotted logarithmically
and analyzed by linear regression (Fig. 5). The mathematical relationship between immune spleen cells and tumor challenge dose producing a
TD_{50} can be illustrated by a linear first-order equation:

$$y = 2.52 \ x \ -10.4$$

where, y is log tumor challenge dose; x is log immune spleen cells
and the coefficient of determination of the regression line (r^2) is
0.95. The slope of the equation, 2.52 indicates that the efficacy
of tumor growth suppression is an exponential function of increasing
numbers of immune spleen cells. A two-fold increment in immune cells
leads to an increased resistance of 5.6-fold in the tumor challenge dose.

The exponential relationship between the numbers of immune lymphoid
cells and doses of tumor suppressed in adoptive immunity is not only
of theoretical interest but also of practical importance. The transferred immune cells may be restimulated and expanded and/or the recip-

ient may be actively immunized by the tumor challenge. Increasing tumor challenge doses would provide increased amounts of antigen and
perhaps a greater immune response which in turn would contribute to the
rejection of the tumor. Thus the rejection of a higher dose tumor
challenge would require proportionally fewer transferred immune cells.
For this hypothesis to be validated, one must demonstrate that
stimulation of a primary immune response in the recipient and/or a
secondary immune stimulation at tumor challenge site are essential

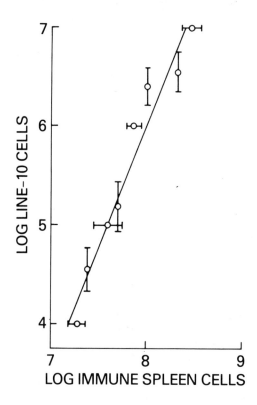

FIG. 5. Logarithmic relationship between immune spleen cells and line-
10 tumor challenge doses producing $TD_{50}s$ in syngeneic recipients.

to tumor suppression by adoptive immunity. In experiments illustrated
in Table 3, we examined whether a systemic immunity developed in guinea
pigs that had rejected a tumor dose by adoptive immunity. In control
animals that each received an iv infusion of immune spleen cells and were
challenged 38 days later with 10^6 line-10 cells each, the TD_{50} doses of
immune cells was 76×10^6. The TD_{50} doses of immune spleen cells in
animals that had rejected the initial challenges of 10^4 and 10^5 line-10

cells were 72 x and 76 x 10^6, respectively. The suppression of the second tumor challenge was a function of transferred immune cells and was independent of rejection of 10^4 or 10^5 line-10 cells. Thus, the rejection of 10^4 or 10^5 line-10 cells by adoptive immunity was not followed by the development of detectable active immunity in the recipients.

TABLE 3. Quantitative analysis of systemic immunity in guinea pigs that had rejected a line-10 challenge by adoptive immunity[a]

| No. of immune spleen cells transferred on day 0 | Tumor incidence at second challenge (10^6) site | | |
| | Rejected line-10 dose (challenged on day 0) | | |
	0	10^4	10^5
0	12/12[b]		
25		9/9	2/2
50	6/6	8/10	7/8
100	1/6	2/11	3/12
TD_{50} dose of immune spleen cells	76 x 10^6	72 x 10^6	76 x 10^6

[a]Each guinea pig received various number of immune spleen cells iv and was challenged id with 10^4 or 10^5 line-10 cells on day 0. At 38 days, tumor-free animals were rechallenged id with 10^6 line-10 cells in the contralateral sides.

[b]No. of animals with tumor at second challenge site/no. tested. Pool data of two experiments.

Failure to demonstrate augmented systemic immunity after tumor rejection by adoptive immunity does not exclude the possible significance of a local immune stimulation of transferred immune cells at the site of tumor challenge. To this end, we determined by titration the number of immune spleen cells required to suppress a line-10 inoculum consisting of a mixture of live and irradiated cells. Irradiated line-10 cells were not tumorigenic but retained tumor specific rejection antigen (1,2) Addition of irradiated cells would provide more antigen than that present in the inoculum without irradiated cells. Table 4 shows that the TD_{50} doses of immune spleen cells in guinea pigs challenged with 10^4 and 10^6 live line-10 cells were 25 x and 71 x 10^6 respectively. The TD_{50} dose of immune spleen cells in guinea pigs challenged with 10^4 live line-10 admixed with 99 x 10^4 irradiated line-10 cells was 18 x 10^6. While these findings suggest that the irradiated cells were not the targets for immune attack, the TD_{50}s of immune cells required to suppress the growth of 10^4 line-10 cells in the absence or in the presence of irradiated line-10 cells were not significantly different. We conclude that local immune stimulation did not significantly contribute to the rejection of tumor by adoptive immunity.

An alternative explanation for the exponential relationship that exists between the numbers of immune spleen cells transferred and the numbers of tumor cells suppressed may be that transferred immune lymphoid cells are specifically attracted to the tumor challenge site and the number of immune cells exponentially increases as a function

of numbers of tumor cells in the challenge site. We therefore designed
experiments to study the skin distribuition of iv injected immune
cells in terms of antitumor activity. Our early experiments revealed
that 100 x10^6 immune spleen cells were sufficient to suppress the
growth of 10^6 but not 10^7 line-10 cells at a single site. If the
limited capacity of the adoptive immunity to reject 10^7 line-10 cells

TABLE 4. Influence of irradiated tumor cells on adoptive immunity

No. of immune spleen cells transferred[a]	Tumor incidence in guinea pigs challenged with line-10 cells		
	10^6 live	10^4 live	10^4 live + 99 x 10^4 irradiated[b]
0	6/6[c]	12/12	12/12
6.25 x 10^6		12/12	12/12
12.5 x 10^6		10/12	12/12
25 x 10^6	6/6	7/12	1/12
50 x 10^6	6/6	0/12	0/12
100 x 10^6	0/6	0/6	0/10
TD_{50} dose of immune spleen cells	71 x 10^6	25 x 10^6	18 x 10^6

[a]Each guinea pig received immune spleen cells iv and was challenged
id with live line-10 cells with or without the addition of irradiated
line-10 cells.

[b]10,000 rads of gamma irradiation

[c]No. of animals with tumor/no. tested; tumor growth was observed
for 38 days.

was due to the lack of specific attraction at the challenge site rather
than due to an insufficient number of immune cells available in the
recipient, one would expect that 10^7 line-10 cells would be rejected
provided that they were divided into multiple small doses and inoculated at separated skin sites. The results of two such experiments
are summarized in Table 5. In guinea pigs receiving 100 x 10^6 immune
spleen cells, the growth of 10^6 line-10 challenge was suppressed
while the growth of 10^7 line-10 challenge at a single site was not
suppressed in eight of the eleven test animals. When the 10^7 line-10
cells were inoculated at ten skin sites (each contained 10^6 cells),
the growth of the majority of the tumor challenge was suppressed.
These findings demonstrate that the skin distribution and expression of
transferred immunity at challenge sites were independent of one another.
The data suggest that there was no specific attraction of transferred
immune cells to the tumor challenge site.

   In a different experimental protocol, we further investigated the
significance of specific attraction and accumulation of iv transferred
immune cells in the skin area of tumor challenge sites. An experiment was designed to test whether a skin challenge of 10^7 line-10
cells could abrogate the adoptive antitumor immunity to 10^6
line-10 cells inoculated adjacent to and distant from the 10^7 line-10
challenge site. To avoid possible growth inhibition or enhancement

of 10^6 line-10 in animals that had extra tumor burden, we also included groups of animals in which 10^7 line-10 inoculation sites were surgically excised three days after the onset of the experiment. The result of this experiment shows that suppression of the growth of 10^6 line-10 cells by adoptive immunity was independent of the presence of 10^7 line-10 cells in the same animal (Table 6). Thus iv trasferred immune cells were not attracted specifically to the site of tumor challenge.

TABLE 5. Expression of tumor immunity in skin of guinea pigs receiving intraveneous injection of immune spleen cells

		Tumor incidence Line-10 challenge (no. of site x dosage)[b]		
Exp.	No. of immune cells transferred[a]	1×10^6	10×10^6	1×10^7
1	0	6/6	6/6	6/6
	100×10^6	0/6	1/5[c]	5/6
2	0	6/6	6/6	6/6
	100×10^6	0/6	1/6[d]	3/5

[a]Each guinea pig received immune spleen cells iv and was challenged id on the same day with line-10 cells.

[b]When ten inoculations were administered, the distance between any two sites was $\geqslant$ 25 mm.

[c]One animal in this group developed tumors at four challenge sites during the course of observation of 42 days.

[d]One animal in this group developed two small papules at sites of tumor challenge.

TABLE 6. Lack of specific attraction of intraveneously injected immune cells at tumor skin challenge site

		Tumor incidence Line-10 challenge dose		
		Left flank[b]	Right flank	
Group	No. of immune spleen cells transferred	10^7	10^6	10^6
1	0		6/6	6/6
2	100×10^6		0/5	1/5
3	0	6/6	6/6	6/6
4	100×10^6	5/5	0/5	1/5
5	0	-[c]	6/6	6/6
6	100×10^6	-	0/5	0/5

[a]Each guinea pig received immune spleen cells iv and was challenged id with line-10 cells on the same day. Tumor growth was observed for 28 days.

[b]10^7 line-10 challenge was inoculated at least 25 mm from 10^6 cell challenge.

[c]10^7 line-10 challenge sites were excised surgically 3 days after inoculation.

From the results of absorption studies and quantitative analyses of adoptive immunity against the syngeneic guinea pig line-10 hepatoma, the following conclusions can be drawn: 1. The protection afforded by adoptive immunization agaisnt challenge with hepatoma cells was tumor line specific, while, in most cases, in vitro cytotoxicity was not. 2. The immune spleen cells mediating cytotoxicity in vitro were functionally distinct from those conveying adoptive protection in vivo. 3. The immune cells possessing receptors for tumor specific rejection antigens reacted with tumor targets specifically. Such interactions, however, did not lead to lysis of the neoplastic cells in vitro in a 48 hour ^{3}H release assay. 4. In adoptive transfer, the number of tumor cells eradicated increased exponentially as a function of the number of immune lymphoid cells. 5. Eradication of 10^4 or 10^5 line-10 tumor cells by adoptive immunity was independent of specific immunity in the recipient thus, under defined conditions, adoptive transfer may provide a quantitative assay for the antitumor activity of lymphoid cells. 6. The transferred immune cells appeared to be distributed randomly throughout the skin of the recipient. There was no evidence indicating that the immune cells were attracted specifically to the tumor challenge site.

REFERENCES

1. Ashley, M.P., Zbar, B., Hunter, J.T., Rapp, H.J., and Sugimoto, T. (1980): Cancer Res., 40:4197-4203.
2. Bartlett, G., and Zbar, B. (1972): J. Natl. Cancer Inst., 48:1709-1726.
3. Burton, R.C., and Warner, N.L. (1977): Cancer Immunol. Immunother., 2:91-99.
4. Borberg, H., Oettgen, H.F., Chondry, F., and Beatti Jr., E.J. (1972): Int. J. Cancer, 10:539-547.
5. Chauvenet, P.H., McArthur, C.P., and Smith, R.T. (1979): J. Immunol., 123:2575-2581.
6. Churchill Jr., W., Rapp, H., Kronman, B., and Borsos, T. (1968): J. Natl. Cancer Inst., 41:13-29.
7. Fernandez-Cruz, E., Halliburton, B., and Feldman, J.D. (1969): J. Immunol., 123:1772-1777.
8. Kleinschuster, S.J., Rapp, H.J., Johnston, A.V., Van Kampen, K.R., Muscoplat, C.C., and Logan, J.B. (1980): Experientia, 36:1239-1240.
9. Mitchison, N.A. (1955): J. Exp. Med., 102:157-177.
10. Oehler, J.R., and Herberman, R.B. (1979): J. Natl. Cancer Inst., 62:525-529.
11. Rapp, H.J., Churchill Jr., W., Kronman, B., Rolley, R.T., Hammond, W.G., and Borsos, T. (1968): J. Natl. Cancer Inst., 41:1-11.
12. Reed, L.J., and Muench, H. (1938): Amer. J. Hyg., 27:493-497.
13. Rosenau, W., and Morton, D.L. (1966): J. Natl. Cancer Inst., 36:825-836.
14. Smith, H.G., Harmel, R.P., Hanna Jr., M.G., Zwilling, B.S., Zbar, B., and Rapp, H.J. (1977): J. Natl. Cancer Inst., 58:1315-1322.

15. Shu, S., Hunter, J.T., Rapp, H.J., and Fonseca, L.S. (submitted for publication).

16. Shu, S., Steerenberg, P.A., Hunter, J.T., Evans, C.H., and Rapp, H.J. (1981): Cancer Res., (in press).

17. Wepsic, H.T., Zbar, B., Rapp, H.J., and Borsos, T. (1970): J. Natl. Cancer Inst., 44:955-963.

18. Zbar, B., Bernstein, I.D., and Rapp, H.J. (1971): J. Natl. Cancer Inst., 46:831-839.

AUDIENCE DISCUSSION

Dr. Truitt: The growth of intradermally inoculated tumor in mice varies with the location on the back where the tumor is injected. Do you see such a variation?

Dr. Shu: In the guinea pig line-10 hepatoma system, the growth of intradermally inoculated tumor has been very consistent during the 4 to 6 weeks that tumor growth was observed.

[Unidentified]: A few years ago, Smith reported that adoptive transfer of immune cells was therapeutically effective in this model. Can you give us any follow up results?

Dr. Shu: In Smith's study, transfer of 200×10^6 unfractionated oil-induced peritoneal exudate cells from hyperimmunized animals eradicated an established skin tumor (about 10 mm diameter) as well as lymph node metastasis. We have found that spleen cells were equally effective.

Dr. Green: It is possible that the reason why 70 times as many cells are needed when given systemically is because that kind of tumor challenge can activate the suppressor mechanism.

Dr. Shu: We considered that possibility. Numerous attempts were made to demonstrate the presence of suppressors by transfer studies at various times after tumor challenge. However, we failed to show any suppressor activity.

The Potential Role of T Cells in Cancer Therapy,
edited by A. Fefer and A. Goldstein,
Raven Press, New York © 1982.

Possible Roles of Interleukin 3 in the Regulation of Lymphocyte Differentiation

James N. Ihle, Andrew Hapel, *Joel Greenberger, John C. Lee, and Alan Rein

*Biological Carcinogenesis Program, Frederick Cancer Research Center, Frederick, Maryland 21701; *Sidney Farber Cancer Center, Boston, Massachusetts 02115*

Lymphokines are known to play a central role in regulating immune responses. Factors such as migration inhibitory factor are important in macrophage localization at sites of inflamation. The macrophage derived factor interleukin 1 (IL-1), also termed LAF, appears to play an essential role by facilitating the production of another lymphokine, interleukin 2 (IL-2), by helper T cells (21,36,37). IL-2 in turn appears to mediate the differentiation and amplification of cytotoxic T cells and is particularly important in current research by virtue of its ability to maintain the growth in tissue culture of cytotoxic T cell lines (9,27,32, 39). In addition to these factors which have been characterized biochemically, a variety of additional factors involved in diverse aspects of immune responses which have not been characterized. These include lymphokines which affect B cells either in allowing the differentiation of an antibody response in vitro or polyclonally activating immunoglobulin production, as well as factors promoting the differentiation and proliferation of myeloid cells or mast cells (10,31). From these observations, it appears reasonable to assume that the majority of the manifestations of humoral and cellular immune responses will be regulated by lymphokines including not only the recruitment of nonantigen-specific components such as macrophages, but also the expansion of potentially antigen-specific components as well.

One of the central regulatory components of an immune response involves an antigen-specific helper T cell. Several lymphokines including MIF, T cell replacing factors in B cell responses, and IL-2 have been shown to be produced by helper T cells under appropriate conditions of antigen stimulation (8,19,34,35). More recently, cloned helper T cell lines have been established from immune mice by antigen stimulation in

vitro and have been shown to produce several lymphokines (10,31). Interestingly, cloned helper T cells have also been shown to mediate a classical delayed type hypersensitivity reaction when put in vivo with the
appropriate antigen, demonstrating the central regulatory role of this
subpopulation of lymphocytes (3). In vitro, antigen-specific helper T
cells mediate classical blastogenic responses. Although this response
had been previously considered to be simply the proliferation of antigen-
specific lymphocytes, recent data has suggested that the response is more
complex (22). In particular, proliferation appears to involve a variety
of lymphocyte subpopulations responding to biochemically distinct
lymphokines produced by an antigen-specific helper T cell. Although the
blastogenic response has been related to a few lymphokines, the vast
majority of the factors and subpopulations involved have not been
characterized.

The factors produced by antigen-stimulated helper T cells clearly
influence the functions of a variety of cell types. Perhaps one of the
most potentially important class of factors, however, are those which
directly influence T cell functions. From a speculative viewpoint it
might be anticipated that antigen-activated T cells would produce factors
which affect many stages of T cell differentiation which would allow the
continued expansion of functional effector cell populations including
helper and cytotoxic cells under conditions of antigen excess. The only
factor to date which has this property is IL-2, and the available data
suggest that this lymphokine only functions at a relatively terminal
stage of cytotoxic T cell differentiation. In the results presented here,
we demonstrate the existence of a second lymphokine which specifically
influences T cell differentiation. This factor promotes a very early
stage of T cell differentiation and in vitro specifically promotes the
differentiation of helper T cells.

MATERIALS AND METHODS

The materials and methods used are described in detail elsewhere (16).

RESULTS

Purification and Biological Characteristics of IL-3

Twenty alpha hydroxysteroid dehydrogenase (20αSDH) was initially
shown by Weinstein (40,41) to be associated with T cells. In particular,
the T cell lineage specificity of 20αSDH was strongly suggested by
the observation that only low levels of activity were observed in
splenic lymphocytes from nu/nu or newborn thymectomized mice. Based on
these observations we initially examined the ability of a variety of
factors to induce the expression of 20αSDH in nu/nu splenic lymphocytes
in vitro. Typical results of these experiments are illustrated in Figure
1. Conditioned media from activated T cells readily induce the expression of 20αSDH in vitro. Activation by Con A or mixed lymphocytes
reactions as well as PHA (not shown) give conditioned media with comparable
activity. The T cell specificity of this response is indicated by the
lack of activity in conditioned media from LPS stimulated splenic lymphocytes. In addition to the above sources, two cell lines were found to
produce a factor inducing 20αSDH. Conditioned media from WEHI-3 cells
were found to be most active. This cell line appears to constitutively

Induction of 20α Hydroxysteroid Dehydrogenase

in nu/nu Splenic Lymphocytes

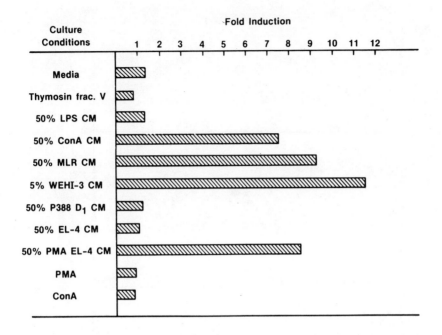

FIG. 1. Splenic lymphocytes were obtained from 4-5 week old BALB/c nu/nu mice and were incubated under the conditions listed for 24 hr at 37°. The lymphocytes were subsequently collected, extracted and assayed for the levels of 20αSDH (33). The fold induction is calculated as the fold increase in enzyme activity relative to untreated splenic lymphocytes.

produce the factor and generally media from 72 hr cultures initially containing 2×10^6 cells/ml produce titers (dilutions giving 50% of maximal induction) of 1:100 whereas the titers of Con A conditioned media are generally approximately 1:5. Last, EL-4 cells can be induced by PMA to produce factor activity under conditions which have previously been shown to induce IL-2 (8).

The factor responsible for the induction of 20αSDH has been purified to homogeneity and has been shown to be biochemically and functionally distinct from a variety of previously defined lymphokines (16). Since the factor is distinct from other lymphokines, is produced by activated T cells and appears to influence T cell differentiation, we have proposed the term interleukin 3 (IL-3). As illustrated in Figure 2, IL-3 can be readily resolved during purification from IL-2 and other lymphokines. In these experiments IL-3 from Con A-conditioned media was initially precipitated with 80% $(NH_4)_2SO_4$, the precipitate resuspended and dialyzed and partially purified on Sephadex G-100 columns. Both IL-2 and IL-3 activity eluted from this column in the 30,000-50,000 dalton region. This fraction was then applied to a DEAE

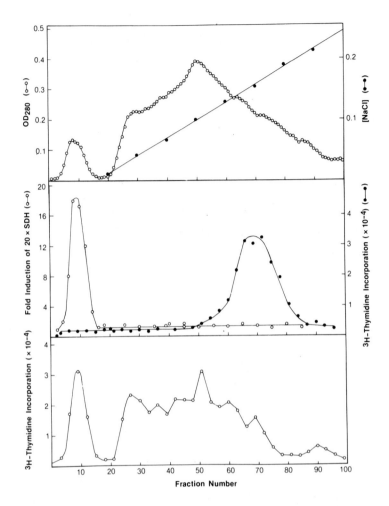

FIG. 2.   DEAE cellulose fractionation of Con A-conditioned media.   The 30,000-50,000 MW fractions from a G-100 Sephadex fractionation of conditioned media were pooled, concentrated, and dialyzed against 0.01 M sodium phosphate buffer, pH 7.0, 0.01 M NaCl.   The sample was then applied to a DEAE cellulose column (1.5 x 30 cm) equilibrated in the same buffer and eluted with a linear NaCl gradient.   Fractions of 5 ml were collected, the optical density at 280 NM (0——0), and the NaCL concentration were determined (●——●), top panel.   The fractions were subsequently assayed for their ability to induce 20αSDH (0——0) and for IL-2 activity (●——●), middle panel or for their ability to induce the proliferation of nylon wool purified splenic lymphocytes (18,24) from MoLV inoculated, preleukemic mice, lower panel.

cellulose column.   As shown in panel B, IL-3 activity elutes from this column in the run through fractions whereas IL-2 binds and elutes in the salt gradient at approximately 0.15 M Nacl.   As illustrated by these results, the fractions containing IL-3 activity have no detectable activity in an IL-2 assay (proliferation in vitro of a cloned cytotoxic T cell line) and conversely IL-2 has no activity in assays for the induction of 20αSDH. Panel C illustrates the results obtained when individual column fractions were assayed in a nonspecific assay for lymphokine activity. This assay is based on the observation that splenic lymphocytes from Moloney leukemia virus inoculated, preleukemic BALB/c mice have a greatly increased frequency of lymphocytes (10-20 fold) capable of responding to a variety of lymphokines in proliferation. As illustrated, using this proliferation assay a variety of peaks of activity were detected including peaks which eluted with IL-3 and IL-2. Interestingly, however, IL-3 and IL-2 appear to represent only a relatively minor components associated with induction of splenic lymphocyte proliferation. The functional significance of the other activities is currently unknown.

Using a combination of standard biochemical techniques IL-3 has been purified to apparent homogeneity (16). The titration curves for preparations at various stages of purification are illustrated in Figure 3. The specific activity (ED_{50}) of the starting material (conditioned media from WEHI-3 cells grown in 1% FCS) is approximately 5 µg/ml whereas homogenous IL-3 after blue-sepharose chromatography has an ED_{50} of approximately 1 ng/ml thus representing a 5000-fold purification. Following blue-sepharose IL-3 is homogenous by SDS-PAGE and has an apparent molecular weight of approximately 41,000 daltons. Preliminary data suggests that IL-3 is a glycoprotein which by isoelectric focusing consists of multiple species differing in pI but which all have comparable specific activities. Experiments are currently in progress to further define the biochemical properties of IL-3.

Several properties of the induction of 20αSDH in nu/nu splenic lymphocytes by IL-3 have been examined (17). The time course for the induction of 20αSDH is shown in Figure 4. The induction of 20αSDH by IL-3 is rapid and after a lag of approximately 6 hr linear increases in 20αSDH occur over the next 24-36 hr. These kinetics strongly suggest that IL-3 is directly promoting differentiation rather than mediating events which secondarily induce 20αSDH. As indicated, the levels of 20αSDH increase 15-20 fold during 24-36 hr strongly suggesting that IL-3 induces 20αSDH expression rather than amplying a population of 20αSDH positive lymphocytes. This aspect has also been suggested by the observation that the precursor is hydrocortisone sensitive whereas the induced population is hydrocortisone resistant (17). Of particular interest for subsequent observations (below) is the specific activity of the induced lymphocyte population. As shown in Figure 4, following induction, the specific activity of 20αSDH reaches levels of approximately 1000 pmoles/hr/10^8 cells. Assuming only approximately 1-10% of the cells are responding to IL-3, the specific activity of these cells would be 10,000-100,000 pmoles/hr/10^8 cells, a level of enzyme activity which has been found in few cloned cells.

The phenotypic characteristics of the lymphocyte subpopulation responding to IL-3 for the induction of 20αSDH expression and in proliferation assays using nylon wool purified splenic lymphocytes have been examined (J.C. Lee and J.N. Ihle, unpublished). Treatment of lymphocytes with complement and antisera against Thy 1.2, Lyt 1, Lyt 2, Ia or Ig does not significantly block either 20αSDH induction or proliferation. Moreover, the phenotype of the lymphocytes after

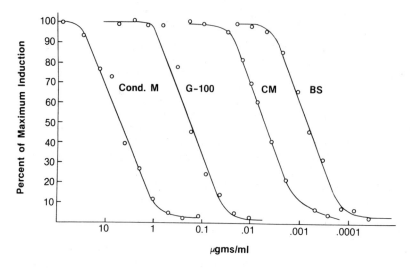

FIG. 3. Titration of samples containing IL-3 during purification. Samples at the indicated steps of purification were assayed for their ability to induce 20αSDH expression as previously described (17). Samples were assayed at the indicated protein concentrations using two-fold dilutions. Protein concentrations were determined by the methods of Lowry et al. (25).

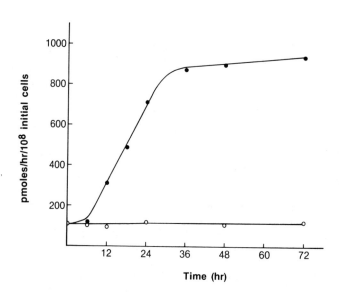

FIG. 4. Time course for the induction of 20αSDH. Nu/nu splenic lymphocytes were incubated in the presence (●—●) or absence (○—○) of IL-3 for the indicated times. The lymphocytes were collected and assayed for the levels of 20αSDH.

responding to IL-3 over a period of 2-3 days remain negative for the above phenotypic markers. Therefore, the exact characteristics of the subpopulation responding to IL-3 are undefined, other than the presence of relatively high levels of 20αSDH.

Production of IL-3 in Antigen-Specific Responses

An essential question concerning the biology of IL-3 involves the normal in vivo sources of IL-3 and more specifically whether the production of IL-3 is associated with immunologically specific reactions. To address this aspect we have examined the cellular immune responses against Moloney leukemia virus antigens in mice regressing MoLV/MSV-induced tumors. The immunological parameters of this response have been examined in considerable detail (7,22). These results have demonstrated that associated with tumor regression are the presence of antigen specific lymphocytes which in vitro respond in blastogenesis to primarily the virion envelope glycoprotein gp70. This proliferative response has been shown to involve the production of blastogenic factors by Thy 1.2[+], Lyt 1[+], 2[-] antigen-specific lymphocytes which induce the majority of the proliferative response by nonantigen specific interactions with a variety of subpopulations of lymphocytes. We, therefore, addressed the question of whether IL-3 was produced in these reactions, the cellular origins of IL-3 and lastly whether IL-3 represented a component of the blastogenic factors responsible for the proliferation observed in vitro.

As illustrated in Table 1, IL-3 activity was readily detectable in cultures of immune lymphocytes stimulated with gp70. The production of IL-3 by these cultures was immunologically specific in that no activity was induced using nonimmune lymphocytes nor was activity detected in cultures of immune lymphocytes incubated with a viral protein, p30, to which the mice do not respond immunologically. Therefore, the production of IL-3-like activity occurs in an antigen-dependent manner using immune lymphocytes. The phenotype of antigen-specific lymphocytes required for the production of IL-3 are also shown by the results in Table 1. Treatment with complement and antisera against Thy 1.2 or Lyt 1 completely abrogated the production of IL-3-like activity whereas antisera against Lyt 2, Ig or Ia had no effect. Therefore, the production of IL-3 in antigen-specific reactions is dependent upon a lymphocyte having the phenotype of helper T cells. Interestingly, the lack of an effect of antisera against Ia and the lack of an effect on IL-3 production by lymphocyte preparations depleted of macrophages (data not shown) demonstrate that IL-3 production in this immune system does not require macrophages for antigen "presentation" or as a source of IL-1.

As indicated above and previously described purified IL-3 has been shown to induce the proliferation of nylon wool purified splenic lymphocytes. Moreover, the induction of 20αSDH has been shown to require proliferation, therefore, the production of IL-3 in antigen-specific reactions strongly indicated that IL-3 may be related to the blastogenic factors shown to be associated with the response to gp70 (22). To examine this possibility, we studied the kinetics of production of IL-3 relative to the general production of blastogenic factors. As shown in Figure 5, the kinetics of production of IL-3 are different from the general production of BF. Maximal production of BF occurred by 24 hr after antigen stimulation, whereas maximal production of IL-3 occurred

TABLE 1. Induction of 20αSDH in nu/nu splenic lymphocytes by factors
in conditioned media from antigen stimulated immune lymphocytes

Culture conditions	pmoles OHP/hr/10^8 lymphocytes	Fold stimulation	% inhibition
Experiment 1[a]			
Media	80	1.0	-
Con A CM	980	12.25	-
gp70/immune CM	840	10.50	-
gp70/nonimmune CM	60	0.75	-
p30/immune CM	70	0.87	-
p30/nonimmune CM	70	0.87	-
Experiment 2[b]			
Media	180	1.0	-
gp70/immune CM +C'	1600	8.89	-
gp70/immune CM α Thy 1 + C'	250	1.39	84%
gp70/immune CM α Lyt 1 + C'	210	1.17	87%
gp70/immune CM α Lyt 2 + C'	1580	8.78	1.2%
gp70/immune CM α Ia + C'	1340	7.44	16.2%
gp70/immune CM α Ig + C'	1570	8.72	1.9%

[a]Nylon wool purified splenic lymphocytes from MoLV/MSV immune or
normal C57BL/6 mice were stimulated for 48 hr with either MoLV gp70
(5 µg/ml) or p30 (5 µg/ml). The conditioned media from these cultures was then tested for their ability to induce 20αSDH at a concentration of 50%.

[b]Immune lymphocytes were used as in a but were initially treated
with the antibodies indicated and C' prior to incubation with gp70
(5 µg/ml). Conditioned media were subsequently assayed as above.

at 48 hr. Therefore, the majority of mitogenic activity produced in
response to gp70 is not associated with IL-3. Consistent with this
we have also observed (data not shown) that mitomycin C treatment of
immune lymphocytes blocks >90% of the IL-3 activity induced by antigen
whereas only approximately 20% of the mitogenic activity is lost.
Therefore, although IL-3 produces lymphocyte proliferation, it represents only a small component of BF activity and is produced in antigen-
stimulated cultures in a pattern distinct from the bulk of BF activity.
Experiments are currently in progress to define more precisely these
differences.

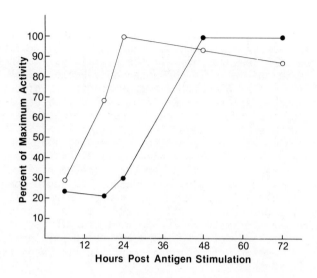

FIG. 5. Time course for the production of blastogenic factors and IL-3 following antigen stimulation. Splenic lymphocytes were obtained from MoLV/MSV-inoculated mice at the peak of tumor regression and purified on nylon wool columns (18,24). They were subsequently incubated with gp70, the conditioned media harvested at the indicated times and the samples assayed for blastogenic factor activity in a lymphocyte proliferation assay (0—0) or for IL-3 by the induction of 20αSDH (●—●).

Establishment of Thy 1.2, Lyt 1$^+$, 2$^-$ Lymphocyte Cell Lines From BALB/c Mice with IL-3

One of the characteristic properties of IL-2 which has allowed its purification and distinction from other lymphokines, is its ability to sustain the growth in vitro of cloned cytotoxic T cell lines (9,27). Since purified IL-3 induced splenic lymphocyte proliferation we reasoned that it may be possible to establish IL-3 dependent cell lines which would in turn allow a more definitive characterization of the responding cell population. For these reasons we examined the ability of IL-3 to support the growth of nylon wool purified splenic lymphocytes in vitro. The ability of IL-3 to support the growth of lymphocytes was initially determined by varying factor concentration, lymphocyte density and media. From these experiments optimal conditions were found to involve plating 2-4 x 10^6 nylon wool purified splenic lymphocytes/cm^3 in RPMI 1640 containing 10% FCS with concentrations of IL-3 giving maximal induction of 20αSDH. The media are changed every 3 days and the cells transferred to fresh wells every 7 days to remove adherent cells. Under these conditions there is a transient period of growth during the first 2-3 days followed by a decrease in cell numbers over the next 10-20 days. After this the cultures increase in growth rate and after 4-6 weeks stable transferable cell lines are established. Using BALB/c splenic lymphocytes the efficiency of establishing lines is approximately 90%, whereas in the absence of IL-3 none have been established. Therefore IL-3 is capable of establishing lymphocyte cell lines reproducibly and efficiently.

The majority of cell lines established from BALB/c mice with IL-3 became independent of exogenously added lymphokines. In this regard they were quite distinct from a number of other cell lines (described below) which required IL-3 for growth. All the cell lines examined could be readily cloned in soft agar in the absense of added lymphokines with cloning efficiencies of 60-90%. The characteristics of several cloned IL-3 derived independent cell lines from BALB/c mice are summarized in Table 2. All of the independent cell lines examined have had a comparable cell surface phenotype of Thy 1.2[+], Lyt 1[+], 2[-]. This phenotype has only been observed with independent lines and has not been observed with any of the IL-3 dependent cell lines (below). A number of the cell lines were also examined for the presence of the T cell associated enzymes TdT (2,14,20) and 20αSDH. As shown none of the lines had detectable TdT by immunofluorescence whereas all the lines examined have had detectable levels of 20αSDH. The levels of 20αSDH have ranged from approximately 100-500 pmoles/hr/10^8 lymphocytes, a relatively low level of activity. The morphology of the cell lines was also examined following Wright's staining. In all cases the cells showed a lymphoblastic morphology.

As noted above, IL-3 very efficiently induces independent Thy 1[+], Lyt 1[+], 2[-] cell lines from BALB/c mice. Moreover, these cell lines proliferate rapidly _in vitro_ and when inoculated i.v. in mice cause disseminated masses suggesting the possibility that some degree of "transformation" may have occurred. Because C-type viruses have been implicated in leukemogenesis and BALB/c mice are known to genetically transmit ecotropic viruses, we examined a number of cell lines for virus expression. As shown in Table 2, both virus positive and negative cell lines were observed. The cell lines A1A and A4A both produced detectable infectious virus. Conversely, the cell lines 3BA2 and 3BA4 were negative for virus expression. Therefore, there currently exists no consistent relationship between virus expression and the establishment of independent cell lines.

Since all the cell lines were independent of exogenously added lymphokines for growth, we examined several for the possible production of IL-3. As shown in Table 2, all the cell lines produced readily detectable IL-3 activity. In general, 48-72 hr conditioned media from cultures initially containing 2 x 10^6 cells/ml gave titers of approximately 1:100, whereas Con A conditioned media normally contain titers of 1:2-1:5. The addition of factors such as PMA or Con A did not enhance IL-3 production. Therefore, all the independent cell lines constitutively produce high titers of IL-3 activity. In preliminary experiments, the biochemical characteristics of the IL-3 produced by these cell lines appears identical to either the IL-3 in Con A conditioned media or WEHI-3 conditioned media based on column elution from G-100, DEAE cellulose and CM cellulose.

Establishment and Characteristics of IL-3 Dependent Cell Lines

In addition to the independent cell lines described above, dependent cell lines have occasionally been established from nylon wool purified splenic lymphocytes. Dependent lines are most often established using lymphocytes from strains other than BALB/c including NIH Swiss and C57BL/6. In addition, dependent cell lines more generally occur, including BALB/c, when cultures are started in normal mouse serum

Table 2. Properties of IL-3 Derived Factor Independent Cell Lines From BALB/c Mice

Properties Examined	Cell Line				
	A1A	A4A	3BA1	3BA2	3BA4
1. Cell Surface Phenotypes					
Thy 1.2	+	+	+	+	+
Lyt 1	+	+	+	+	+
Lyt 2	-	-	-	-	-
2. T Cell Associated Enzymes					
TdT	-	-	-	-	-
20αSDH (pmoles/hr/10^8)	214	160	363	ND	ND
3. C-type Virus Expression					
FFU virus/10^4 cells	>10^3	10^3	ND	0	0
4. Lymphokine Production					
IL-3 (units/ml)	100	100	100	100	100

and IL-3 rather than FCS. The basis for this difference is not well understood but several possibilities are considered in the discussion section.

The characteristics and strain of origin of three IL-3 dependent cell lines are shown in Table 3. The titration curves for proliferation of these cell lines in response to IL-3 and IL-2 have been examined. The three cell lines showed comparable responses to increasing concentrations of purified IL-3. Moreover, the ED$_{50}$ for proliferation was identical to the ED$_{50}$ for the induction of 20αSDH strongly suggesting that a single factor is active in both assays. As summarized in Table 3, the three IL-3 dependent cell lines had comparable cell surface phenotypes being Thy 1.2$^+$, Lyt 1$^-$, 2$^-$. The lines could, however, be distinguished on the basis of morphology. Both 8S and C were heavily granulated cells whereas the C cell line was lymphoblastic in morphology. The granulated cell lines also stained positive with toluidine blue suggesting the possibility that they were mast cell lines. Interestingly, Nabel et al. (29,30) have previously demonstrated that lectin depleted Con A conditioned media contains a factor which allows the isolation and growth of mast cells, which appear to have characteristics similar to the 8S and C cell lines. In preliminary experiments (G. Nabel, personal communication) purified preparations of IL-3 have been found to support the proliferation of the cloned mast cell lines with titration curves comparable to those for induction of 20αSDH. Therefore, these preliminary results suggest that IL-3 may contribute to the proliferation and perhaps the differentiation of mast cells. One distinction between the mast cell lines isolated by Nabel et al. (29,30) and the 8S and C lines, however, is that their mast cell lines are Thy 1.2$^-$. The significance of these differences, however, is currently not known.

Table 3. Characteristics of IL-3 Dependent Cell Lines Established From Splenic Lymphocytes

Properties Examined	Cell Line		
	8S	B	C
1. Strain of Origin	NIH Swiss	C57BL/6	C57BL/6
2. Cell Surface Phenotype			
Thy 1.2	+	+	+
Lyt 1	−	−	−
Lyt 2	−	−	−
3. T Cell Associated Enzymes			
TdT	−	ND	ND
20αSDH (pmoles/hr/10^8 cells)	196	ND	558
4. Production of IL-3			
units/ml	<1	<1	<1
5. Morphology/Histochemistry			
Wright's	granulated	granulated	lymphoblastic
toluidine	+	ND	ND

Some of the IL-3 dependent cell lines were also examined for the expression of TdT and 20αSDH (Table 3). As shown, the 8S line was negative for TdT by immunofluorescence, whereas 8S and C were found to have detectable but low levels of 20αSDH. Last, as expected, none of the cell lines constitutively produced any IL-3 activity when cultured in lymphokine free media.

The above cell lines were established using nylon wool purified splenic lymphocytes and purified IL-3. However, a number of cell lines have previously been established from bone marrow using culture conditions containing glucocorticoids and WEHI-3 conditioned media (11,12,13). Since, as noted above, the WEHI-3 cell line constitutively produces high levels of IL-3, and a number of the lines were dependent on CM from WEHI-3 for growth, we have examined the response of several of these lines to IL-3. One such cell line, initially described by Dexter et al. (6) and established from bone marrow, is dependent on WEHI-3 CM for growth. Moreover, growth of this cell line was found to not be dependent on classically defined CSF from L cells, suggesting that WEHI-3 cells produced a unique factor. The response of one of these cell lines, the FD line, to purified IL-3 is shown in Figure 6. As shown, purified IL-3 induced proliferation of these cells with a dose response identical to the dose response curve for the induction of 20αSDH, suggesting that a single factor was active in both assays. To determine whether IL-3 uniquely was capable of supporting the growth of FD cells, we examined the ability of various fractions of a DEAE-cellulose column of Con A conditioned media to induce proliferation. As noted above, such columns resolve a variety of factors which induce proliferation of lymphocytes from preleukemic mice. Only those fractions containing IL-3 activity

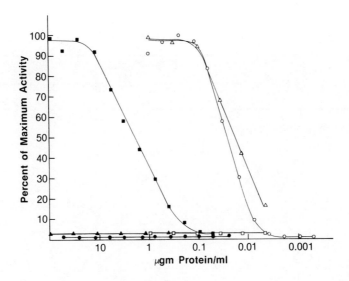

FIG. 6. Response of FD cells to purified IL-2 and IL-3. The proliferative response of FD cells to purified IL-3 (0——0) and IL-2 (●——●) was determined using the indicated protein concentrations and a standard proliferation assay. For comparison the ability of IL-3 to induce proliferation of a cloned cytotoxic T cell line, CT6, (□—□) and to induce 20αSDH (△—△) are also shown. Similarly, the ability of IL-2 to induce 20αSDH (▲—▲) and to promote the proliferation of CT6 cells (■——■) are shown for comparison.

induced proliferation of the FD cell line (not shown). Of particular interest is the observation that the fractions containing IL-2 activity did not promote proliferation. In additional experiments the ability to induce proliferation of FD cells was found to copurify in all steps of purification with IL-3 activity. Therefore, the maintenance of FD cell growth appears to represent a unique characteristic of IL-3.

In addition to the FD cell line, we have also examined a number of bone marrow cell lines established by one of us (J.G.) (11-13) which are dependent on WEHI-3 CM for growth. As above, these cell lines were found to proliferate in response to purified IL-3 with dose responses identical to the induction of 20αSDH. Experiments are currently in progress to determine whether the ability to promote growth of these cell lines uniquely copurifies with IL-3 activity.

To determine the relationship of bone marrow derived, IL-3 dependent cell lines to the cell lines established from splenic lymphocytes, we examined the cell surface phenotypes of several of the lines. As indicated in Table 4, by Wright's staining, all of the cell lines had a lymphoblastic morphology and specifically did not resemble the mast cell like lines such as 8S and C. By cell surface markers two phenotypes were observed. Both the FD and B6Sut cell lines were strongly positive for Thy 1.2 with 100% of the cells being positive. These cell lines, however, were Lyt 1⁻ and Lyt 2⁻. In contrast, the other cell lines were Thy 1.2⁻, Lyt 1⁻, 2⁻. The cell lines were also examined for the

Table 4. Characteristics of IL-3 Dependent Cell Lines Established
From Bone Marrow Cultures

Properties Examined	Cell Line					
	$C3H_5$	32-DCL	Rotundi	B6D2F1(D)	FD	B6Sut
1. Cell Surface Phenotype						
Thy 1.2	–	–	–	–	+	+
Lyt 1	–	–	–	–	–	–
Lyt 2	–	–	–	–	–	–
2. Morphology						
Wright's stain	lym.	lym.	lym.	lym.	lym.	lym.
3. 20αSDH Level pmoles/hr/10^8 cells	90,000	20,000	335	690	466	247

levels of 20αSDH. As indicated two phenotypes were observed. Most
of the cell lines contained levels of 20αSDH consistent with that
observed in the lines derived from splenic lymphocytes. In contrast
to these, two cell lines with a Thy 1.2-, Lyt 1-, 2- phenotype had
levels of 20αSDH 20-100 fold higher than previously observed in any
T cell lines. Additional characteristics of these cell lines are
currently being examined.

DISCUSSION

The biochemical and biological properties of IL-3 clearly distinguish
this lymphokine from a variety of previously characterized factors. The
unique and distinguishing characteristic of IL-3 is its ability to
induce 20αSDH in nu/nu splenic lymphocytes in vitro. Although the
exact significance of this induction to lymphocyte differentiation is
not presently known as discussed below, a number of characteristics of
the assay are important and unique relative to most assays for lymphokine activity. First, induction occurs rapidly in vitro. Unlike the
majority of assays which examine the promotion of functionally active
lymphocytes and require cultures of 4-5 days or longer, induction of
20αSDH starts with a lag of only approximately 6 hr and is maximal
by 24-36 hr. This is particularly important when using complex
lymphocyte populations where a variety of "secondary" events might be
anticipated. The rapidity of induction strongly suggests that the
increases of 20αSDH are directly due to interactions of IL-3 with a
responding subpopulation. Second, the induction of 20αSDH is unique in
not requiring the generation of functional activity. Therefore, it is
possible that early steps of differentiation may be measured which
precede and perhaps are required for the generation of functional
activity. For example, generation of cytotoxic T cells clearly requires
IL-2; however, since CTLs are 20αSDH positive, optimal generation of
CTLs may require both IL-3 and IL-2. Similar types of events may be
required for generation of helper T cells and perhaps other lineages.
Last, in our experience the induction of 20αSDH has been a highly

reproducible and sensitive assay. Titration of samples over long periods of time have given identical response curves indicating little variability in the response of different preparations of lymphocytes. From studies with homogenous IL-3, the sensitivity of the assay is extremely good such that concentrations of IL-3 at 0.1 ng/ml can be detected. Because of the rapidity of the response, the reproducibility and the sensitivity, the induction of 20αSDH would appear to provide an important and convenient assay to study lymphocyte differentiation.

The biochemical characteristics of IL-3 distinguish it from a variety of lymphokines. Purified IL-3 has an apparent molecular weight of 30,000-50,000 on Sephadex columns under nondenaturing conditions and an apparent molecular weight of 41,000 by SDS-PAGE under denaturing conditions. IL-3 can be readily resolved from IL-2 and other lymphokines including CSF (38) by virtue of its elution from DEAE cellulose columns. In our experience, using Con A-conditioned media, the run through fractions from DEAE cellulose contain primarily if not exclusively IL-3. In particular, these fractions on continued purification steps fail to give rise to additional activities detectable in the more nonspecific assay of induction of proliferation of preleukemic splenic lymphocytes.

IL-3 is similar to several other lymphokines in that it is primarily the product of activated helper T cells. Conditions such as Con A or PHA stimulation as well mixed lymphocyte reactions give rise to relatively high levels of IL-3. Conditioned media from such reactions are commonly used as a source of IL-2 without additional purification and some of the affects ascribed to IL-2 may well be due to IL-3 or "other factors" detected in Con A conditioned media unassociated with IL-2 or IL-3 but detectable in assays for induction of proliferation of preleukemic splenic lymphocytes. More importantly, however, IL-3 is also a product of antigen-specific reactions and is dependent upon an antigen-specific Thy 1.2^+, Lyt 1^+ 2^- helper-like T cell subpopulation. Similarly all the Thy 1.2^+, Lyt 1^+, 2^- lymphocyte lines we have developed constitutively produce IL-3 whereas a variety of other phenotypes including cytotoxic lines do not (data not shown). These observations strongly implicate IL-3 as a physiological component of cellular immune responses. Conversely, IL-3 is not apparently produced by B cell mitogens or by nonspecific activation of macrophages or macrophage cell lines similar to IL-1. With regard to the production of IL-3, the most unusual observation was the constitutive production of lymphokine at high titers by the WEHI-3 cell line, since this line was considered to be a monocyte-macrophage line. The derivatives we have examined, however, have phenotypes more characteristic of lymphocytes. In particular, they have a lymphoblast morphology, are negative for Ia or nonspecific esterase and are strongly Thy 1 positive although they express no detectable Lyt 1 or 2. Experiments are currently in progress to assess additional properties of these cells. Moreover, the constitutive production of IL-3 clearly distinguishes the WEHI-3 line from other monocyte lines such as P388D₁.

Perhaps one of the most important questions, however, concerns the role of 20αSDH induction and IL-3 in lymphocyte differentiation. The observations that 20αSDH levels in nu/nu splenic lymphocytes and in lymphocytes from newborn thymectomized mice are very low and strongly implicate 20αSDH expression in lymphocyte differentiation. Moreover, the observation that 20αSDH is uniquely expressed in a variety of T cell lines but not B cells, macrophages, erythrocytes, fibroblasts, etc. again suggests a specific relationship to T cell differentiation. Our initial observations (17) that 20αSDH was induced in an initially Thy 1⁻ lymphocyte which stayed Thy 1⁻ after induction suggested that IL-3 was promoting a relatively early T cell precursor prior to the expression of Thy 1. Clearly, it now becomes important to more definitively establish the relationship of this type of lymphocyte to more mature, functional lymphocytes. In this regard, two of the cells derived from bone marrow and dependent on IL-3 for growth may be of particular interest. Specifically, during the induction of 20αSDH in nu/nu splenic lymphocytes, specific activities of 1500-2000 pmoles/hr/10^8 lymphocytes are often observed. Since it is unlikely that IL-3 is inducing greater than 10% of the cells and probably significantly less, the specific activity of the subpopulation responding to IL-3 would have to be extremely high. As noted in the results, the majority of functionally differentiated T cells have considerably lower specific activities, suggesting that high levels of activity may be characteristic of an early IL-3 responsive population. This phenotype was observed in the bone marrow derived IL-3 dependent lines. The phenotype of these cell lines is, therefore, consistent with the possibility that they represent the primary IL-3-induced population.

The implications from the above observations are that as a consequence of an ongoing cellular immune response, IL-3 would be produced and induce 20αSDH expression. In turn, the physiological effect of these events might be anticipated to include a transient decrease in circulating progesterone levels, during the period of circulation of the high 20αSDH type intermediate. This may have relevance to the immune response since progesterone has been found to be immunosuppressive both in vivo in allograft rejection (4,26) and in vitro in mitogen responses (28). In contrast, 20α dihydroxyprogesterone the reduced derivative produced by 20αSDH, is not immunosuppressive (40). Experiments are currently in progress to more directly assess these relationships in vivo, and to better define the mechanisms by which progesterone mediates immunosuppression.

In addition to induction of 20αSDH, our results demonstrate that several phenotypes of lymphocytes require IL-3 for growth in vitro. In this regard IL-3 is similar in biological properties to IL-2 which is known to be required for the growth in vitro of cytotoxic T cells (9,27). However, the diversity of phenotypes which require IL-3 for growth is unusual. The majority of the cell lines were lymphoblastic but variably expressed the Thy 1 antigen. In the absence of any apparent functional activities, the relationship of these phenotypes to lymphocyte differentiation is uncertain. The only cell lines with apparant "functional" activities are those with the properties of mast cells. Somewhat unexpectedly most of these cell lines were Thy 1 positive. How this phenotype is related to T cell differentiation is at present uncertain. Perhaps the most important point to be raised relative to these observations is that the property of requiring IL-3 for growth may help to define a specific lineage of lymphocytes. By using additional factors in attempts to promote in vitro differentiation of these lines it may well be possible to define precisely the interrelationship of these phenotypes.

The ability of IL-3 to promote the establishment of independent, Thy 1+, Lyt 1+, 2- cell lines from nylon wool purified splenic lymphocytes was unexpected. Previous studies have not detected an influence of IL-3 on this phenotype of lymphocyte. As noted in the results, the establishment of these lines requires 4-6 weeks in tissue culture and, therefore, could be the culmination of a sequence of events promoted by IL-3. Our results suggest that the establishment of these lines does not require C-type virus expression, but whether somatic changes are involved and required for "transformation" cannot be excluded. The cell surface phenotype of all the independent cell lines suggest a relationship to helper T cells, similarly the production of IL-3 and IL-2 (15) is consistent with this interpretation. Moreover, the constitutive production of IL-3 suggests that if they are helper T cell clones they are clonally "activated". Experiments are in progress to better define the events required for establishment of these cell lines. However, because the lines grow independently, are stable over many generations and proliferate rapidly they provide a convenient source of IL-3 as well as several other lymphokines.

In summary, IL-3 represents a unique lymphokine with a variety of biological effects in vitro. The characteristic property of this lymphokine is the ability to induce 20αSDH in nu/nu splenic lympho-cytes. In addition, however, it is clear that IL-3 is required for the growth in vitro of a variety of phenotypes of lymphocytes. Although it is currently difficult to interrelate these activities, continued studies into the biology of IL-3 should provide new insights in lymphocyte differentiation and regulation.

ACKNOWLEDGEMENTS

The authors are greatly indebted to Jonathan Keller and Linda Rebar for their excellent technical assistance and to Linda Fawley for help in preparation of the manuscript. We also would like to thank Dr. E. Scolnick of the National Cancer Institute for kindly providing the FD cell line.

REFERENCES

1. Adelman, N.E., Ksiazek, J., Yoshida, T., and Cohen, S. (1980): J. Immunol., 124:825.

2. Barton, R., Goldschneider, I., and Bollum, F.J. (1976): J. Immunol., 116:462.

3. Bianchi, A.T.J., Hooijkaas, H., Benner, R., Tees, R., Nordin, A.A., and Schrier, M.H. (1981): Nature, 290:836.

4. Bilder, G.E. (1976): Imm. Comm., 5:163.

5. David, J.R., and David, R.A. (1972): In: Progress in Allergy, edited by P. Kallos, B.H. Waksman, and A. deWeck, p. 300. S. Karger, Basel.

6. Dexter, J.M., Garland, J., Scott, D., Scolnick, E., and Metcalf, D. (1980): J. Exp. Med., 152,1036.

7. Enjuanes, L., Lee, J.C., and Ihle, J. N. (1979): J. Immunol., 112:665.

8. Farrar, J.J., Mizel, S.B., Fuller-Farrar, J.J., Farrar, W.L., and Hilfiker, M.L. (1980): J. Immunol., 125:793.

9. Gillis, S., and Smith, K.A. (1977): J. Exp. Med., 146:468.

10. Glasebrook, A.L., Quintans, J., Eisenberg, L., and Fitch, F.W. (1981): J. Immunol., 126:240.

11. Greenberger, J.S. (1980): J. Supramol. Struct., 13:501.

12. Greenberger, J.S., Newburger, P., Karpas, A., and Moloney, W. (1978): Cancer Res., 38:3340.

13. Greenberger, J.S., Gans, P.J., Davisson, P.B., and Moloney, W.C. (1979): Blood, 53:987.

14. Gregoire, K.E., Goldschneider, I., Barton, R.W., and Bollum, F.J. (1977). Proc. Natl. Acad. Sci. USA, 74:3993.

15. Hapel, A.J., Lee, J.C., Farrar, W.L., and Ihle, J.N. (1981). Cell, (in press).

16. Ihle, J.N., Keller, J., Lee, J.C., Farrar, W.L., and Hapel, A.J. (1981): In: Lymphokine and Thymic Factors and Their Potential in Cancer Therapeutics, edited by A.L. Goldstein and M. Chirigo. Raven Press, New York, (in press).

17. Ihle, J.N., Pepersack, L., and Rebar, L. (1981): J. Immunol., 126:2184-2189.

18. Julius, M.H., Simpson, E., and Herzenberg, L.A. (1973): Eur. J. Immunol., 3:645.

19. Kuhner, A.L., Cantor, H., and David, J.R. (1980): J. Immunol., 125: 1117.

20. Kung, P.C., Silverstone, A.E., McCaffrey, R.P., and Baltimore, D. (1975): J. Exp. Med., 141:855.

21. Larsson, E.L., Iscove, N.N., and Coutinho, A. (1980): Nature, 283:664.

22. Lee, J.C., Enjuanes, L., Cicurel, L., and Ihle, J.N. (1981): J. Immunol., 127:78-83.

24. Lipsky, P.E., and Rosenthal, A.S. (1976): J. Immunol. 117:1594.

25. Lowry, O.H., Rosebrough, N.J., Farr, A.L., and Randall, R.J. (1951): J. Biol. Chem., 193:265.

26. Monroe, J.S. (1971): J. Reticuloendothelial Soc., 9:361.

27. Morgan, D.A., Ruscetti, F.W., and Gallo, R. (1976): Science, 193: 1007.

28. Mori, T., Kobayashi, H., Nishimura, T., Mori, T.S., Fumii, G., and Inou, J. (1975): Imm. Comm. 4:519.

29. Nabel, G., Fresno, M., Chessman, A., and Cantor, H. (1981): Cell, 23:19.

30. Nabel, G., Galli, S.J., Dvorak, A.M., Dvorak, H.F., and Cantor, H. (1981): Nature 291:332.

31. Nabel, G., Greenberger, J.S., Sakakeeny, M.A., and Cantor, H. (1981). Proc. Natl. Acad. Sci. USA, 78:1157.

32. Nabholz, M., Conselman, A., Acuto, O., North, M., Haas, W., Pohlit, H., von Boehmer, H., Hengartner, H., Mach, J.P., Engers, H., and Johnson, J.P. (1980): Immunol. Rev., 51:125.

33. Pepersack, L., Lee, J.C., Enjuanes, L., and Ihle, J.N. (1980): J. Immunol., 124:279.

34. Schimpl, A., and Wecker, E. (1972): Nature (New Biol.), 237:15.

35. Shaw, J., Caplan, B., Paefkau, V., Pilarski, L.M., Delovitch, T., and McKenzie, I.F.C. (1980): J. Immunol. 124:2231.

36. Smith, K.A., Gilbride, K.J., Favata, M.F. (1980): Nature, 287:836.

37. Smith, K.A., Lachman, L.B., Oppenheim, J.J., and Favata, M.F. (1980): J. Exp. Med., 151:1551.

38. Stanley, E.R., and Guilbert, L.J. (1981): J. Immunol. Methods, 42:253.

39. Watson, J., Gillis, S., Marbrook, J., Mochizuki, D., and Smith, K.A. (1979). J. Exp. Med., 150:849.

40. Weinstein, Y. (1977): J. Immunol., 119:1223.

41. Weinstein, Y., Linder, H.R., and Eckstein, B. (1977). Nature, 266:632.

AUDIENCE DISCUSSION

[Unidentified]: How do you know that a single factor is involved in the various activities you've described for IL-3.

Dr. Ihle: The specific activity of purified IL 3 is around a nanogram per milliliter. The assays have been done with preparations having a minimal specific activity of 5-10 ng/ml. In addition, we always do titration curves to make sure that they have the same slope. We, therefore, believe that IL 3 is common to all the activities.

Dr. Herberman: Do you know if IL 3 is species restricted? Have you looked at the various IL 3-dependent lines for natural killer cell activity?

Dr. Ihle: We have not looked for natural killer cell actiivty. Cantor is now looking at the effect of IL 3 on NK cells. Secondly, mouse IL 3 induces proliferation of human lymphocytes.

<u>Dr. Warner</u>: Will other Thy-1 positive mouse macrophage lines produce this? WEHI-3 is inducible by a variety of agents. Does its production of IL 3 change? Have you looked at any human AMNLs for source of IL 3?

<u>Dr. Ihle</u>: We have not found a human cell line that produces IL 3 that can be measured in a mouse assay. With regard to WEHI-3, PHA and Con A doesn't alter induction. Other monocyte cell lines, like the P388D1, did not produce detectable IL 3.

<u>Dr. Matheson</u>: Does this cell have any relationship to the cells that have been described as the target cells for Moloney virus induction?

<u>Dr. Ihle</u>: We don't know. We have not yet used any of the antisera to type the primary cell induced by IL 3.

<u>Dr. Matheson</u>: Have you fractionated bone marrow to see whether you can induce particular kinds by IL 3?

<u>Dr. Ihle</u>: No.

<u>Dr. Gillis</u>: Does the 24-hour proliferative assay for activity work on just naive spleen cells, spleen cells from virus primed animals or spleen cells from preleukemic mice?

<u>Dr. Ihle</u>: In a standard blastogenic assay nude splenic lymphocytes yield 5-10,000 counts, normal splenic lymphocytes (nylon wool purifed) yield less than 2,000 and preleukemic 30-40,000. There's a dramatic difference between the preleukemic and normal spleen.

The Potential Role of T Cells in Cancer Therapy,
edited by A. Fefer and A. Goldstein,
Raven Press, New York © 1982.

The Effects of Interleukin 2 on Primary *In Vivo* Immune Responses

Paul J. Conlon, Steven H. Hefeneider, Christopher S. Henney, and Steven Gillis

Program in Basic Immunology, The Fred Hutchinson Cancer Research Center, Seattle, Washington 98104

The important immunoregulatory roles of several cell-derived factors (cytokines) have recently been documented. One such class, T-cell growth factor (Interleukin 2 or IL-2), has been shown to enhance a variety of immunological responses in vitro. These include: the generation of cytotoxic T cells from athymic animals (9); production of antibody producing cells from T cell-depleted lymphocyte systems (4,21); sustained proliferation of long term helper and cytolytic T cell lines (1,7,20,21); and recently, natural killer (NK) cell activity (11,12). However, no direct evidence exists documenting the in vivo significance of IL-2. Given the availability of highly purified preparations (14), it has now become possible to determine if indeed IL-2 is involved in the modulation of immune reactivity in vivo.

The present investigation was designed to elucidate the effects of in vivo administration of IL-2 on cytotoxic effector cell function. We therefore examined: (i) the lytic reactivity of alloantigen directed cytolytic T-lymphocytes (CTL), harvested from alloimmunized animals, and (ii), natural killer cell function in normal mice following systemic administration of highly purified, murine IL-2. We found that both CTL and NK responses were enhanced approximately two-fold in mice that received IL-2 as compared with control animals receiving only saline and carrier protein. These in vivo data substantiate the contention put forth from in vitro evidence, suggesting that IL-2 is an important immunoregulatory protein. Furthermore, the ability of IL-2 to augment in vivo immune responses bodes well for the possible effectiveness of this lymphokine as an immunotheraupetic drug.

MATERIALS AND METHODS

Animals: BALB/c (H-2^d) male mice were obtained from the central animal facility at the Hutchinson Cancer Research Center. CBA/J (H-2^k) males were purchased from the Jackson Laboratories, Bar Harbor, Maine. Mice were 6-8 weeks old at the time of each experiment.

Tumor cells: The murine thymoma, EL4 (C57BL/6 origin) was maintained as an ascites tumor by weekly passage in syngeneic mice (10^6 cells/animal). Viable tumor cells were harvested by peritoneal aspiration. SL-3 (H-2^k), YAC-1 (H-2^a), L5178Y (clone 27v) and an NK insusceptible variant (designated clone 27 av) (3) were maintained in in vitro cultures in RPMI 1640 medium supplemented with 10% fetal calf serum (FCS), and were kindly provided by Dr. Colin G. Brooks.

Reagents and antiserum: Anti-thy 1.2 antibody was produced by a rat/mouse hybridoma cell line. The derivation of this antibody and its specificity have previously been described (15). Rabbit anti-asialo-GM$_1$ serum was kindly provided by Dr. David Urdal. The specificity of this serum has been described in detail elsewhere (22). Treatment of effector cells was carried out by incubating 2×10^6 cells (100 μl) and equal volume of either anti-thy 1.2 (1/50 dilution of hybridoma culture supernate) or anti-Asialo-GM$_1$ (1/100 dilution) for 60 minutes on ice. 100 μl of guinea pig complement (1:40 final dilution) was then added to the cell suspension and the incubation continued for 45 minutes at 37°C. Cells were then washed in Hank's Buffered Salt Solution (HBSS, Grand Island Biological Co., Grand Island, New York) and resuspended in RPMI 1640-2% FCS. Depletion of adherent cells from peritoneal exudates (PEC) was performed using Sephadex G-10.(13).   Twenty-five million PEC were layered onto a 3ml Sephadex G-10 column equilibrated in RPMI-1640 and 5% FCS. The cells were allowed to enter the column and were incubated for 30 min at 37°C.   The non-adherent cell population was collected by elution with 2 column volumes of RPMI-1640 5% FCS and resuspended to an appropriate concentration for cytotoxic assays (2-4×10^6 cells/ml).

IL-2 production and purification: Murine IL-2 was purified from tissue culture medium conditioned by 1% PHA stimulation of cloned LBRM-33-5A4 lymphoma cells. Methods for purification of IL-2 including sequential ammonium sulfate precipitation, gel-exclusion, ion exchange and hydrophobic affinity chromatography and preparative flatbed isoelectric focusing have been previously described in detail (14).   IL-2 fractions used in the in vivo trials contained no detectable colony stimulating factor, interleukin-1, or interferon. IL-2 titer of the material used was determined in the standard bioassay, testing the capacity of the material to maintain cloned T cell proliferation as assessed by T-cell incorporation of tritiated thymidine (8).

Immunization/in vivo IL-2 administration:

A. Alloimmune CTL: BALB/c mice (3/group) were immunized intraperitoneally (ip) with 2×10^7 viable, allogeneic EL-4 tumor cells. Animals also received either intravenously (iv) or ip, at varying time periods after allo-immunization, either a 1 ml solution of bovine serum albumin (BSA, 1mg/ml) in physiological saline (Saline-BSA) or 100 units (U) of IL-2 together with 1 mg BSA in 1 ml of saline (IL-2 BSA). BSA was used throughout these studies as a source of carrier protein to insure stability of purified IL-2 throughout manipulation during and prior to in vivo use.

B. NK cells: CBA/J mice (2/group) were injected ip with 1ml solution of either saline-BSA or IL-2-BSA (25, 50, or 100 U/ml).

Harvesting of effector cell populations:

A. Alloimmune CTL: At varying time intervals after EL4 immunization (5-10 days), animals were sacrificed, spleen and PEC populations harvested and pooled.   These cell populations were tested for lytic reactivity against ^{51}Cr labeled tumor target cells in standard 4 hr lymphocyte-mediated cytolysis (LMC) assays.

B. NK cells: Forty-eight hours after IL-2 administration, animals were sacrificied and splenic effector cell cytotoxicity determined.

LMC Assays: The cytolytic activity of spleen and PEC populations was assessed using a standard microcytoxicity assay employing ^{51}Cr-labeled target cells. Methods used for conducting LMC assay have been described elsehwere (15). The cultures were incubated at 37°C for 4 hr. An aliquot of cell-free supernate was collected at the end of the 4 hr incubation and the amount of ^{51}Cr-released determined by gamma scintillation counting. Percent specific lysis was calculated using the following equation:

```
CPM liberated in experimental culture -
CPM liberated in spontaneous release medium culture
```

```
CPM liberated in maximum released (detergent) culture -
CPM liberated in spontaneous release culture
```

RESULTS

Based on well-documented experimentation demonstrating that IL-2 is required for the in vitro differentiation of alloreactive CTL (4, 15, 16, 18, 19), we questioned whether administration of highly purified IL-2 might have beneficial effect on the generation of alloreactive killer cells in vivo. Using an in vivo immunization regimen previously shown to produce CTL (10), we observed that ip innoculation of BALB/c (H-2^d) mice with 100 U of purified IL-2, together with live allogeneic tumor cells (EL4-H-2^b) resulted in approximately a two-fold augmentation of effector cell lytic activity when assessed 10 days following immunization. Both PEC and spleen cell populations exhibited an increased anti-EL4 lytic activity as compared to effector cells harvested from alloimmunized donors receiving saline-BSA (Figure Ia and Ib). In ^{51}Cr-release assays we observed a modest degree of cytotoxicity (36% at an effector/target cell ratio of 200/1) mediated by PEC harvested from animals receiving EL4 tumor cells and saline BSA. In contrast, in vivo administration of IL-2 resulted in PEC which mediated 62% specific release at the same effector/target cell ratio. We further established that IL-2 induced augmentation of CTL reactivity was specific for the immunizing antigen, in that an inappropriate tumor cell target (SL3-H-2^k) was not lysed by animals receiving EL4 tumor cells and either saline BSA or IL-2 BSA (data not shown).

While EL4 tumor cells have been shown to be insensitive to NK-cell attack, we felt it necessary to further characterize the effector cell population which mediated augmented cytolytic reactivity in vivo. Table I demonstrates that the effector cell population responsible for enhanced lytic reactivity was indeed of the T cell lineage. Passage of PEC over a Sephadex G-10 column (13) (followed by subsequent testing of the non-adherent cell population's lytic reactivity) did little to reduce the cytolytic activity of PEC harvested from IL-2 treated mice. Furthermore, treatment of PEC populations with anti-asialo GM1 serum (directed against a neutral glycolipid surface marker found on NK cells) (22) and complement resulted in only slight diminution of effector cell function (23% reduction). However, cytolytic reactivity mediated by PEC following treatment with anti-Thy 1.2 antibody and complement was virtually abolished (90% reduction).

Although the in vivo administration of IL-2 substantially enhanced cytotoxic activity of PEC and spleen cells harvested from animals 10 days following alloimmunization, we questioned whether the lymphokine might also alter the kinetics of CTL development. To assess this, groups of BALB/c mice were immunized with EL4 tumor cells and treated simultaneously with either saline

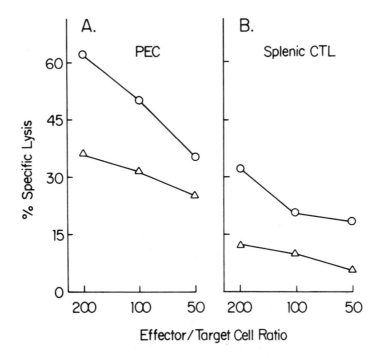

FIG. I. The ability of purified IL-2 to augment alloreactive cytotoxic activity.

BALB/c mice were immunized ip with 2×10^7 EL4 tumor cells.   Identical cohorts of mice were treated ip with Iml of either saline BSA (▲) or 100 U of IL-2 in saline BSA (◯). Ten days later PEC (a) and splenic effector cells (b) were removed and their cytotoxic activity against EL-4 targets determined in standard 4 hr ^{51}Cr-release assay.

BSA or IL-2-BSA. Mice were then sacrificed 5, 7 and 10 days after immunization and the CTL activity in both spleen and PEC populations measured. As seen in Figure 2, no significant differences in the rate of CTL appearance were observed between effector cell populations harvested from saline BSA and IL-2 BSA treated animals. Both 5 and 7 days after immunization, negligible CTL activity was present in cells harvested from either the spleen or PEC pool from mice in either group. However, by day 10, a significant level of augmented lytic reactivity was observed in immune cell populations taken from animals in-noculated with IL-2.   Thus, <u>in vivo</u> IL-2 administration did not appear to significantly alter the rate of development of alloreactive CTL.

Based on earlier observations that IL-2 responsiveness requires prior ligand activation (17), we questioned whether changing the timing of <u>in vivo</u> lymphokine adminstration (after injection of the allogeneic tumor cells) might increase the level of IL-2 augmented responsiveness. To this end, groups of BALB/c mice were injected with 2×10^7 EL4 cells.   Purified IL-2 (100 U) was also administered either at the time of alloimmunization or 48 hr later. As seen in Table II, <u>in vivo</u> treatment with IL-2 48 hr after allogeneic tumor cell injection

Table I. Characterization of PEC-CTL responsible for augmented cytolytic reactivity observed ten days after in vivo administration of purified IL-2

PEC harvested from[a] allo-immunized mice treated with	PEC treatment[b]	% Reduction in in cytotoxic activity (50/1)[c]
Experiment I.		
Saline-BSA	G-10 passage	35%
IL-2-BSA	G-10 passage	15%
Experiment II.		
IL-2-BSA	NMS+C	0%
IL-2-BSA	Anti-AsialoGM$_1$+C	23%
IL-2-BSA	Anti-thy 1.2+C	87%

[a]BALB/c mice (3 animals/group) were immunized with 2×10^7 EL-4 tumor ip and either 1 ml saline-BSA (1mg/ml) or 100 Units of IL-2 in 1mg of saline BSA.
[b]Ten days later PEC were recovered. 25×10^6 cells layered over a Sephadex G-10 column, incubated for 30' at 37°C, the resulting non-adherent cells collected, and the cytotoxic activity determined. In the case of antibody treatment, 2×10^6 PEC were treated with either normal mouse serum (NMS), anti-thy 1.2 hybridoma supernate (1/50 dilution), or anti-asialo Gm$_1$ (1/100) serum for 1 hr at 0° C. An equal value of guinea pig complement (1/40) was then added and the cell suspension incubated for 30' at 37°C. The cells were washed once, resuspended to their original volume, and their cytotoxicity determined in a standard 4h ^{51}Cr-release assay.

[c]% reduction $= 1 - \dfrac{\text{\% lysis mediated by experimental group}}{\text{\% lysis mediated by untreated control group}} \times 100$

was slightly more efficacious in augmenting PEC-CTL reactivity observed on day 10. Such augmentation was over and above that mediated by effector cells harvested from EL4 immunized mice that received IL-2 BSA on day zero. That is, PEC harvested from BSA treated animals generated 27.4% target cell lysis at an effector/target cell ratio of 100/1; while PEC harvested from similarly allo-immunized mice that received IL-2 on day zero demonstrated 60.6% lysis at an identical effector/target cell ratio. However, if the IL-2 injection was delayed for 48 hrs after alloimmunization we witnessed a slight but reproducable increase in CTL activity (72% specific lysis at an effector/target ratio of 100/1). Further delay in IL-2 administration (5 or 8 days after alloimmunization) was not as effective in augmenting PEC-CTL activity in comparison to animals given IL-2 at the time of alloantigen sensitization (data not shown).

Finally, based on the ability of ip IL-2 treatment to augment splenic CTL responses (fig. 1) we examined what effect iv lymphokine administration would have on CTL activity. As detailed in Table III, iv and ip IL-2 treatment on day 0 (100U/animal) significantly augmented the lytic activity of spleen cells harvested from BALB/c mice 10 days after EL4 immunization. Although the level of lysis achieved by splenic CTL was substantially less than that observed in experiments using PEC effector cells (Figure 1, Tables I and II), the ability of systemic IL-2 treatment to augment alloimmune splenic CTL reactivity further testified to the capacity of the purified lymphokine to function in a physiological setting in vivo.

Based on the recent demonstration that in vitro exposure of normal or nude mouse spleen cell populations to purified IL-2 results in a significant increase in NK responses (11, 12), we questioned whether in vivo administration of IL-2

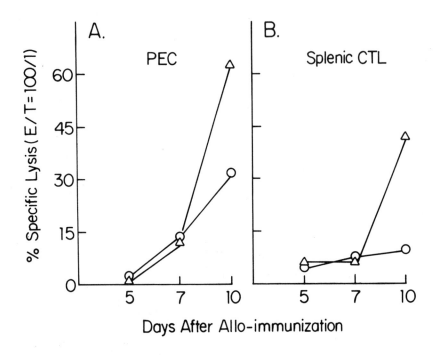

FIG. 2. Kinetics of IL-2 augmented alloreactive CTL responses.

Five, 7 and 10 days following alloimmunization and treatment with either saline BSA (**O**) or IL-2 BSA (**△**), PEC and spleen cell populations were removed and tested for lytic reactivity against ^{51}Cr-labeled EL4 tumor target cells.

would have a similar potentiating effect on NK cytotoxicity. To examine this possibility CBA mice were injected ip with either saline BSA or 100 U of purified IL-2 in saline BSA. 48 hr later spleen cells were removed and NK activity determined using a standard 4 hr ^{51}Cr-release assay. As shown in figure 3, in vivo administration of IL-2 resulted in a significant augmentation of splenic cytotoxic cell activity. At an effector/target cell ratio of 100/1, cytolytic activity increased from 4.8% in animals receiving saline BSA to 21.5% in animals receiving IL-2 in saline BSA.

In an attempt to establish what cell type was in fact responsible for the boosted lytic responses following in vivo IL-2 administration, we examined the specificity of the augmented reactivity. This was approached by assaying the capacity of spleen cells from IL-2 treated mice to lyse two NK sensitive targets (YAK-1 and L5178Y-clone 27v) as well as the NK insusceptible target (L5178Y-clone 27 av) (13). As seen in Table IV, IL-2 induced augmentation of splenic cytotoxic activity resulted in appreciable lysis of NK susceptible targets but had no effect on the NK resistant clone 27 av tumor. It should be stressed that previous studies have shown that both clone 27 v and av cells are equally susceptible to alloimmune directed CTL activity (3). From these data it appeared that in vivo administration of IL-2 resulted in potentiation of NK cell

Table II. Kinetics of IL-2 administration.

Treatment	Day of treatment after alloimmunization[a]	%specific lysis effector/target cell ratio		
		100/1	50/1	25/1
Saline-BSA	0	27.4	13.5	5.9
IL-2-BSA	0	60.6	36.0	20.9
IL-2-BSA	2	72.0	45.6	34.9

[a]At varying times after alloimmunization on Day 0 with 2×10^7 viable EL-4 cells, BALB/c animals received either saline-BSA or IL-2 BSA i.p. Ten days later, PEC were removed and their cytotoxic activity measured in a 4 hour ^{51}Cr-release assay.

activity.

We further examined the precise amount of IL-2 which was required for optimal augmentation of NK responses. Table V shows that animals receiving mock IL-2 (a fraction from the final preparative isoelectric focusing gel, which contained no IL-2 activity (as assessed by its inability to sustain the growth of an IL-2 dependent T cell line) did not augment NK cell activity above levels observed in animals receiving saline-BSA. In addition, in vivo administration of 25 units of IL-2 did not result in augmentation of splenic cytolytic activity, whereas treatment of animals with either 50, 100, or 150 units resulted in a significant increase in NK responses. From these data, 50-100 units of purified IL-2, when administered ip, appeared to result in optimal augmentation of NK cell activity.

Table III. Effect of route of IL-2 administration on enhanced splenic effector cell allo-reactive CTL activity.

Alloimmunized mice treated with	Route of Administration[a]	% specific lysis		
		50/1	50/1	12.5/1
Saline-BSA	IP	4.9	3.1	2.8
IL-2-BSA	IP	18.6	16.3	14.3
Saline-BSA	IV	17.6	10.4	9.6
IL-2-BSA	IV	27.0	24.6	17.4

[a]BALB/c animals received either saline-BSA or IL-2 (100 U) in saline-BSA either ip or iv. Ten days later the mice were sacrificed, splenocyte cytotoxic reactivity measured.

DISCUSSION

The work presented here describes the in vivo augmentation of cytolytic responses following administration of the T-cell derived growth factor, IL-2.

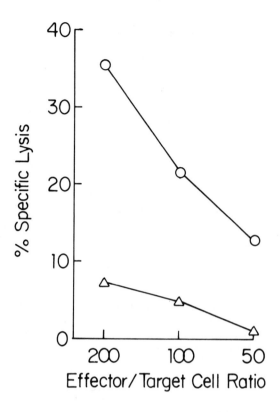

FIG. 3. Ability of purified IL-2 to augment natural killer cell activity.

CBA/J mice received either saline-BSA (**△**) or IL-2 in saline BSA (**O**), 48 hrs prior to evaluation of splenic NK activity in a standard 4 hr ^{51}Cr-release assay, using YAC-I targets.

Injection of purified preparations of IL-2 concomitantly or shortly after immunization with allogeneic tumor cells resulted in the enhancement of allo-specific CTL activity in both the spleen and PEC responder populations (Fig. 1). Cytotoxic cells were not retained on columns of Sephadex G-10 yet were sensitive to pretreatment with anti-Thy 1.2 antibody and complement (Table 1). Moreover this response was specific for the immunizing antigen arguing against polyclonal expansion of CTL by IL-2. Thus, as previously demonstrated in vitro in T cell deficient systems (4, 15, 19), IL-2 facilitates the production of cytotoxic T cells in vivo by normal animals.

  IL-2 has previously been shown to enhance T lymphocyte proliferation, differentiation, and function in a variety of immunological responses (1, 4, 7-9, 15-21). This lymphokine is produced by antigen or mitogen activated Lyt 1+ T cells (16, 18, 19), but can also be generated by Lyt 2+ lymphocytes under certain conditions (H-2^k and/or H-2^d region mixed lymphocyte culutre disparity) (15).

Table IV. IL-2 dependent in vivo augmentation of NK cell activity.

| Treatment[a] | Target[b] | % specific lysis Effector/target cell ratio | | |
		200/1	100/1	50/1
Saline-BSA	YAC-1	14%	11.2%	6.2%
IL-2-BSA	YAC-1	36.4%	22.5%	14.7%
Saline-BSA	Clone 27v	8.4%	3.9%	3.0%
IL-2-BSA	Clone 27v	27.9%	11.4%	9.5%
Saline-BSA	Clone av	0	0	1.6%
IL-2-BSA	Clone av	0	0	0

[a]CBA/J mice (2 mice/group) received either saline-BSA or 100 units IL-2 in saline-BSA 48 hrs prior to evaluation of splenocyte cytolytic activity in a standard 4 hr ^{51}Cr-release assay.
[b]YAC-1 (H-2^a) and clone 27 v (L5178Y) are NK sensitive targets while clone av (25178Y) is NK insusceptible (3).

However in all instances, the target cell appears to be an antigen or mitogen activated T cell. Once activated, T cells express receptors which bind IL-2 (17). Such lymphokine receptor interactions then subsequently induce proliferation. Non-activated (resting) T cells, immature thymocytes, as well as non-T cells (B cells or monocytes) are incapable of binding IL-2 and do not proliferate in response to in vitro stimulation with IL-2 (17). Thus, from in vitro evidence, IL-2 appears to be produced by antigen and/or mitogen activated T cells and is bound by other activated T lymphocytes resulting in their proliferation.

If such a hypothesis were extended to the in vivo system described in this communication, one would suspect that in vivo, alloantigen primed T cells would bind the IL-2 administered in vivo and be stimulated to divide. This then could lead to the enhanced cytotoxic response observed. Such an augmented response may be at the expense of memory CTL, the increased expansion of antigen activated T lymphocyte, or the result of the accelerated differentiation of precursor CTL into mature cells. At present the exact mechanism behind the in vivo action of this immunoregulatory protein is unknown. Interestingly, if IL-2 is given prior to allo-immunization (48 hrs earlier) no augmentation in CTL activity is observed (personal observation).   This temporal restriction suggests that antigen-activation must occur prior to administration of the lymphokine, in order to obtain an enhanced CTL response.

Alternatively, the injection of IL-2 may induce the production of another cell or factor (5), which is responsible for the observed increase in effector cell reactivity. However, it should be noted that the preparations of IL-2 used in these investigations has been found to be free of the following contaminating biological activities: interleukin-1, colony stimulating factor, and immune interferon.

The data presented above have also described for the first time the in vivo augmentation of NK cell activity by purified IL-2. A single ip injection of 100 units of IL-2 resulted in an almost two-fold increase in splenic NK cell activity. The augmented cytolytic activity was mediated by NK cells as further estab-

Table V. Effect of IL-2 dose-response on augmentation of splenic NK cell activity.

Treatment[a]	200/1	% specific lysis Effector/target cell ratio 100/1	50/1
Experiment # 1			
Saline-BSA	18.4	14.8	10.3
Mock IL-2[b]	22.3	12.8	11.3
IL-2-BSA			
25 units	18.3	10.9	8.8
50 units	37.6	23.4	16.3
Experiment #2			
Saline-BSA	14.0	11.6	6.4
IL-2-BSA			
100 units	36.3	22.4	14.7
150 units	30.8	16.1	11.3

[a]CBA/J mice (2 mice/group) received a single ip injection of either saline-BSA or IL-2 in saline-BSA 48 hrs prior to testing of spleen cell cytotoxic activity in a standard 4 hr ^{51}Cr-release assay (YAC-1 target).
[b]IEF fraction, obtained during preparation purification of IL-2, which lacks IL-2 activity as assessed by its inability to sustain growth of IL-2 dependent T-cells.

lished by the effector cell population's specificity of killing (Table IV). Recently, the ability of purified IL-2 to augment NK cell activity in vitro was reported by Henney and co-workers (11,12). Such an enhancement of cytolytic reactivity appeared to be independent of interferon. Previous reports (2,6) have documented the ability of interferon inducers (poly IC for one) to augment NK cell activity both in vitro and in vivo. In the in vivo system detailed above the mechanism of action of IL-2 remains to be established. It is conceivable that the IL-2 induced augmentation of NK cell activity is interferon mediated. Alternatively, IL-2 may act directly on NK cells resulting in the enhanced cytolytic activity observed. Studies aimed to determine the mechanism of action behind in vitro and in vivo IL-2 dependent augmentation of NK activity are currently underway.

In summary, the experiments presented above have demonstrated the beneficial effect of in vivo administration of purified IL-2 on two distinct in vivo responses; CTL generation and NK cell activity. While both responses are similar (the effector function is a lytic one), they are strikingly different in their specificities, memory, and effector cell populations. However, both cytolytic activities are markedly enhanced following exposure to highly purified preparations to IL-2. These preliminary experiments reveal the immunoregulatory potential of IL-2. As such, the immunotheraupetic value of this lymphokine in treating immunodeficiencies and other immune disorders is only now being recognized.

References

1.   Baker, P.E., Gillis, S., Ferm, M.M., and Smith, K.A. (1978). J. Immunol. 121:2168-2174.
2.   Djeu, J.Y., J.A. Heibaugh, H.T. Holden, and R.B. Herberman. 1979. J. Immunol. 122:175.
3.   Durdik, J.M., B.N. Beck, E.A. Clark, C.S. Henney. 1980. J. Immunol. 125:683-689.
4.   Farrar, J.J., P.L. Simon, W.L. Farrar, J. Koopman, and J. Fuller-Bonar. 1980. Ann. N.Y. Acad. Sci. 332:303.
5.   Farrar, W.L., Johnson, H.M., and Farrar, J.J. 1981. J. Immunol.: 1120-125.
6.   Gidlund, M., A. Orn, H. Wigzell, A. Senik, and I. Gressar. 1978. Nature 273:759.
7.   Gillis, S. and Smith K.A. 1977. Nature 268:154-156.
8.   Gillis, S., Ferm, M.M., Ou, W., and Smith K.A. 1978. J. Immunol. 120:2027-2023.
9.   Gillis, S., Union, N.A., Baker, P.E., and Smith, V.A. 1979. J. Exp. Med. 149:1460-1476.
10.   Henney, C.S. 1971. J. Immunol. 107:1558-1566.
11.   Henney, C.S., K. Kuribayashi, D.E. Kern, and S. Gillis. 1981. Nature 291:335.
12.   Kuribayaski, K., S. Gillis, D.E. Kern, and C.S. Henney. 1981. J. Immunol. 126:2321.
14.   Mochizuki, D., Watson, J., and Gillis, S. 1980. J. Immunol. 125:2579-2583. Okada, M. and Henney, C.S. 1980. J. Immunol. 125:300-307.
16.   Shaw, J. Caplan, B., Paetkau, V., Pilarski, P.L.M., Delovitch, T.L., and McKenzie, I.F.C. 1980. J. Immunol. 124:2231-2239.
17.   Smith, K.A., S. Gillis, P.E. Baker, D. McKenzie, and F.W. Ruscetti. 1979. Ann. N.Y. Acad. Sci. 332:423.
18.   Wagner, H. and M. Rollinghoff. 1978. J. Exp. Med. 148:1523-1536.
19.   Wagner, H., Rollinghoff, M., Pfizenmaier, K., Hardt, C., and Johnscher, G. 1980. J. Immunol. 124:1058-1067.
20.   Watson, J. 1979. J. Immunol. 150:1510-1519.
21.   Watson, J., Gillis, S., Marbrook, J., Mochizuki, D., and Smith, K.A. 1979. J. Exp. Med. 150:849:861.
22.   Young, W.W., Hakomori, S., Durdik, J.M. and Henney, C.S. 1980. J. Immunol. 124:199-205.

AUDIENCE DISCUSSION

Dr. Goldstein: The last molecular weight you've indicated is about 15,000, which is smaller than the 21 and 26,000 mentioned previously.
Dr. Gillis: The 15,000 mw band is from Jurket human leukemia cells. IL 2 from peripheral blood cells is about 15,000. In the mouse system, it is 26,000 and 21,000 molecular weight. This material is predominantly from the murine IL 2 species with a PI of 4.9. The gel patterns from the PI 4.3 mouse IL 2 species reveal molecular weights of 15,000 to 28,000.
Dr. Goldstein: Have you attempted partial proteolysis to see whether the various molecules represent fragments of one another, or is there any selective activity? Now that you have an antibody, have you at-

tempted to look at specificity? Have you seen if you can inhibit with other lymphokines or other biological response modifiers?

Dr. Gillis: We have not done any tryptic digests or any other proteolysis to look for smaller active molecular weight species. The antibody we've tested does not inhibit IL 1. We're doing collaborative experiments with Frank Fitch to see if it has any capacity to react with colony stimulating factor.

Dr. Rosenberg: Will a partially purified IL 2 enhance the generation in vivo of cytotoxic cells as measured in a short-term chromium release assay?

Dr. Gillis: The least pure material we've used to generate in vivo responses has been through a 5-stage purification, the last step of which was isolectric focusing. That material works.

Dr. Rosenberg: So the material prior to elution from STS gels will enhance in vivo generation?

Dr. Gillis: Yes. But that material as well has been through a 5-step purification.

Dr. Rosenberg: Have you looked at the half-life of material in vivo?

Dr. Gillis: No. It's another reason why we need high specific activity IL 2.

Dr. Rosenberg: We've taken highly active T cell growth factor, that is about 300 fold purified and determined that following injection into syngeneic mice it has a half-life of only about 90 seconds in vivo. It is not destroyed by mouse serum.

Dr. Gillis: You're describing its half-life in those cases as the ability to get back biologic activity from the serum. That's the reason why we're trying to generate a radioimmunoassay. In our hands, mouse serum itself is tremendously inhibitory for IL 2-dependent cell line proliferation. Hermann Wagner's recently did many experiments to look for and purify the inhibitor present in mouse serum.

Dr. Rosenberg: I've not seen mouse serum inhibit TCGF reactivity. Granted, you can't measure TCGF reactivity in mouse serum alone, but so long as one has another heterologous serum source, TCGF is highly active in vitro.

Dr. Mitchell: Speculate about the physiological in vivo role. Lyt 1 positive cells are the predominant source of Interleukin 2 and some of the information we heard this morning suggests that this is the method by which inducer cells induce. Would you comment on that?

Dr. Gillis: We must be cautious in attributing effects to IL 2. A few years ago Con A supernatant was synonomous with migration inhibition factor and now may be synonomous with IL 2. We also have to abandon the idea that a single phenotype cell produces only one factor or a single cloned tumor cell line only produces one factor, because clones of cells may produce a multitude of lymphokines.

Dr. Bonavida: You showed that co-culture of NK cells with IL 2 for 24 hours results in NK activation. What happens if co-culture is less than 24 hours?

Dr. Gillis: There is a hint of enhanced reactivity in about 12 hours which peaks at 24. It's impossible to rule out that the mechanism of action of IL 2 in my experiments may be by induction of interferon. I've heard that Barry Bloom's lab has found that IL 2 and interferon may indeed act on separate subpopulations of NK cells.

Dr. Bonavida: Does the anti-IL 2 monoclonal antibody affect the NK activity as measured in vitro or in vivo?

Dr. Gillis: We haven't done a neutralization experiment with just anti-IL 2 Ig G. We've only done the immune precipitation.

Dr. Greenberg: Did you demonstrate that the enhanced cytotoxicity generated when you gave IL 2 in vivo was a reflection of antigen specific CTL?

Dr. Gillis: Yes. Those cells don't kill irrelevant tumor. Also, one can eliminate their reactivity by pretreatment with anti-Thy 1 serum and complement.

Dr. Greenberg: That would imply that in an allo response, help is what is limiting. Have you therefore looked at whether or not IL 2 would be active in primed mice or if you adoptively transferred help?

Dr. Green: Did you administer anti-IL 2 antibodies in vivo?

Dr. Gillis: No.

Dr. Herberman: Do you see any indication for heterogeneity of IL 2 in your studies with neutralization by monoclonal antibody?

Dr. Gillis: We have used the monoclonal antibody to immune percipitate biosynthetically labeled IL 2 from the PI 4.9 species. From this species we can precipitate both of the two bands showed. Experiments with other molecular weight species are ongoing.

The Potential Role of T Cells in Cancer Therapy,
edited by A. Fefer and A. Goldstein,
Raven Press, New York © 1982.

Specific Adoptive Therapy of Murine Leukemia with Cells Secondarily Sensitized *In Vitro* and Expanded by Culture with Interleukin 2

Martin A. Cheever, Philip D. Greenberg, Steven Gillis, and Alexander Fefer

Department of Medicine, Division of Oncology, University of Washington School of Medicine, and Medical Oncology and Basic Immunology Programs, The Fred Hutchinson Cancer Research Center, BB1015 Health Sciences RK-25, Seattle, Washington 98195

Since T lymphocytes can lyse tumors in vitro, it seems reasonable that adoptive transfer of specifically immune T lymphocytes would provide benefit in tumor therapy. However, although adoptive transfer of immune cells provides the potential of unique antitumor specificity, it has been limited in its ability to cope with established tumors. Although lymphocytes which can lyse tumor in vitro can also prevent tumor growth in vivo if administered with the inoculation of tumor, therapy with lymphocytes alone is, with rare exceptions, ineffective once tumor has become established (26). In order to better define and overcome the problems involved in eradicating established tumors with adoptively transferred immune lymphocytes, we have developed several murine models in which advanced disseminated leukemia can be cured by combining chemotherapy and specifically immunized T lymphocytes (9). The leukemias employed were chosen because they have well-defined antigenicity and they have proven to be susceptible to immune manipulation. These models might not be precisely duplicated in the clinical setting, however, they are extremely well suited for developing and testing certain new approaches to specific immunotherapy.

One such approach is to manipulate immune lymphocytes in vitro to augment therapeutic efficacy and increase the number of donor cells for therapy. This report will summarize our initial attempts to explore the feasibility of secondarily sensitizing immune cells in vitro and culturing them long-term with T cell growth factor, now termed Interleukin 2 (24), to generate large numbers of specifically cytotoxic effector cells for tumor therapy. Data will be reviewed demonstrating that lymphocytes secondarily sensitized in vitro and expanded in number by culture in Interleukin 2 (IL 2) are able to mediate specific adoptive tumor therapy and the efficacy of such IL 2-dependent cells can be augmented by in vivo inoculation of purified IL 2. The mechanisms by which long-term cultured T lymphocytes eradicate tumor in vivo will be compared to those of noncultured immune lymphocytes.

Adoptive Chemoimmunotherapy Model

FBL-3, a syngeneic Friend virus-induced leukemia of C57BL/6 origin was utilized for study. This tumor is antigenic and sensitive to spec-ific immune attack (23,33). If injected intraperitoneally (i.p.), as few as 100 FBL-3 cells grow progressively and kill 100% of adult mice. In the adoptive chemoimmunotherapy model (9), adult C57BL/6 mice are inoculated i.p. with 5×10^6 FBL-3 cells on day 0 and treated on day 5 with a combination of chemotherapy plus donor lymphocytes. At the time of therapy, mice have ascites, and disseminated tumor is detectable in both blood and spleen (17). The results of the adoptive chemoimmuno-therapy model are exemplified by the cumulative results of 4 consecutive experiments presented in Figure 1 (4). Mice receiving FBL-3 on day 0 and no treatment all died by day 14. Treatment with a single injection of cyclophosphamide (CY) i.p. (180 mg/kg) approximately doubles median survival time (MST), but all mice eventually died with tumor.

Immune spleen cells for therapy ($C57_{\alpha FBL}$) were derived from syngeneic C57BL/6 mice rendered immune by i.p. inoculation with irradiated FBL-3 6 to 8 weeks prior to therapy. Treatment on day 5 with $C57_{\alpha FBL}$ alone was totally ineffective. However, as an adjunct to CY, such cells had a significant dose-dependent effect. Thus, CY plus 5×10^6 $C57_{\alpha FBL}$ pro-longed the MST to day 31 (P<0.01) and CY plus 2×10^7 $C57_{\alpha FBL}$ cells prolonged the MST to day 64 and cured 41% of mice (P<0.01). Larger dose of immune cells would have cured an even greater percentage of mice. In contrast, normal nonimmune C57BL/6 spleen cells ($C57_{normal}$) were in-effective as an adjunct to CY.

To be effective in therapy, donor cells must be immune since therapy with CY and normal nonimmune spleen cells was no more effective than therapy with CY alone. Additionally, donor cells must contain T lympho-cytes. The T lymphocyte subpopulation responsible for the majority of the antitumor efficacy following infusion on noncultured immune donor spleen cells is a noncytotoxic Lyt 1^+2^- T lymphocyte (18). Noncultured immune lymphocytes for therapy can be derived from peripheral blood or spleens of immune mice and cells inoculated intravenously or intraperi-toneally are equally as effective. Noncultured immune cells must be capable of proliferating in the host to be effective and must survive in the host for greater than 2 weeks for maximal benefit in therapy (17).

Specificity of Chemoimmunotherapy

The specificity of adoptive chemoimmunotherapy with immune cells was confirmed by utilizing EL-4(G-) as a control (4). El-4(G-) is a subline of EL-4, a chemically-induced tumor of C57BL origin, and is negative for Gross cell surface antigens and mouse endogenous virus-associated surface antigen 1 and is antigenically distinct from FBL-3 and other tumors induced by Friend, Moloney, and Rauscher viruses (20). Treatment of mice bearing advanced FBL-3 with CY plus cells from C57BL/6 mice immune to EL-4 (C57$_{\alpha EL-4}$) was no more effective than was treatment with CY alone (Figure 1). Specificity was confirmed in reciprocal experiments for the chemoimmunotherapy of advanced EL-4(G-) to be presented later (Figure 7).

Therapeutic Efficacy of Cells
Secondarily Sensitized In Vitro

In the preceding chemoimmunotherapy experiments advanced disseminated FBL-3 was successfully treated with CY plus in vivo immunized cells. This same model was used to examine the ability of in vitro sensitization (2,3) and long-term culture techniques (5) to generate specifically immune T lymphocytes capable of in vivo therapy. The purpose of primary sensitization in vitro is to render ineffective cells effective without exposing the donor to tumor material. On the other hand, since the tumor-bearing host has already been exposed to tumor, the purpose of secondary sensitization in vitro is to increase the quantity of effector cells and bypass mechanisms operative in vivo such as tumor-induced immunosuppression (10,11) or blocking factors (19) which might limit effective sensitization in vivo. We have shown that both primary (7) and secondary in vitro sensitization (2,3) can generate cells capable of tumor therapy; however, only the results of secondary in vitro sensitization will be reviewed.

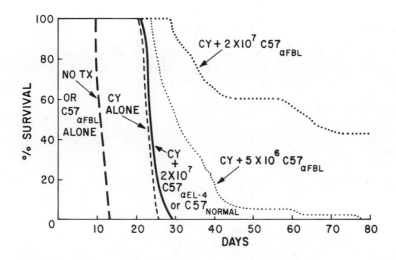

FIG. 1. Adoptive chemoimmunotherapy of FBL-3 with noncultured immune cells. C57BL/6 mice inoculated i.p. on day 0 with 5 x 10^6 FBL-3 received either no therapy (No Tx) or treatment on day 5 with cyclophosphamide (CY Alone) at 180 mg/kg, or 2 x 10^7 cells from mice immune to FBL-3 (C57$_{\alpha FBL}$ Alone), or CY plus 5 x 10^6 or 2 x 10^7 C57$_{\alpha FBL}$ or CY plus 2 x 10^7 cells from normal nonimmune mice or from mice immune to EL-4(G-), denoted as C57$_{normal}$ and C57$_{\alpha EL-4}$, respectively. The cumulative results of four experiments are represented with 32 mice per treatment group.

For secondary in vitro sensitization, spleen cells from mice immune to FBL-3 were cultured for 5 days with γ-irradiated FBL-3. Secondary sensitization was confirmed by measuring direct antitumor cytotoxicity in vitro in a standard 4-hour chromium release assay (Figure 2) (3). Immune spleen cells tested directly without prior culture demonstrated no measurable cytotoxicity, whereas immune cells cultured with secondary tumor stimulation developed marked antitumor cytolytic reactivity and were significantly more cytotoxic than were cells cultured with control syngeneic spleen cells. The specificity of the cytolytic reactivity induced by culturing in vivo primed cells with tumor was confirmed by testing these cells against EL-4(G-) (Table I).

These same cultured spleen cells were concurrently tested in vivo in tumor therapy (Figure 3) (3). Mice inoculated with FBL-3 and treated on day 5 with CY had a median survival of 26 days. As an adjunct to CY, cells from mice immunized in vivo with FBL-3, $C57_{\alpha FBL}$ (noncultured), prolonged the median survial time to day 35. Immune cells which were secondarily sensitized in vitro by culture with tumor, $C57_{\alpha FBL} \cdot (FBL)_x$, were significantly more effective and prolonged the median survival to day 52. In contrast, immune cells cultured without tumor, $C57_{\alpha FBL} \cdot (C57)_x$, were significantly less effective and prolonged median survival time only 2 days to day 27. Normal cells cultured with tumor (not depicted) were ineffective. Thus, noncultured cells that were effective in

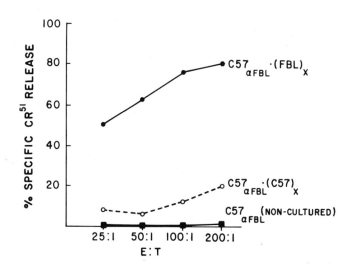

FIG. 2. In vitro cytotoxicity of cells secondarily sensitized in vitro. Spleen cells from C57BL/6 mice immunized in vivo to FBL-3 [$C57_{\alpha FBL}$ (noncultured)] were cultured for 5 days with x-irradiated FBL-3 [$C57_{\alpha FBL} \cdot (FBL)_x$] or x-irradiated C57BL/6 spleen cells [$C57_{\alpha FBL} \cdot (C57)_x$] and were tested for cytotoxicity to tumor in a 4-hour chromium release assay at variable effector-to-target (E:T) ratios.

therapy were rendered more effective by secondary sensitization in vitro
(P<0.01) and immune cells cultured without secondary sensitization were
less effective (P<0.01).

Effect of Culture-Induced Suppressor Cells On Therapy

Two problems which limit the efficacy of this culture system have been
identified. First, culture-induced suppressor cells which are generated
during the sensitization period coexist with antitumor effector cells
and are capable of inhibiting their in vivo therapeutic efficacy (16).
The second is inefficient expansion of effector cells (25) due in part
to progressive cell loss during culture. Although cells secondarily
sensitized in vitro for 5 days are therapeutically more effective on a
cell-for-cell basis than are noncultured primed cells, less than 30% of
cells remain viable, and therefore the net change in therapeutic benefit
is minimal (6).

Culture-induced suppressor cells have been described by others as
radio-sensitive T lymphocytes generated during in vitro culture of
normal spleen cells which nonspecifically suppress in vitro allogeneic
responses (21). We have shown that tumor immune cells cultured in vitro
with or without tumor for 5 days contain similar nonspecific suppressor
cells (16).

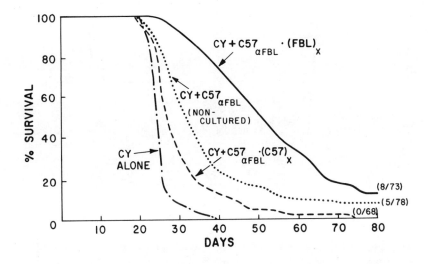

FIG. 3. Therapeutic efficacy of cells secondarily sensitized in vitro.
C57BL/6 mice inoculated i.p. with 5×10^6 FBL-3 on day 0 were treated on
day 5 with cyclophosphamide (CY Alone) at 180 mg/kg or with CY plus
5×10^6 noncultured immune cells ($C57_{\alpha FBL}$) or CY plus 5×10^6 immune
spleen cells cultured for 5 days with x-irradiated FBL-3 or x-irradiated
C57BL/6 spleen cells denoted as $C57_{\alpha FBL} \cdot (FBL)_x$ and $C57_{\alpha FBL} \cdot (C57)_x$,
respectively. Numbers represent number of mice surviving 80 days/total.

The effect on therapy of suppressor cells generated during secondary sensitization in vitro of tumor immune cells could not be directly tested in mixing experiments because of the coexisting antitumor effector cells. However, the effect of cultured normal cells on therapy was determined (Figure 4) (16). Therapy with CY plus cells secondarily sensitized in vitro prolonged the MST to day 64. However, their efficacy ficacy was diminished by the concurrent inoculation at a separate i.p. site of an equal number of cultured normal cells. Thus, secondarily sensitized cells were made less effective in therapy by the in vivo presence of culture-induced suppressor cells.

Thus, although secondary in vitro sensitization renders immune spleen cells more effective in therapy, this culture system also generates culture-induced suppressor cells; and the in vivo therapeutic effect of the secondarily sensitized cells is diminished by concurrent inoculation of similar culture-induced suppressor cells. Whether or not the in vivo efficacy of secondarily sensitized cells can be increased by the elimination of coexisting suppressor cells is being investigated.

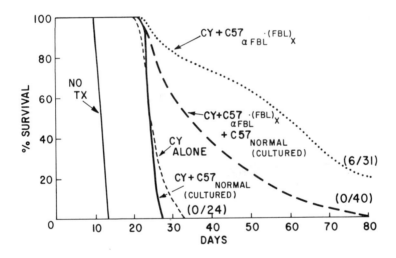

FIG. 4. Adoptive chemoimmunotherapy of FBL-3 with cells secondarily sensitized in vitro: effect of culture-induced suppressor cells. C57BL/6 mice inoculated i.p. on day 0 with 5×10^6 FBL-3 received either no therapy (No Tx), treatment on day 5 with cyclophosphamide (CY Alone) at 180 mg/kg, or treatment with CY plus 5×10^6 primed cells secondarily sensitized in vitro by culture for 5 days with x-irradiated FBL-3 $[C57_{\alpha FBL} \cdot (FBL)_x]$, 5×10^6 normal spleen cells cultured for 5 days $[C57_{normal}$ (cultured)] or both 5×10^6 secondarily sensitized cells and 5×10^6 cultured normal cells. Fractions represent number of mice surviving 80 days/total.

Long-Term Growth of Tumor Immune Lymphocytes in Interleukin 2

To overcome the problem of inefficient expansion of effector cells during secondary in vitro sensitization, we initiated studies to test the efficacy of cells numerically expanded in vitro by culture with IL 2. Culture with IL 2 offers the means for generating large numbers of specifically reactive T lymphocytes in different functional sub-classes.

IL 2 is a soluble protein produced by stimulated amplifier T lymphocytes (30,34) which regulates T lymphocyte function, at least in vitro, through control of clonal expansion (12,13,28). Activated T lymphocytes are induced to proliferate in vitro by IL 2 and can be maintained continuously even without the continued presence of activating antigen

TABLE 1. Specific Cytolytic Reactivity of Noncultured Immune Cells and Immune Cells Following Secondary Sensitization In Vitro For 7 Days and Following Long-Term Culture to Day 19

Responder	Stimulator	Day of Culture	% Specific Lysis			
			FBL-3		EL-4(G-)	
			20:1	5:1	20:1	5:1
$C57_{normal}$	Noncultured	0	-1	0	-1	0
$C57_{\alpha FBL}$	Noncultured	0	-1	-1	-2	-1
$C57_{\alpha EL-4}$	Noncultured	0	-1	0	1	0
$C57_{normal}$	$(C57)_x$	7	2	1	1	1
$C57_{normal}$	$(FBL)_x$	7	5	2	2	1
$C57_{normal}$	$(EL-4)_x$	7	7	3	5	2
$C57_{\alpha FBL}$	$(C57)_x$	7	1	1	1	1
$C57_{\alpha FBL}$	$(FBL)_x$	7	38	16	0	-3
$C57_{\alpha FBL}$	$(EL-4)_x$	7	4	1	4	2
$C57_{\alpha EL-4}$	$(C57)_x$	7	1	1	1	0
$C57_{\alpha EL-4}$	$(FBL)_x$	7	4	3	2	1
$C57_{\alpha EL-4}$	$(EL-4)_x$	7	3	-2	26	9
$C57_{\alpha FBL}$	$(FBL)_x$	19	61	40	13	7
$C57_{\alpha EL-4}$	$(EL-4)_x$	19	10	8	34	22

Spleen cells from normal nonimmune C57BL/6 mice ($C57_{normal}$), or from C57BL/6 mice which had been immunized in vivo with FBL-3 ($C57_{\alpha FBL}$) or with EL-4(G-) ($C57_{\alpha EL-4}$) were cultured for 7 days with irradiated $(C57)_x$, $(FBL)_x$, or $(EL-4)_x$. Then selected groups were further cultured to day 19 and induced to proliferate by supplementing media with Con A supernatants containing Interleukin 2. Cytotoxicity against FBL-3 and EL-4(G-) was determined on days 0, 7 and 19 in a standard 4-hour chromium release assay at effector-to-target ratios of 20:1 and 5:1. The data represent the means of 2 experiments.

(1,31). By continually supplementing cultures with IL 2, activated
lymphocytes can be serially grown in vitro to large numbers (12,27).
Lymphocytes cytotoxic to tumors (12,29,35) have been maintained long-
term in such cultures, some for greater than one year.

Although long-term cultured T lymphocytes have been shown to be
cytotoxic to tumor in vitro and have been shown to inhibit the growth of
syngeneic tumors in a Winn assay, in which tumor and lymphocytes are
mixed together in vitro and inoculated together in vivo (32), it had not
been demonstrated that all the requisite subpopulations required for
successful adoptive therapy survived long-term culture and thus that
such cells were capable of mediating tumor therapy.

Since only activated T lymphocytes grow in response to IL 2, in vivo
immunized lymphocytes were first activated (5). To activate tumor
immune lymphocytes, spleen cells from mice immune to FBL-3 were cultured
with irradiated FBL-3 for 7 days and cells from mice immune to EL-4 were
cultured with irradiated EL-4 for 7 days. Specific activation was
confirmed by measuring cytotoxicity in vitro in a standard 4-hour chromium release assay (Table 1). Cells immune to FBL-3 and cultured with

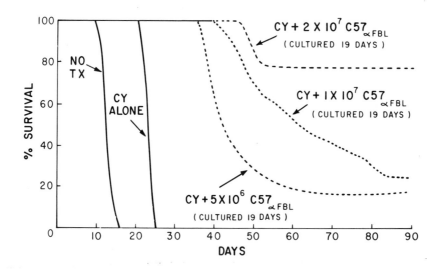

FIG. 5. Efficacy of long-term cultured T lymphocytes in the adoptive
chemoimmunotherapy of FBL-3. C57BL/6 mice inoculated i.p. on day 0 with
5×10^6 FBL-3 received either no therapy (No Tx), treatment on day 5
with cyclophosphamide (CY Alone) at 180 mg/kg, or treatment with CY plus
variable dose of long-term cultured T lymphocytes from mice sequentially
immunized in vivo to FBL-3, secondarily sensitized in vitro and numerically expanded by culture through day 19 with Interleukin 2, denoted as
$C57_{\alpha FBL}$ (cultured 19 days). The cumulative results of two experiments
are represented with 16 mice per treatment group.

irradiated FBL-3 became specifically cytotoxic to FBL-3 and cells immune to EL-4 and cultured with irradiated EL-4 became specifically cytotoxic to EL-4.

Following culture for 7 days, cells were harvested, washed, recultured and induced to proliferate through day 19 by repeated supplementation of media with supernatants from Con-A stimulated lymphocytes containing IL 2. Following a lag period of several days, cells grew progressively and expanded in number by greater than 700%. Growth remained exquisitely dependent on repeated addition of IL 2, since cells similarly cultured without IL 2 supplementation progressively died and less than 1% remained viable on day 19. Following culture for 19 days the expanded cell populations remained specifically cytotoxic to the immunizing tumor (Table 1).

These long-term cultured cells, denoted as $C57_{\alpha FBL}$ (cultured 19 days) and $C57_{\alpha EL-4}$ (cultured 19 days) were concurrently tested for efficacy (Figure 5) and specificity (Figures 6 and 7) in adoptive chemoimmunotherapy (5).

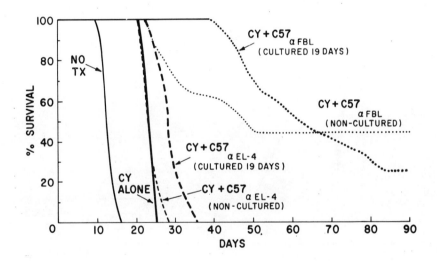

FIG. 6. Specificity of the adoptive chemoimmunotherapy of FBL-3 with long-term cultured T lymphocytes. C57BL/6 mice inoculated i.p. on day 0 with 5 x 10⁶ FBL-3 received either no therapy (No Tx), treatment on day 5 with cyclophosphamide (CY Alone) at 180 mg/kg, or treatment with CY plus 1 x 10⁷ cells from mice immunized in vivo to FBL-3 or EL-4(G-), denoted as $C57_{\alpha FBL}$ (noncultured) and $C57_{\alpha EL-4}$ (noncultured), respectively or treatment with CY plus 1 x 10⁷ long-term cultured T lymphocytes from mice sequentially immunized in vivo to FBL-3 or EL-4(G-), secondarily sensitized in vitro to the immunizing tumor and numerically expanded by culture through day 19 with Interleukin 2, denoted as $C57_{\alpha FBL}$ (cultured 19 days) and $C57_{\alpha EL-4}$ (cultured 19 days), respectively. The cumulative results of two experiments are represented with 16 mice per treatment group.

Therapeutic Efficacy and Specificity of Long-Term Cultured T Lymphocytes

To test the therapeutic efficacy of long-term cultured T lymphocytes immune to FBL-3, mice receiving FBL-3 on day 0 were treated on day 5 with CY plus variable doses of $C57_{\alpha FBL}$ (cultured 19 days). As an adjunct to CY, therapy with 5×10^6 cultured cells prolonged median survival to day 42, 1×10^7 cultured cells prolonged median survial to day 62 and 2×10^7 cultured cells further prolonged survival and cured 80% of mice. Thus, following in vitro manipulation for 19 days the resultant cells were expanded in number and were able to mediate in vivo therapy and efficacy was dependent upon the dose of infused cells.

To test for specificity of therapy, the efficacy of $C57_{\alpha FBL}$ (cultured 19 days) at a dose of 1×10^7 cells per mouse was compared to the efficacy of $C57_{\alpha EL-4}$(cultured 19 days) in both the therapy of FBL-3 and El-4(G-) (Figures 6 and 7). As an adjunct to CY, therapy of FBL-3 with

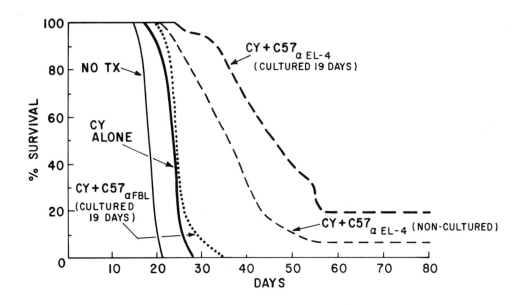

FIG. 7. Specificity of adoptive chemoimmunotherapy of EL-4(G-) with long-term cultured T lymphocytes. C57BL/6 mice inoculated i.p. on day 0 with 2×10^5 EL-4(G-) received either no therapy (No Tx), treatment on day 5 with cyclophosphamide (CY Alone) at 180 mg/kg, or treatment with CY plus 2×10^7 cells from mice immunized in vivo to FBL-3 [$C57_{\alpha FBL}$(noncultured)] or EL-4(G-) [$C57_{\alpha EL-4}$ (noncultured)] or CY plus 2×10^7 similar cells sequentially immunized in vivo, secondarily sensitized in vitro and numerically expanded by culture through day 19 with Interleukin 2, denoted as [$C57_{\alpha FBL}$ (cultured 19 days)] and [$C57_{\alpha EL-4}$ (cultured 19 days)], respectively. The cumulative results of two experiments are represented with 16 mice per treatment group.

C57$_{\alpha FBL}$ (cultured 19 days) prolonged MST to day 62 and cured 1 of 16 mice (Figure 6). Noncultured C57$_{\alpha EL-4}$ were totally ineffective and C57$_{\alpha EL-4}$ (cultured 19 days) demonstrated only a small effect. Reciprocal specificity was confirmed by treating mice bearing advanced EL-4 rather than FBL-3 (Figure 7). As an adjunct to CY, C57$_{\alpha EL-4}$ (cultured 19 days) were effective and C57$_{\alpha FBL}$ (cultured 19 days) were ineffective, being no more effective than CY$^{\alpha}$alone.

Comparisons of Noncultured Immune Cells and
Long-Term Cultured T Lymphocytes in Therapy

In the EL-4 and the FBL-3 models, both long-term cultured cells and noncultured immune cells were effective in therapy (Figures 6 and 7). In the FBL-3 model we have begun to contrast the mechanisms of action of these effector populations and have thus far identified four differences: 1) the kinetics of tumor elimination, 2) the influence of route of administration, 3) the sensitivity of effector cells to irradiation, and 4) the response to exogenously administered IL 2.

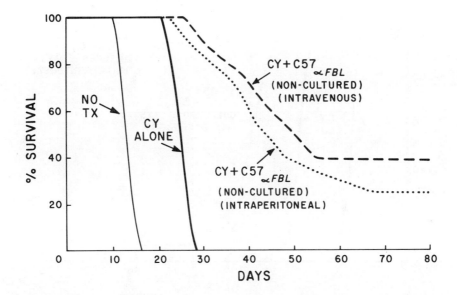

FIG. 8. Adoptive chemoimmunotherapy of FBL-3 with noncultured immune cells: influence of route of administration. C57BL/6 mice inoculated i.p. on day 0 with 5 x 10^6 FBL-3 received either no therapy (No Tx) or treatment on day 5 with 180 mg/kg cyclophosphamide (CY Alone) or CY plus 5 x 10^6 noncultured immune cells, C57$_{\alpha FBL}$ (noncultured), inoculated either intraperitoneal or intravenous. The cumulative results of these experiments are represented with 24 mice per treatment group.

First, the kinetics of tumor elimination were markedly different as reflected by the shapes of the survival curves following therapy with long-term cultured T lymphocytes and noncultured immune spleen cells (Figure 6). Treatment with long-term cultured T lymphocytes significantly (P=0.03) prolonged the median survival but this prolonged early survival was not reflected in prolonged late survival or cure rate (5). We have previously published in this model that following curative therapy with immune cells, tumor elimination is not completed immediately but rather occurs over an extended period of time exceeding two weeks (17). The ability of long-term cultured cells to relatively prolong median survival might then reflect an enhanced early antitumor cytotoxic response and the relative inability of cultured lymphocytes to mediate late survival could reflect a failure of cultured cells to survive in vivo.

The second difference noted is the influence of route of administration. In the previous experiment immune cells were inoculated i.p. Noncultured in vivo immunized cells are equally effective whether inoculated i.p. or i.v. (Figure 8). In contrast, long-term cultured lymphocytes which are effective i.p. are significantly less effective when inoculated i.v. (Figure 9), implying abnormalities in the ability to traffic to sites of tumor.

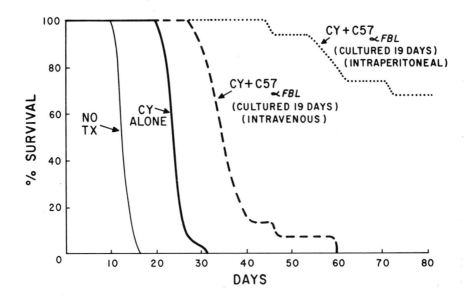

FIG. 9. Adoptive chemoimmunotherapy of FBL-3 with long-term cultured T lymphocytes: influence of route of administration. C57BL/6 mice inoculated i.p. on day 0 with 5×10^6 FBL-3 received either no therapy (No Tx) or treatment on day 5 with 180 mg/kg cyclophosphamide (CY Alone) or CY plus 1×10^7 long-term cultured T lymphocytes inoculated intraperitoneal or intravenous. The cumulative results of two experiments are represented with 16 mice per treatment group.

The third difference noted is the sensitivity of effector cells to
γ-irradiation. Noncultured immune cells are not cytotoxic to tumor at
the time of therapy and must proliferate in vivo to be effective in
therapy. If such cells are irradiated with 1200 rad they do not proliferate or become cytotoxic in response to secondary sensitization
in vitro and are ineffective in tumor therapy (Figure 10). By contrast,
long-term cultured T lymphocytes are cytotoxic to tumor at the time of
therapy. If such cells are irradiated with 1200 rad they do not proliferate but remain specifically cytotoxic to tumor in a 4-hour chromium
release assay (8) and their efficacy in therapy is diminished but not
abolished (Figure 10). Thus, long-term cultured cells which are cytotoxic at the time of therapy can mediate a significant antitumor effect
without further proliferation.

The fourth difference noted is the response of adoptively transferred
cells to the administration of exogenous IL 2. Since the ability of
long-term cultured T lymphocytes to proliferate and survive, at least

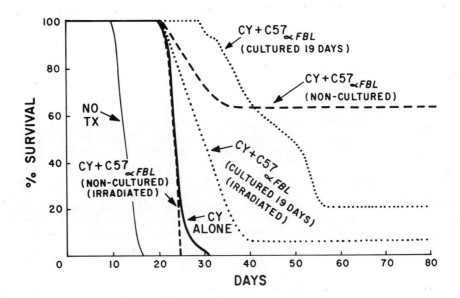

FIG. 10. Chemoimmunotherapy of FBL-3 with noncultured immune cells or
long-term cultured T lymphocytes: effect of donor cell irradiation.
C57BL/6 mice inoculated with FBL-3 on day 0 received either no therapy
(No Tx), treatment on day 5 with CY Alone at 180 mg/kg or treatment with
CY plus 5 x 10⁶ noncultured cells from mice immunized in vivo to FBL-3,
C57$_{\alpha FBL}$ (noncultured), or CY plus 5 x 10¹⁰ cells from mice sequentially
immunized in vivo to FBL-3, secondarily sensitized in vitro and numerically expanded by culture through day 19 with IL 2, C57$_{\alpha FBL}$ (cultured 19
days) or noncultured immune cells or long-term cultured T lymphocytes
following 1200 rad x-irradiation. The cumulative results of two experiments are represented with 16 mice per treatment group.

in vitro, is exquisitely dependent upon repeated exposure to IL 2, their ability to proliferate and survive in vivo, and thus their effectiveness in therapy is likely to be dependent upon the availability of IL 2 in vivo. The in vivo distribution and availability of endogenous IL 2 is unknown, since it is not readily detectable in serum by bioassay and no radioimmunoassay for its presence has been reported. However, since the availability of endogenous IL 2 might limit the therapeutic efficacy of adoptively transferred long-term cultured T lymphocytes, the efficacy of exogenously administered IL 2 in adoptive chemoimmunotherapy was examined (8).

In the preceding studies supernatants from Con A stimulated mouse spleen cells which had been only partially purified were utilized for cell culture in vitro. Con A supernatants contain not only IL 2 but other lymphokines and monokines such as colony stimulating factors, Interleukin 1 and immune interferon as well as cell breakdown products and small amounts of residual lectin (22). Since the end-point of culture was the growth of activated T lymphocytes and since Con A supernatants supported growth well, the presence of these impurities was acceptable. However, such crude supernatants are inappropriate for testing the effect of IL 2 in vivo since the presence of impurities would render results uninterpretable. In fact, in preliminary experiments partially purified Con A supernatants had a small direct antitumor effect in therapy. Thus, to determine the pharmacological antitumor effect of IL 2 in vivo, we used purified IL 2 which had been produced by the lymphoma cell line LBRM 33 (14) and isolated by successive ammonium sulfate precipitation, gel exclusion chromotography (G-100), ion exchange chromotography (DEAE), preparative isoelectric-focusing and SDS-poly acrylamide gel electrophosis (electroelution). This preparation migrates as a single band upon secondary SDS-poly acrylamide gel electrophoresis and contains no known functional activity other than those postulated to be associated with IL 2. It has been functionally screened and is negative for interferon, colony stimulating factor, Interleukin 1, and burst promoting activity (15).

The cumulative data of 2 therapy experiments examining the in vivo efficacy of purified IL 2 are presented in Figure 11. Mice inoculated with FBL-3 on day 0 and given no treatment (No Tx) had a median survival time (MST) of 11 days. Treatment with IL 2 alone, 80 U/day, on days 5-9 had no effect on survival. Therapy on day 5 with CY alone or with CY plus IL 2 on days 5-9 prolonged the MST to day 24. Thus, IL 2 had no detectable antitumor effect either by itself or as an adjunct to CY.

Therapy on day 5 with CY plus 5×10^6 $C57_{\alpha FBL}$ (cultured 19 days) further prolonged the MST to day 38 but no mice were cured. In contrast, therapy on day 5 with CY plus 5×10^6 $C57_{\alpha FBL}$ (cultured 19 days) plus 80 U/day of IL 2 on days 5-9 cured 11 of 16 mice. Thus, as an adjunct to CY, long-term cultured T lymphocytes were effective in tumor therapy and their efficacy was significantly ($p<0.01$) augmented by inoculation of exogenous IL 2.

In contrast, the efficacy of noncultured immune cells was not augmented by the IL 2 regimen (Figure 11). Therapy on day 5 with CY plus 5×10^6 noncultured immune cells, $C57_{\alpha FBL}$ (noncultured), prolonged the MST to day 30 and cured 5 of 32 mice ($p<0.01$). Similarly, therapy on day 5 with CY and $C57_{\alpha FBL}$ (noncultured) plus IL 2 on days 5-9 prolonged the MST to day 30 and cured 1 of 16 mice. Thus, although noncultured immune cells were effective in tumor therapy, their efficacy was not enhanced by exogenous IL 2.

Since exogenous IL 2 promotes continued proliferation and prolonged survival of long-term cultured T lymphocytes in vitro, exogenous IL 2 in vivo may augment the therapeutic efficacy of such cells by performing a similar function in vivo. However, this mechanism of action has not yet been established by quantitating in vivo proliferation of cultured cells in response to IL 2. The reasons for the inability of IL 2 to augment the in vivo efficacy of noncultured immune cells have not yet been determined but may relate to multiple factors (8) such as donor cell subtype, the timing of IL 2 administration or the presence of serum inhibitions to IL 2 function following therapy with noncultured immune spleen cells but not following therapy with long-term cultured T lymphocytes. Although exogenous IL 2 was unable to augment the therapeutic efficacy of noncultured immune cells under the conditions tested, further examination of these models to determine the mechanisms responsible for allowing and/or disallowing exogenous IL 2 to function in vivo may offer the possibility that pharmacologic IL 2 can be used to control other T cell reactions in vivo.

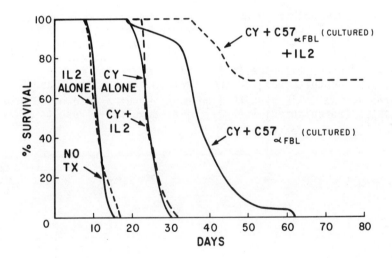

FIG. 11. Chemoimmunotherapy of FBL-3 with long-term cultured T lymphocytes: enhancement of efficacy with IL 2 in vivo. C57BL/6 mice inoculated i.p. on day 0 with 5×10^6 FBL-3 received either no therapy [No Tx], therapy on days 5-9 with Interleukin 2 i.p. at a dose of 80 U/day [IL 2 Alone], treatment on day 5 with cyclophosphamide at a dose of 180 mg/kg [CY Alone], treatment on day 5 with CY plus treatment on days 5-9 with IL 2 [CY + IL 2], treatment on day 5 with CY and 5×10^6 long-term cultured T lymphocytes [CY + C57$_{\alpha FBL}$ (cultured)], or treatment on day 5 with CY and 5×10^6 long-term cultured T lymphocytes plus IL 2 on days 5-9, [CY + C57$_{\alpha FBL}$ (cultured) + IL 2]. The cumulative results of two experiments are represented with 16 mice per treatment group.

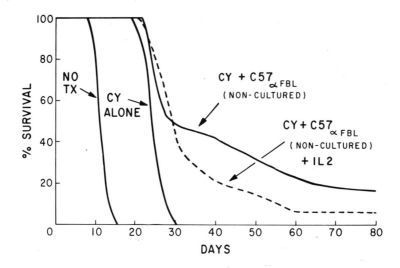

FIG. 12. Chemoimmunotherapy of FBL-3 with noncultured immune cells: failure of IL 2 *in vivo* to enhance therapeutic efficacy. C57BL/6 inoculated i.p. on day 0 with 5 x 10⁶ FBL-3 received either no therapy [No Tx], treatment on day 5 with CY [CY Alone], treatment on day 5 with CY and 5 x 10⁶ noncultured cells from mice immune to FBL-3, [CY + C57$_{\alpha FBL}$ (noncultured)] or treatment on day 5 with CY and 5 x 10⁶ noncultured immune cells plus IL 2 on days 5-9 at a dose of 80 U/day (CY + C57$_{\alpha FBL}$ (noncultured) + IL 2)]. The cumulative results of two experiments are represented.

In summary, the studies presented demonstrate that *in vivo* immunized lymphocytes activated by secondary sensitization *in vitro* and grown to large numbers with IL 2 can mediate specific adoptive tumor therapy. However, the mechanisms by which these long-term cultured T lymphocytes eradicate tumor *in vivo* are qualitatively and/or quantitatively distinct from those of noncultured immune cells.

Acknowledgements

The authors wish to thank M. Bolton, S. Emery, and B. Keniston for expert technical assistance; and J. Hoak and M. Lund for preparation of the manuscript.

REFERENCES

1. Bonnard, G.D., Yasaka, K. and Jacobson, D.(1979): J. Immunol. 123:2704.
2. Cheever, M.A., Kempf, R.A. and Fefer, A. (1977): J. Immunol. 119: 714.
3. Cheever, M.A., Greenberg, P.D. and Fefer, A. (1978): J. Immunol. 121:2220.
4. Cheever, M.A., Greenberg, P.D. and Fefer, A. (1980): J. Immunol. 125:711.
5. Cheever, M.A., Greenberg, P.D. and Fefer, A. (1981): J. Immunol. 126:1318.
6. Cheever, M.A., Greenberg, P.D. and Fefer, A. (1981): J. Natl. Cancer Inst. 67:169.
7. Cheever, M.A., Greenberg, P.D. and Fefer, A. (1981): Ca. Res. 41:2658.
8. Cheever, M.A., Greenberg, P.D. Fefer, A. and Gillis, S. (1982): J. Exp. Med., in press.
9. Fefer, A., Einstein, Jr., A.B., Cheever, M.A. and Berenson J.R. (1976): Ann N. Y. Acad. Sci. 276:573.
10. Friedman, H., Spector, S., Kamo, I. and Katelye, J. (1976): Ann N. Y. Acad. Sci. 276:417.
11. Fujimoto, S., Greene, M.I. and Sehon, A.H. (1976): J. Immunol. 116:800.
12. Gillis, S. and Smith, K.A. (1977): Nature 268:154.
13. Gillis, S., Ferm, M.M., Ou, W. and Smith, K.A. (1978): J. Immunol. 120:2027.
14. Gillis, S., Scheid, M., and Watson, J. (1980): J. Immunol. 125: 2570.
15. Gillis, S. and Mochizuki, D. (1981): Immunol. Rev., in press.
16. Greenberg, P.D., Cheever, M.A. and Fefer, A. (1979): J. Immunol. 123:515.
17. Greenberg, P.D., Cheever, M.A. and Fefer, A. (1980): Cancer Res. 40:4428.
18. Greenberg, P.D., Cheever, M.A. and Fefer, A. (1981): J. Exp. Med. 154:952.
19. Hellström, K.E., and Hellström, I. (1974): Adv. Immunol. 18:209.
20. Herberman, R.B., Aoki, T., Nunn, M., Lavrin, D.H., Soares, N., Gazdar, A., Holden, H. and Chang, K.S.S. (1974): J. Natl. Cancer Inst. 53:1103.
21. Hodes, R.J., Nadler, L.M. and Hathcock, K.S. (1977): J. Immunol. 119:961.
22. Lafferty, K.J., Warren, H.S., Woolnough, J.A., and Talmage, D.W. (1978): Blood Cells 4:395.
23. McCoy, J.L., Fefer, A. and Glynn, J.P. (1967): Cancer Res. 27: 1743.
24. Mizel, S.B. and Farrar, J.J. (1979): Cell Immunol. 48:433.
25. Plata, F. and Jongeneel, C.V. (1977): J. Immunol. 119:623.
26. Rosenberg, S.A. and Terry, W.D. (1977): Adv. Cancer Res. 25:323.
27. Rosenberg, S.A. Schwarz, S. and Spiess, P.J. (1978): J. Immunol. 121:1951.
28. Ruscetti, F.W., Morgan, D.A. and Gallo, R.C. (1977): J. Immunol. 119:131.

29. Ryser, J.-E., Cerottini, J.-C. and Brunner, K.T. (1979): <u>Eur. J.
     Immunol.</u> 9:179.
30. Shaw, J., Caplan, B., Paetkau, V., Pilarski, L.M., Delovitch, T.L.,
     and McKenzie, I.F.C. (1980): <u>J. Immunol.</u> 124:2231.
31. Smith, K.A., Gillis, S., Baker, P.E., McKenzie, D. and
     Ruscetti, F.W. (1979): <u>Ann N. Y. Acad. Sci.</u> 332:423.
32. Smith, K.A., Gillis, S., and Baker, P. (1979): <u>Proc. of Am. Assoc.
     Ca. Res.</u> 20:93 (abstract).
33. Ting, C.C. and Bonnard, G.D. (1976): <u>J. Immunol.</u> 116:1419.
34. Wagner, H. and Rollinghoff, M. (1978): <u>J. Exp. Med.</u> 148:1523.
35. Zarling, J.M. and Bach, F.H. (1979): <u>Nature</u> 280:685.

AUDIENCE DISCUSSION

<u>Dr. Bortin</u>: How is primary sensitization <u>in vitro</u> working as opposed to
primary sensitization <u>in vivo</u> with restimulation <u>in vitro</u>?

<u>Dr. Cheever</u>: In the FBL-3 chemoimmunotherapy model, we have not been
able to generate therapeutically effective cells by primary <u>in vitro</u>
sensitization. A major problem may be the concurrent generation of
culture-induced suppressor cells along with antitumor effector cells.
The presence of culture-induced suppressor cells is potentially a greater
problem for a weak primary response than for a stronger secondary response. In a different model, the chemoimmunotherapy of a Moloney
virus-induced leukemia (LSTRA) in syngeneic BALB/c mice, we have demonstrated that spleen cells are effective in therapy following primary
sensitization <u>in vitro</u>. However, we have not yet attempted to culture
these cells long-term in IL 2.

<u>Dr. Bortin</u>: Have you tested long-term cultured cells generated follow-
ing primary <u>in vitro</u> sensitization in your EL-4 model?

<u>Dr. Cheever</u>: The majority of our therapy experiments with EL-4(G-) in
which primary <u>in vitro</u> sensitization techniques were utilized have been
in F_1 hybrid mice so as to allow the examination of the specificity of
both tumor-associated antigens and major histocompatibility antigens.
We have not attempted to culture these cells long-term in IL 2.

<u>Dr. Oldham</u>: Do you get cytotoxicity following primary <u>in vivo</u> sensi-
tization?

<u>Dr. Cheever</u>: Dr. C.C. Ting reported that low levels of cytolytic react-
ivity to FBL-3 were detected in an 18 hour [125]IUdR release assay several
weeks after primary <u>in vivo</u> immunization. However, in a standard 4-hour
chromium release assay we have been unable to consistently demonstrate
that cells are cytotoxic to tumor following primary sensitization
<u>in vitro</u>.

<u>Dr. Warner</u>: Do you know the phenotype of the effector cells in the 19
day culture?

<u>Dr. Cheever</u>: The T lymphocyte and subpopulation responsible for the
majority of the antitumor effect following infusion of <u>noncultured</u>
immune donor spleen cells is a noncytotoxic Lyt 1^+2^- T <u>lymphocyte</u>. In
contrast, day 19 cultured cells are cytotoxic to tumor at the time of
therapy. We have not yet determined the Lyt phenotype of the cell
subpopulation responsible for therapeutic efficacy <u>in vivo</u>. Thus, it is
unknown whether the increased efficacy of long-term cultured T lymphocytes results from the generation of cytotoxic effector cells or from an
expansion of the noncytotoxic cell subpopulation.

Dr. Herberman: You stressed that the IL 2 material used for in vivo treatment was more purified than that used for cell culture. Do you have any indications that purification is necessary? Have you tested the cruder Con A supernatants in vivo?

Dr. Cheever: Yes. Crude Con A supernatants worked extremely well in vivo -- much better than purified IL 2. The crude supernatants contained a variety of lymphokines and monokines as well as cell break-down products and residual lectin. In addition, such supernatants have a direct antitumor affect. Thus, the efficacy in vivo cannot be attributed solely to the effects of IL 2 on host or donor T lymphocytes.

Dr. Herberman: Have you examined recipient spleen cells for cytolytic reactivity in a situation in which you are demonstrating an increase in in vivo efficacy following IL 2 therapy.

Dr. Cheever: No, not yet. It is the next obvious experiment.

Dr. Kedar: Have you tried to repeatedly inject your cultured T cells to determine whether you can get a better therapeutic effect? Have you noticed any clinical toxicity or graft-versus-host disease from long-term cultured T lymphocytes in cyclophosphamide pretreated mice.

Dr. Cheever: We have not noticed any toxicity from long-termed cultured T lymphocytes even at high doses. We have not yet tested multiple inoculations of cultured T lymphocytes in vivo. However, since the outcome of therapy is related to the dose of a few cells, such a regimen should be effective.

Dr. Grimm: Have you tested cured mice for immunity to tumor? Do they resist another challenge of FBL-3?

Dr. Cheever: When we treat with in vivo sensitized cells, cured mice are immune, their spleen cells are effective in therapy and they resist tumor challenge. We have not yet tested cells from mice following cure with long-term cultured T lymphocytes.

Dr. Ihle: The effect you demonstrated with IL 2 in vivo is quite striking considering the fact that you use only 80 units. Have you tested BSA alone as a control?

Dr. Cheever: We are initiating such experiments. However, interpretation of the results of therapy following inoculation of BSA or any other biological substance unrelated to IL 2 may be difficult. The only parameter measured in vivo is the outcome of therapy and the outcome of therapy can presumably be affected by a variety of mechanisms. Long-term cultured T lymphocytes require IL 2 in vitro for both survival and proliferation. Confirmation that a similar mechanism is responsible for their augmentation by exogenous IL 2 in vivo will require actual quantitation of either donor cells or donor cell divisions in the host rather than an evaluation of the therapeutic efficacy of other substances.

Dr. Gillis: The therapeutic results were obtained with 80 units a day for 5 days for a total of 400 units of IL 2 rather than 80 units total.

Dr. Cheever: The dramatic effect demonstrated might be the result of the very sensitive assay system for detecting the in vivo effects of exogenous IL 2.

Dr. Ihle: The BSA has a lot of funny effects too; that's why control data are extremely important.

Dr. Green: I agree that an incredibly small amount of IL 2 is having an effect. Have you considered Bob Stout's demonstration that an adherent cell in culture inhibits secretion of IL 2? If your donor cells contain such inhibitory cells, they might inactivate the endogenous production of IL 2 by the recipient. If that cell can be removed prior to therapy, the need for IL 2 might be less.

<u>Dr. Cheever</u>: Dr. Altman made an excellent point yesterday. When mice are treated with cells from bulk cultures, many of the donor cells have been activated by culture and thus express IL 2 receptors but are irrelevant to therapy. Such cells might potentially absorb out endogenous IL 2, which would otherwise be available <u>in vivo</u>.

The Potential Role of T Cells in Cancer Therapy,
edited by A. Fefer and A. Goldstein,
Raven Press, New York © 1982.

Enhancement of Anti-Tumor Immune Responses with Interleukin 2

Verner Paetkau, Gordon B. Mills, and R. Chris Bleackley

Department of Biochemistry, University of Alberta, Edmonton, Alberta, Canada T6G 2H7

INTRODUCTION

Tumor Immunotherapy

Tumor immunotherapy is an appealing approach because in theory it offers the prospect of continuing active surveillance against tumor cells. The immune system, with its innate capacity to recognize and neutralize a wide array of recognizably foreign antigens, seems to be well suited to the eradication of tumor cells, which are often antigenically different from their normal counterparts. The immune system could inactivate metastatic cells independent of their growth rate or cell cycle state, thus complementing chemotherapy. Early hopes that tumor immunity can easily be demonstrated have generally been disappointed, however. Even the relatively tractable tumors favored by experimental tumorologists show an impressive versatility in escaping "immune surveillance". Recent advances in understanding and manipulating immune responses suggest that it may be time to examine tumor immunotherapy in more sophisticated ways.

An approach which has renewed appeal is the nonspecific, positive stimulation of the immune system when it is already involved in an anti-tumor response. The theory behind this approach (if there is one) is that the immune system already has the specifity to recognize tumor cells, but may have been paralyzed by demonstrable suppressive mechanisms, such as the generation of inhibitory factors (20,24), or the "blinding" of effector cells or molecules with tumor antigen. In that case, a nonspecific stimulatory factor might overcome the inhibition and allow the system to function properly.

Interleukin 2

One useful immunostimulatory factor is the lymphokine Interleukin 2 (IL2). Originally described by different laboratories on the basis of different bioassays (5,8,15,23), IL2 is presently thought to be a single kind of molecule, albeit one showing microheterogeneity. Its properties are described elsewhere (14,16) and will only be summarized. Murine IL2

is an acidic, Ia⁻ protein (probably glycosylated), normally isolated as
a 32,000 MW structure (16,19), but apparently consisting of chains
approximately half this MW (2). It is a product of T lymphocytes of the
"helper" type (19) and is elicited from them by appropriate molecular
signalling, involving Interleukin 1 (a product of activated macrophages)
and antigen (16). Its most characteristic biological property is the
stimulation of T lymphocyte growth (8). IL2 stimulates cytotoxic lymphocyte responses in 2 ways; during the inductive phase, when it probably
acts by eliciting interferon production (7), and subsequently, during
clonal expansion. In addition, it enhances antibody-forming-cell
responses by B lymphocytes. That all 3 activities are induced by a
single molecule is supported by classical purification studies from
several labs (cf Ref. 23). A definitive answer awaits development of
molecular genetic approaches, a subject to be touched on here.

Mastocytoma P815

In applying IL2 to the manipulation of anti-tumor immune responses,
our interest was attracted by the work of Takei, Levy and Kilburn on the
mastocytoma P815 of DBA/2 mice (20). Although this tumor grows rapidly
and disseminates widely, resulting inevitably in the death of its syngeneic host, a transient cellular immune response can be demonstrated
about 8-10 days after tumor administration. This response wanes, and
tumor growth, which had stopped, resumes without further interruption
(20). In other words, the immune system does indeed recognize and react
to the tumor. Can the positive, transient, reaction be converted to an
effective anti-tumor response, and immunity established, using the
immunostimulatory properties of IL2?

THE GENERATION AND PROPERTIES OF LYMPHOCYTES CYTOTOXIC TO P815

Specific Antitumor CL

Spleen cells from P815-bearing DBA/2 mice have a demonstrable, but
very low level of cytotoxic lymphocytes (CL) directed against P815 cells
(20). When such spleen cells were cultured with optimal levels of IL2
and (inactivated) tumor, their CL activity increased dramatically over
5-6 days (Figure 1; Ref. 13). The CL activity generated from the
spleens of tumor-bearers was significantly higher than that seen with
normal spleen cells, indicating that the former carried a high, but
cryptic, responsiveness. This is consistent with the idea that the
tumor-bearing animal suffers, not from a failure to recognize the tumor,
but from suppression (20). The sharp decline in CL activity after day 6
(Figure 1) is due to depletion of IL2, as addition of further IL2 at
this time leads to increased CL activity (data not shown).
The requirements for CL production are outlined in Table 1 (see also
Ref. 13). Although different experiments gave different absolute levels
of activity, as illustrated by experiments A and B, the pattern was the
same. High levels of CL activity were obtained when spleen cells from
tumor-bearing animals were stimulated with both antigen (P815) and IL2.
Surprisingly, the potential CL activity was highest at fairly late
stages of tumor growth (mice with subcutaneous P815 die by day 30). A
typical allogeneic CL response is also shown in Table 1, for comparison
(CBA-anti-H-2^d). The maximal CL activity against syngeneic tumor was
20-25% as high as the allogeneic response.

Other experiments (13) indicated that the cytotoxic activity resided in T lymphocytes and was reasonably specific, although other H-2^d (syngeneic) tumors were also lysed, to a lesser extent than P815.

Anti-P815 CL are Effective in Mice

The CL generated in vitro from the spleen cells of tumor-bearing DBA/2 mice were injected into DBA/2 mice bearing intraperitoneal (i.p.) P815 tumors. These mice were monitored for tumor clearance by following the elimination of radiolabelled P815 cells (3). Their survival was also followed (Table 2). Both parameters were significantly enhanced under appropriate conditions. The time of survival of 30% of the mice given P815 i.p. was extended by 50% if CL were administered on the same day as tumor, but by separate injection (Table 2; see also Ref. 12).

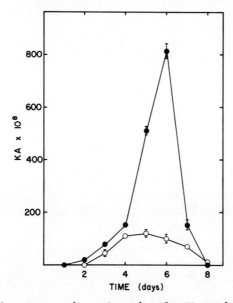

FIG. 1. Generation of anti-P815 CL activity from spleen cells. Spleen cells (1.25 x 10^6/ml) from either normal (O) or P815-bearing DBA/2 (●) mice were incubated in RPMI 1640 medium with 6.2 x 10^4 gamma-irradiated P815 cells per ml and 15 U/ml IL2. CL activity was monitored on ^{51}Cr-labelled P815 cells and expressed as Killing Activity (KA). This parameter is derived from the relationship (11): F = 1- exp(-N·KA·t), where F is the fraction of cells specifically killed (^{51}Cr released) in t hours by cytotoxic cells derived from N lymphocytes placed into culture on day 0. A KA value of 200 x 10^{-8} corresponds to 10% specific lysis in 5 hours when 10^4 P815 are exposed to CL derived from 10^4 spleen cells. Tumor-bearing mice had been given 10^3 P815 cells subcutaneously 19 days before their spleen cells were harvested. Other experimental details are given in Ref. 13.

TABLE 1. Generation of lymphocytes cytotoxic to mastocytoma P815[a]

Presence during culture:		$KA \times 10^8$				
			Source of spleen cells			
		Normal DBA/2	Tumor-bearing DBA/2			Normal CBA/J
P815	IL2		Day 11	Day 21	Day 26	
Expt.	A					
−	−	<5	23	30	15	<5
−	+	70	82	140	<5	30
+	−	<5	<5	15	<5	500
+	+	295	390	1230	230	4855
Expt.	B					
−	−	<5	<5	6	nd	<5
−	+	<5	14	28	nd	<5
+	−	<5	<5	<5	nd	163
+	+	36	40	280	nd	1587

[a]*Spleen cells from DBA or CBA mice, as indicated, were cultured for 5 days. Other conditions were as described in the legend to Figure 1.*

TABLE 2. Survival after treatment with cytotoxic lymphocytes[a]

CL given:	30% survival (days)
None	19.5
Day 0	30.5
Day 1	27.5
Day 2	29.5
Day 5	20.5
Day 10	26.0
Day 15	25.5

[a]*DBA/2 mice were injected with 2×10^4 P815 cells i.p. on day 0. Cytotoxic lymphocytes (CL) were generated by culturing spleen cells from P815-bearing mice with IL2 and irradiated P815 cells for 5 days, as described in the text and Figure 1. In this experiment, the i.p. tumors were given on different days, so that the CL could all be taken from the same pool, and administered on the same day.*

The effectiveness of CL waned with time of administration up to day 5, but then increased again by day 10. The refractoriness of mice to treatment 4-5 days after tumor was noted in every case, and also occurred during treatment with IL2 itself (below). On the other hand, the ability to affect survival 10 or 15 days after tumor is encouraging, as the mice carried palpable tumors by this time, and died by 19-20 days (Figure 3).

Another measure of efficacy is the ability to enhance tumor clearance (Figure 2). CL were injected 2 days after tumor, and resulted in more rapid clearance of labelled P815 from the mice (see also Ref. 12). Furthermore, two out of 5 mice in the treated group survived indefinitely, with no sign of tumor. When a group of 10 surviving, CL-treated mice was examined up to 2 years after being "cured" by administered CL, all mice were fully resistant to tumor. Their spleens also contained a higher anti-P815 CL activity than those of normal mice (unpublished data). In short, they appeared to be tumor-immune.

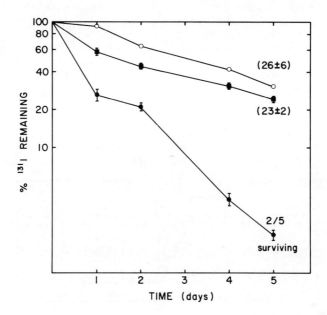

FIG. 2.   Clearance of P815 tumor by mice treated with CL.   DBA/2 mice were injected with 10^6 ^{131}I-iododeoxyuridine-labelled P815 cells on day -2 (i.e. 2 days before CL).   On day 0, they were given 10^7 spleen cells i.p. as the source of CL. The CL were derived by incubating (see Figure 1) spleen cells from 21 day tumor-bearing mice for 5 days with: no additions, or with irradiated P815 (results the same as untreated controls (O)); IL2 alone (■); or with IL2 and P815 (●).   Radioactivity remaining in the mice was assessed by whole body counting (3).   Survival times are given in parenthesis.   The last group (●) contained 2 mice which survived indefinitely (more than 1 year), and which were tumor-immune.

The mechanism of Anti-P815 Action is Unclear

It might be supposed that the tumor immunity observed in some mice after treatment with high levels of CL resulted simply from tumor reduction. This is probably not the case. Data presented elsewhere (12) indicate that reducing the tumor mass does not lead to enhanced clearance. Nor is it likely that the administered CL colonize the animal and provide cellular immunity, since the CL themselves are dependent on IL2 for viability. Indeed, most of the administered cells were rapidly eliminated from the recipient mice (12). Also, CL were ineffective if given 2 days before tumor, but did lead to enhanced clearance if, given after tumor, they were irradiated to block their proliferation (12). Admittedly, the mechanism of action of CL is far from understood, but the facts are consistent with an active host response being required.

Another aspect of host-tumor relationship is illustrated in Figure 3. Cyclophosphamide (CY), given in high doses, partly or completely eliminates P815 tumor. However, the "cured" mice show no sign of tumor immunity, probably because this agent has profoundly inhibitory effects on the immune system. Indeed, we are presently trying to restore immunity to CY-treated mice, by various immunotherapeutic means (CL and IL2). So far, we have been unable to influence the tumor response of CY-treated mice with CL or IL2. This further supports the notion that, in the absence of an active host immune function, treatment with CL is ineffective.

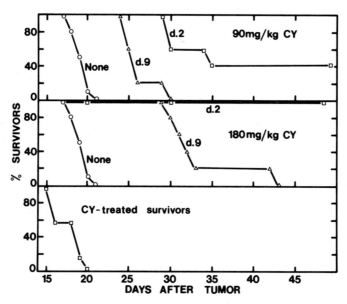

FIG. 3. *Treatment of P815 tumor with cyclophosphamide (CY). Mice carrying P815 tumors i.p. were injected with 90 or 180 mg/kg CY (i.p.) on day 2 or 9. Control mice died by day 21. Survivors from the 90 or 180 mg/kg regimens were challenged with P815 tumor between days 50 and 70, with the results shown in the bottom panel.*

DIRECT IMMUNOTHERAPY WITH IL2

Pharmacokinetics

A different approach to tumor immunotherapy is offered by the availability of large quantities of murine IL2 derived from certain lymphoid
tumor cell lines (6,9). We have prepared IL2 from the EL4 variant line
described by Farrar and colleagues (6). Although we have purified this
material to a specific activity of 2000 units/µg as measured by the T
Cell Growth Factor (TCGF) assay, the experiments described here were
performed with Fraction 3 IL2, of specific activity about .5 U/µg. (One
unit/ml produces 1/3 the maximal proliferation under standard assay
conditions; cf Ref. 16). The question is, whether IL2 injected directly
into tumor-bearing mice has any anti-tumor activity.

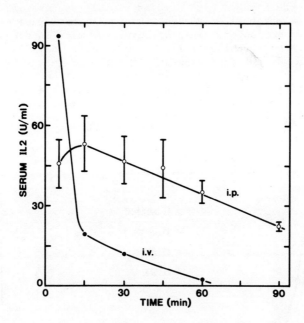

FIG. 4. *Pharmacokinetics of IL2. Fraction 3 IL2
was prepared from the EL4 cell line described
elsewhere (6), and 3000 units injected either
i.p. or i.v. into normal DBA/2 mice. Mice were
bled and their serum IL2 levels determined in the
TCGF assay (8) by titration, using the T cell
line MTL2.8.2 (Bleackley et al., in preparation).
Serum was assayed for IL2 by titration between 10
and 0.1%. In a separate experiment, IL2 was
added to whole mouse blood, incubated at 37°, and
assayed after dilution to 0.3%. The activity in
the assay at 60, 90 and 240 minutes was .56, .63,
and .58 of maximal response, where the expected
value at this dilution was .56. Thus, there was
no loss of activity by 4 hours in whole blood.*

A dose of 3000 units of IL2, given i.v. to normal DBA/2 mice, was rapidly cleared from the circulation (Figure 4). The rapid clearance was due neither to instability in blood, nor to the reported inhibitory activity of mouse serum (22). (Inhibition was noted only at 10% serum. When incubated in whole blood at 37°, IL2 activity was unchanged in 4 hours, indicating that it is stable in blood.)

IL2 injected i.p. was apparently released into the circulation more slowly than IL2 given i.v., and a reasonable level of blood IL2 was present for at least 90 minutes (Figure 4). This route of injection is both more convenient and more effective than intravenous injection.

Antitumor Effects of IL2

DBA/2 mice bearing P815 tumors for various times were injected i.p. with 5000 units of Fraction 3 IL2, with the results shown in Figure 5. Although most of the treated mice died as rapidly as control, tumor-bearing animals (average life 19 days), a significant fraction of IL2-treated mice survived longer. This was true for mice injected with IL2 immediately after tumor (day 0 or 1), or much later (day 10), at a time when tumor growth was increasing again after the plateau (20). By contrast, treatment beginning on day 5 was uniformly without effect in 3 series of experiments, reminiscent of the refractory state at this time when CL were used (Table 1). Higher doses of IL2 must now be used, to try to increase the effects already seen.

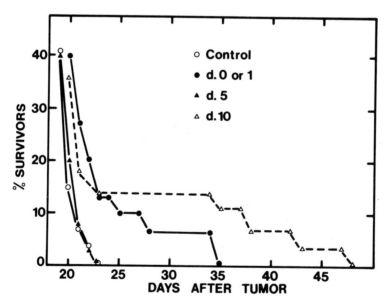

FIG. 5. Immunotherapy with IL2. DBA/2 mice with P815 tumors were injected with Fraction 3 IL2, at the times shown. These results were pooled from several experiments, in which 5,000 or 8,000 units of IL2 were injected i.p. (no significant difference was seen between these levels).

CLONAL APPROACHES

Molecular Biology of IL2

The EL4 variant cell line alluded to earlier (6) produces about 1000 times as much IL2 as mouse spleen cells, when properly stimulated. It appeared to be a useful starting point for an attempt to isolate mRNA coding for IL2, a first step in the molecular cloning of the lymphokine. Poly A$^+$ mRNA was therefore prepared from the EL4 variant line stimulated with phorbol myristate acetate (PMA), and microinjected into Xenopus oocytes. The product of 48 hours' protein synthesis in this system contained IL2 activity, as determined in the TCGF bioassay. Water-injected oocytes produced no activity, as did oocytes injected with mRNA from unstimulated EL4 cells (1). The poly A$^+$ mRNA coding for IL2 had a sedimentation coefficient of about 11.5 S (Figure 6), slightly less than that of Kappa light chain mRNA, which encodes 24,000 daltons of protein.

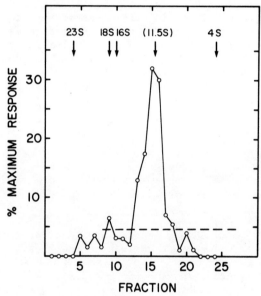

FIG. 6. *Sedimentation of IL2 mRNA on a sucrose gradient. Poly A$^+$ RNA was prepared from the EL4 variant cell line (6) by the method of Reference 18, using 2 cycles of chromatography on oligo dT cellulose. It was loaded onto a 10-28% sucrose gradient and centrifuged at 35,000 rpm (SW 41 rotor) at 4° for 19 hours. RNA in each fraction was precipitated with ethanol and injected into Xenopus oocytes (10). The oocytes were homogenited after 48 hours and the crude extracts assayed for IL2 in the TCGF assay. RNA worked up from unstimulated EL4 cells, and subjected to gradient centrifugation gave no detectable activity under these conditions (values were below the dotted line at 4.5%). Other details are reported in Ref. 1.*

Besides showing that IL2 activity undoubtedly resides in protein, these
experiments indicate that molecular cloning should be possible along the
lines successfully followed with interferon mRNA (4). A "library" of
cDNA clones from the 11-12S region of a gradient like the one in Figure
6 is now in hand, and is being screened for IL2 sequences by the Hybrid-
Arrest-of-Translation method (17). A clonally-defined source of IL2
would directly answer the question of whether all the biological activities ascribed to it are carried by one molecule. Also, it may open the
way to the controlled production of large amounts of murine, and human,
IL2, free of other eukaryotic products.

Clones of Anti-P815 Lymphocytes

A centrally-important question in this work is whether the effects of
administered CL are due to classical cytotoxic T lymphocytes, or to
another type of cell which has been carried through the protocol (e.g.
T lymphocytes of the "helper" type or "Natural Killer" cells). A clear
answer would be provided by cloned CL directed against P815. Such cells
are now available, but not yet in sufficient numbers to carry out the
desired experiments. The method of their production is similar to
approaches reported elsewhere, with a few novel aspects (Figure 7). In
outline, spleen cells from DBA/2 mice bearing subcutaneous P815 tumors
for 19 days were grown in culture with IL2 (15 U/ml) and, initially,

P815 injected subcutaneously.

 ↓ 19 days

Spleen cells into culture at 10^6/ml with 15 U/ml
IL2 + 50,000 irradiated P815/ml.

 ↓ Change medium, add IL2, for 70 days;
   test CL activity throughout

Cells seeded into microtiter wells at 0.5/well,
with 10^4 mitomycin-treated P815 + 15 U/ml IL2.

 ↓ Medium changed each 2-3 days.
   Mitomycin-treated P815 added each
   7 days.

In about 2 weeks, clearing of P815 target cells
in 12/96 wells.

 ↓ Continue clonal expansion with IL2,
   test for rapidity of killing mito-
   mycin-P815.

Pick 5 clones with high killing activity for
further growth.

FIG. 7. *Protocol for clonal, anti-P815 CL.*

with gamma-irradiated P815 cells. After numerous passages and several assays to ensure that anti-P815 activity had persisted, CL were cloned by limiting dilution (0.5 cells/well). Mitomycin c-inactivated P815 cells were added as feeders and also to indicate CL activity. (These were also added at weekly intervals, since they disappear in a few days even from negative cultures). After 2 weeks, 12/96 wells were positive, as shown by the rapid clearance of the P815 indicator (target) cells. Several of the most active clones are now being grown up in larger numbers.

CONCLUSIONS AND PROSPECTS

The potency and variety of effects on immune responses elicited by IL2 (8,16,23) has generated some hope that this lymphokine may have useful anti-tumor capabilities. Our studies suggest the following conclusions regarding IL2 and the P815 tumor of DBA mice:

(i) Tumor-bearing mice have a high level of potential anti-P815 CL activity, but this activity is revealed only by incubation with IL2 and antigen.

(ii) The activity elicited by the in vivo to in vitro protocol increases tumor clearance, enhances survival, and in some cases leads to complete control of the tumor. In the last case, the mice are rendered tumor-immune.

(iii) Moderately high levels (5-10,000 units) of IL2, injected i.p., expose the animal to saturating IL2 in the blood (50-100 U/ml) for about 1 hour.

(iv) Intraperitoneally-injected IL2 leads to extended survival of a small fraction (10-15%) of tumor-bearing mice.

(v) Tumors are sensitive to CL or IL2 treatment at early times (days 0 or 1), or later, when tumor growth is rapid (day 10). They are refractory to both agents at days 4 or 5.

(vi) IL2 is encoded in an mRNA perhaps 1000 nucleotides long, and IL2 mRNA can be translated into biologically active IL2 protein in oocytes.

(vii) Clones of T cells able to kill P815 tumor cells can be obtained from extended cultures of spleen cells taken from tumor-bearing animals.

Experiments to study the effects of higher levels of CL or IL2, or combinations of the two, are indicated. The efficacy of anti-P815 CL in blocking or reversing tumor growth in vivo will be known once sufficient numbers of cloned cells are available.

The immunotherapy protocols described here offer some interesting possibilities, particularly because they are effective as late as 10-15 days after tumor administration. However, they are primarily designed to counteract metastatic spread. Ideally, they should be coupled to a method of reducing primary tumor mass, such as surgery or chemotherapy. An interesting problem in this context is how to overcome the immunosuppressive effects of CY, which bears some relevance for the treatment of human tumors with this drug.

Although the results given here were obtained with the P815 tumor, other tumors show similar results, such as enhanced anti-tumor CL generated by the in vivo-in vitro protocol described for P815. Preliminary experiments with the DBA tumor CaD_2, of mammary gland epithelial origin (21), show how combined surgery plus CL treatment can be used. Subcutaneous CaD_2 tumors were treated either with CL generated in vitro by co-culture of spleen cells from tumor-bearing mice with antigen and IL2, or by surgical resection, or both. Compared to controls, which died at 27 ± 3 days, surgery (day 20) extended average survival to 44 ± 19 days. Treatment with CL extended average survival to 48 ± 8 days; 1 mouse out of 4 in this group recovered completely. Most significantly, surgery plus CL cured 4 out of 4 mice.

In summary, IL2-related procedures offer two effective routes to control of certain syngeneic tumors in mice, either by generating high levels of CL directed against the tumor, or by injection of moderate levels of IL2 into tumor-bearing animals. We expect to find that these protocols are most effective when used in conjunction with other methods such as surgery or chemotherapy, to reduce the primary tumor mass. Questions of mechanism will probably be answerable soon, since molecularly cloned IL2 and clones of CL will likely be available before long.

ACKNOWLEDGEMENTS

This work was supported by grants from MRC and NCI of Canada, and the Alberta Heritage Trust Fund. We thank T. Lee, C. Havele and R.G. Ritzel for their help in this work.

REFERENCES

1. Bleackley, R.C., Caplan, B., Havele, C., Ritzel, R.G., Mosmann,T.R., Farrar, J.J., and Paetkau, V. (1981): J. Immunol., (in press).
2. Caplan, B., Gibbs, C., and Paetkau, V. (1981): J. Immunol., 126:1351-1354.
3. Carlson, G.A., and Terres, G. (1978): J. Immunol., 121:1752-1759.
4. Derynck, R., Content, J., DeClerq, E., Volchaert, G., Tavernier, J., Devos, R., and Fiers, W. (1980): Nature, 285:542-547.
5. DiSabato, G., Chen, D.-M., and Erickson, J.W. (1975): Cell Immunol., 17:495-504.
6. Farrar, J.J., Fuller-Farrar, J., Simon, P.L., Hilfiker, M.L., Stadler, B.M., and Farrar, W.L. (1980): J. Immunol., 125:2555-2558.
7. Farrar, W.L., Johnson, H.M., and Farrar, J.J. (1981): J. Immunol., 126:1120-1125.
8. Gillis, S., Ferm, M.M., Ou, W., and Smith, K. (1978): J. Immunol., 120:2027-2032.
9. Gillis, S., Scheid, M., and Watson, J. (1980): J. Immunol., 125:2570-2578.
10. Gurdon, J.B. (1974): The Control of Gene Expression in Animal Development., Harvard University Press, Cambridge.
11. Miller, R.G., and Dunkley, M. (1974): Cell. Immunol., 14:284-302.
12. Mills, G.B., Carlson, G., and Paetkau, V. (1980): J. Immunol., 125:1904-1909.
13. Mills, G.B., and Paetkau, V. (1980): J. Immunol., 125:1897-1903.
14. Möller, G., editor (1980): Immunol. Rev., Vol. 51.
15. Paetkau, V., Mills, G.B., Gerhart, S., and Monticone, V. (1976): J. Immunol., 117:1320-1324.
16. Paetkau, V., Shaw, J., Mills, G.B., and Caplan, B. (1980): Immunol. Rev., 51:157-175.
17. Parnes, J.R., Velan, B., Felsenfeld, A., Ramanathan, L., Ferrini,V., Appella, E., and Seidman, J.G. (1981): Proc. Natl. Acad. Sci. USA., 78:2253-2257.
18. Przybyla, A.E., MacDonald, R.J., Harding, J.D., Pictet, R.L., and Rutter, W.J. (1979): J. Biol. Chem., 254:2154-2159.

19. Shaw, J., Caplan, B., Paetkau, V., Pilarski, L.M., Delovitch, T.L., and McKenzie, I.F.C. (1980): J. Immunol., 124:2231-2239.
20. Takei, F., Levy, J.G., and Kilburn, D.G. (1976): J. Immunol., 116:288-293.
21. Talmage, D.W., Woolnough, J.A., Hemmingsen, H., Lopez, L., and Lafferty, K.J. (1977): Proc. Natl. Acad. Sci. USA, 74:4610-4614.
22. Wagner, H., Hardt, C., Heeg, K., Pfizenmaier, K., Solbach, W., Bartlett, R., Stockinger, H., and Röllinghoff, M. (1980): Immunol. Rev., 51:215-255.
23. Watson, J., Aarden, L.A., Shaw, J., and Paetkau, V. (1979): J. Immunol., 122:1633-1638.
24. Yu, A., Watts, H., Jaffe, N., and Parkman, R. (1977): N. Engl. J. Med., 297:121-127.

AUDIENCE DISCUSSION

Dr. Altman: How is it that you generate such a low level of cytotoxicity in the presence of viable tumor?

Dr. Paetkau: The cytotoxic reactivity dies away after challenge. It's possible that we weren't optimally culturing them.

Dr. Altman: How does your definition of a unit of IL 2 activity compare with that of Gillis?

Dr. Paetkau: It's close. Initially we thought about calling it 1 over E which is 37 percent and, on Jim Watson's suggestion, I settled for one-third maximal. Our definition pertains to an assay in which long-term cytotoxic T cells lines from a clone are maintained in a microwell and assayed after 24 hours for DNA synthesis and the level of IL 2 which will give one-third of that maximal stimulation we considered to be 1 unit per ml.

Dr. Gillis: It's close but some numbers are different. We usually use 50 percent but I think we must eventually speak in terms of activity per microgram protein. Incidentally, you showed that animals successfully treated with cytotoxic lymphocytes cultured in IL 2 retain the capacity to reject a lethal tumor inoculum over a year later. What type of cell is responsible for that long-term immunity? Is it possible to grow those cells and maintain them in long-term culture?

Dr. Paetkau: We don't know the cell type responsible and have not been able to grow them in long-term culture.

Dr. Greenberg: Do you have any evidence that having IL 2 present during culture in any way enhanced the generation of the cell population that was effective in therapy? Were cells without IL 2 less effective? At the time when you examined cultures for the generation of cytotoxicity one would not expect much cytolytic activity in cultures growing without IL 2. Have you looked at earlier time points to see if you generated cytotoxicity equally as high in cultures without IL 2?

Dr. Paetkau: No. We know only that if any of the components were left out of culture we got no effect. The cytotoxicity generated is optimal around 5 to 6 days.

The Potential Role of T Cells in Cancer Therapy,
edited by A. Fefer and A. Goldstein,
Raven Press, New York © 1982.

Adoptive Transfer of Lymphoid Cells Expanded in T-Cell Growth Factor: Murine and Human Studies

S. A. Rosenberg, T. Eberlein, E. Grimm, A. Mazumder,
and M. Rosenstein

Surgery Branch, National Cancer Institute, National Institutes of Health, Bethesda, Maryland 20205

A major limitation to the development of successful adoptive immunotherapy for the treatment of cancer has been the development of techniques
to provide sufficiently large numbers of lymphoid cells with appropriate
specific antitumor reactivity (13). The development of techniques for the
long term expansion of T-lymphoid cells to large numbers in vitro as well
as the development of methods for growing large numbers of lymphoid cells
from single cloned starting cells have provided potential methods for
overcoming these limitations (3,8-12).

We and others have demonstrated that lymphoid cells expanded in vitro
in T-cell growth factor (TCGF) maintain specific cytotoxic reactivity
after prolonged growth and that single reactive cells can be cloned into
large populations with maintenance of cytotoxic specificity (3,5,9,11,
12). The large numbers of lymphoid cells that can be generated in vitro
are illustrated by the data in Table 1 which presents the growth rate of
a specific culture of murine splenocytes. Beginning with 10^4 lymphoid
cells, over 26 kilograms of cells could be generated in less than 2
months if all of the cells resulting from the exponential growth of
these cultures were saved.

TABLE 1. Growth of cells in TCGF

Days in Culture	Days to Split to 10^4/Well[a]	Cell Increase[b] (from 10^4/Well Split)	Total Potential Cell number[c]
		no.	
8	8	1.9×10^5	1.9×10^5
13	5	1.2×10^5	2.3×10^6
17	4	1.8×10^4	4.1×10^7
21	4	7.5×10^4	3.1×10^8
25	4	1.2×10^5	3.7×10^9
30	5	1.1×10^5	4.1×10^{10}
34	4	2×10^4	8.1×10^{10}
38	4	3.6×10^4	2.9×10^{11}
42	4	6.2×10^4	1.8×10^{12}
47	5	1.2×10^4	2.2×10^{12}
51	4	1.2×10^5	2.6×10^{13}

[a]Cells always cut-back to 10^4 cells/well into fresh medium and growth
medium.
[b]10^4 cells/well seeded in culture.
[c]if all cells were saved.

Though cells expanded in TCGF maintained specific cytotoxic reactivity, we have previously demonstrated that these cells traffic in an abnormal fashion when they are reinjected into the intact mouse (4). An unusually large number of cells distribute initially to the lung with most cells ultimately distributing to the liver by 24 hours after injection. This abnormal pattern of cell distribution has led to concerns that these cells might not function appropriately in vivo and thus be ineffective in mediating the rejection of tumors.

We have attempted to develop models for studying the in vivo effects of cells grown and expanded in TCGF. In this review we will discuss studies of the ability of cytotoxic lymphoid cells grown in TCGF to mediate the accelerated rejection of allogeneic skin grafts and to cure C57BL/6 mice with a disseminated syngeneic lymphoma. Also discussed are our attempts to develop specific cytotoxic cells reactive with chemically induced murine tumors and spontaneous human tumors in an effort to develop populations of lymphoid cells that may be effective in the adoptive immunotherapy of spontaneous human tumors.

LYMPHOID CELLS EXPANDED IN T-CELL GROWTH FACTOR CAN

MEDIATE THE ACCELERATED REJECTION OF ALLOGENEIC SKIN GRAFTS

To study the ability of lymphoid cells expanded in TCGF to mediate the rejection of allogeneic skin grafts we have used the skin allograft assay described by Sugarbaker et al. (17). Skin grafts from B10·BR mice were placed on recipient B6AF1 mice. These allogeneic skin grafts are routinely rejected at 12-14 days, though the adoptive transfer of in vivo sensitized cells can accelerate the graft rejection to 7-9 days. We have utilized this system to test the ability of in vitro sensitized B6AF1 anti-B10·BR lymphocytes expanded in TCGF to mediate the accelerated rejection of these allogeneic skin grafts (16). A typical experiment is shown in Figure 1 taken from the work of Rosenstein, et al. in our laboratory (16). As can be seen, 3×10^7 specifically sensitized lymphoid cells expanded in TCGF can mediate the accelerated rejection of this allogeneic graft. Irradiation of these cells abrogates their effect implying that some proliferation of these adoptively transferred cells is necessary in vivo to exert their immunologic effects. Rosenstein, et al. have further shown that the accelerated rejection of allogeneic grafts is immunologically specific and that non-immunized cells grown in TCGF or cells immunized against irrelevant antigens and grown in TCGF are not capable of accelerating this graft rejection (16).

ADOPTIVE TRANSFER OF SPECIFICALLY SENSITIZED CELLS GROWN

IN T-CELL GROWTH FACTOR CAN CURE MICE OF THE SYNGENEIC FBL-3 LYMPHOMA

We next attempted to determine whether cells expanded in T-cell growth factor were capable of mediating rejection of a syngeneic tumor. For these studies we selected the model of Fefer and his co-workers who have demonstrated that the adoptive transfer of immune lymphoid cells given in conjunction with cyclophosphamide are capable of curing

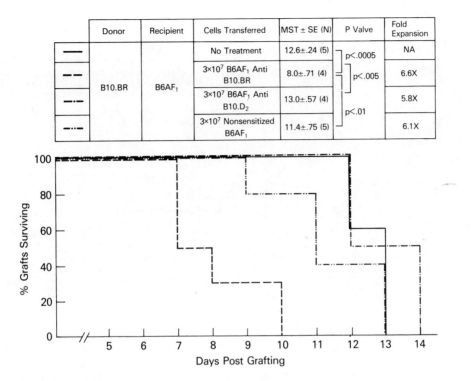

	Donor	Recipient	Cells Transferred	MST ± SE (N)	P Valve	Fold Expansion
——			No Treatment	12.6±.24 (5)	p<.0005	NA
– –	B10.BR	B6AF₁	3×10⁷ B6AF₁ Anti B10.BR	8.0±.71 (4)	p<.005	6.6X
—·—			3×10⁷ B6AF₁ Anti B10.D₂	13.0±.57 (4)	p<.01	5.8X
—··—			3×10⁷ Nonsensitized B6AF₁	11.4±.75 (5)		6.1X

FIG. 1. Specificity of the acceleration of skin allograft rejection after the adoptive transfer of nonsensitized B6AF1 lymphocytes or B6AF1 lymphocytes sensitized to the relevant B10·BR or irrelevant B10·02 allo-antigen and subsequently expanded in LF-TCGF. Only the specifically sensitized lymphoid cells expanded in LF-TCGF were capable of accelerating skin graft rejection.

mice with the disseminated FBL-3 lymphoma (2). In our preliminary studies Eberlein, et al. confirmed that in vivo sensitized as well as in vitro boosted cells were capable of curing mice with disseminated FBL-3 lymphoma (1). Mice were treated with cyclophosphamide intraperitoneally followed 5 hours later with immune cells 5 days after the intraperitoneal injection of the FBL-3 tumor. Using this model Eberlein, et al. then attempted to treat mice with disseminated lymphoma with immune cells grown in TCGF (1). For these studies mice were immunized by two intraperitoneal injections with irradiated FBL-3 cells. Spleens from these mice were then boosted in vitro with the FBL-3 tumor and then expanded for up to 2-1/2 months in TCGF. These cells were then utilized in adoptive transfer experiments and were given to mice in conjunction with cyclophosphamide 5 days after intraperitoneal injection of FBL-3 tumor. As can be seen in Figure 2, specifically sensitized lymphoid cells expanded in TCGF were capable of significantly improving the survival of mice with disseminated FBL-3 lymphoma compared to treatment of mice with either cytoxan alone or cytoxan plus nonimmunized cells expanded in TCGF (1).

Eberlein, et al. have further been able to demonstrate that cytotoxic cells cloned from individual starting cells can be isolated and grown for long periods in TCGF with maintenance of high levels of specific cytotoxic reactivity (1). These clones are now being tested for their ability to prolong the survival of mice with disseminated FBL-3 lymphoma.

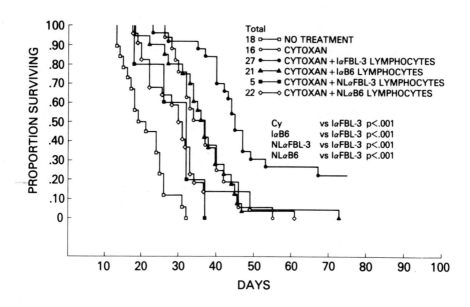

FIG. 2. Survival of mice with disseminated syngeneic FBL-3 lymphoma treated with <u>in vitro</u> sensitized cells expanded up to 10-fold in LF-TCGF for 6 days. Treatment with immune lymphocytes resensitized to FBL-3 tumor and then expanded in LF-TCGF conferred significant survival benefit when compared to treatment with cytoxan alone, cytoxan plus immune lymphocytes sensitized to normal C57BL/6 stimulators and then expanded in LF-TCGF or cytoxan plus non-immune lymphocytes sensitized to normal stimulators or FBL-3 tumor and then expanded in LF-TCGF.

THE GENERATION OF HUMAN LYMPHOID CELLS CYTOTOXIC FOR FRESH

AUTOLOGOUS HUMAN TUMOR

The results described above demonstrate that lymphoid cells expanded in TCGF are capable of mediating immunologic effects in vivo and have provided a strong stimulus to develop human cells cytotoxic for autologous human tumor that can be expanded to large numbers for use in the adoptive immunotherapy of human tumors. Three methods have been developed in our laboratory for generating human lymphoid cells cytotoxic to autologous fresh tumor target cells in 4 hour chromium release cytotoxicity assays (6,7,14). The three methods we have studied for generating these human cytotoxic lymphoid cells are presented in Table 2. Human lymphoid cells cytotoxic for fresh autologous tumor can be generated by growth of peripheral blood lymphoid cells in TCGF (6), by lectin activation of peripheral blood lymphoid cells (7), and by allosensitization of peripheral blood lymphoid cells to a pool of allogeneic stimulator lymphoid cells (14).

TABLE 2. Methods for Generating Human Peripheral Blood Lymphoid

Cells Lytic for Fresh Autologous Human Tumor Cells*

1. Growth in TCGF or lectin-free TCGF.

2. In vitro sensitization to a pool of allogeneic donor lymphocytes.

3. Activation by T-cell mitogens.

*Measured in a 4-hour ^{51}Cr-release assay in vitro.

Growth of autologous lymphoid cells in T-cell growth factor

generates cells cytotoxic to fresh autologous human tumor

In earlier studies Yron, et al. in our laboratory, demonstrated that
the growth of murine splenocytes in TCGF or lectin-free TCGF led to the
generation of cytotoxic reactivity directed against fresh autologous
murine sarcoma cells (18). Lotze et al. (6) and Grimm et al. (unpublished observations) in our laboratory, extended these findings to demonstrate that the growth in TCGF of peripheral blood lymphoid cells from
the human resulted in the generation of cytotoxic cells lytic to fresh
autologous human tumor (see Fig. 3) (6). Human peripheral lymphoid cells
expanded in TCGF or lectin-free TCGF are capable of lysing fresh target
cells that themselves have never been exposed to culture or any xenogeneic serum. These cytotoxic cells are capable of killing fresh autologous tumor but not fresh autologous lymphoid cells (6). The lytic capacity of these cells is not limited to tumor targets since autologous
cultured normal fibroblasts, as well as autologous cultured tumor, are
killed. Peripheral lymphoid cells expanded in TCGF appear to be capable
of killing virtually any cultured target cell. To the degree to which
it has been checked, however, the lysis of fresh target cells is limited
to tumor cells. The lysis of fresh autologous tumor extends to lysis of
allogeneic tumor but not to the killing of allogeneic fresh lymphoid
cells. This lysis appeared to be generated after only three days of
culture in TCGF or lectin-free TCGF (Grimm et al., unpublished data).

Activation of peripheral lymphoid cells by lectin generates cells

cytotoxic for fresh autologous tumor

Mazumder et al. in our laboratory, has studied the ability of human
peripheral lymphoid cells activated by a variety of lectins to lyse fresh
autologous tumor and normal target cells (7). Mazumder et al. have demonstrated that activation of lymphoid cells by T-cell mitogens, such as
phytohemagluttinin or conconavalin A can give rise to lymphoid cells
cytotoxic for fresh autologous tumor (Fig. 4). These lymphoid cells
are not lytic for fresh autologous lymphoid cells or for fresh autologous
Con-A induced lymphoblasts despite the equal lysability of each of these
three target cell populations (7). These lytic cells are generated
within two days and lose much of their lysis by five days after culture.
The generation of these cells is dependent on the presence of adherent
cells though the lytic cells themselves are not adherent. Irradiation

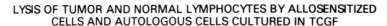

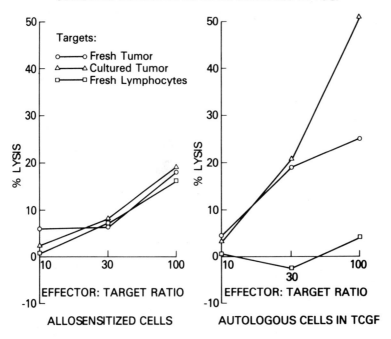

FIG. 3: (Right panel) Lysis of autologous fresh tumor, cultured tumor, and fresh peripheral blood lymphocytes by autologous lymphocytes cultured in T-cell growth factor as measured in the 4-hour chromium release assay. Fresh and cultured tumor are lysed but fresh autologous lymphocyte targets are not lysed. (Left panel) A normal individual was sensitized in vitro to the lymphocytes of the cancer patient. These allosensitized lymphocytes were used as effector cells against fresh tumor, cultured tumor, and fresh lymphocyte target cells from the patient. All three of these targets were equally lysable when used as targets for these allosensitized cells.

of these peripheral lymphoid cells prior to lectin activation does not inhibit the appearance of cells lytic for fresh autologous tumor. We have recently begun a phase I clinical trial to study the effects of these lectin activated cells when administered intravenously to patients with cancer.

Sensitization to a pool of allogeneic lymphoid cell generates

lymphocytes cytotoxic for fresh autologous human tumor

Zarling et al. have previously demonstrated that pool sensitization of human peripheral lymphoid cells is capable of generating cells cytotoxic for fresh autologous leukemic cells (19). We have extended these ob-

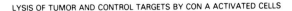

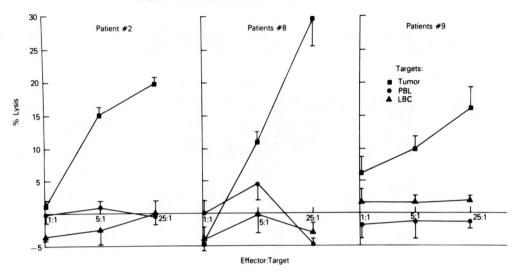

FIG. 4: Lysis of fresh autologous tumor, peripheral blood lymphocytes, and Con-A induced lymphoblasts by Con-A activated cells from
three different cancer patients as measured in a 4-hour chromium release assay. In each case, only fresh autologous tumor was lysed
and not autologous peripheral blood lymphocytes or lymphoblasts.

servations to a variety of fresh human solid tumors (14). Strausser et al.,
in our laboratory, has demonstrated that pool sensitization of human
peripheral blood lymphoid cells generates cells cytotoxic for fresh
autologous human target cells but not for autologous fresh lymphocytes
or fresh Con-A lymphoblast target cells. Sensitization to a single
allogeneic donor also often gives rise to cells cytotoxic for fresh
autologous tumor though most often this lysis is less potent than when a
pool of allogeneic stimulator cells are used (see Fig. 5)(14).

The three methods that we have described (see Table 2) for generating cytotoxic cells directed against fresh autologous tumor targets are
currently under active investigation. The nature of the effector cell
in this cytotoxicity and the nature of the target antigen recognized by
these cytotoxic cells are not yet known. Our observations suggest that
activation of peripheral lymphoid cells in the human is capable of
giving rise to cells cytotoxic for cell surface components on fresh
human tumors as well as a variety of cultured cell lines. It is likely
that several different forms of lysis are involved and we are currently
attempting to separate cell subpopulations with different lytic specificities. It should be noted that neither of these three techniques
generates cytotoxic cells specific for only the fresh autologous tumor
targets. We are also continuing studies of in vitro sensitization and
cloning, analogous to our studies in the mouse, to attempt to generate
appropriate lymphoid cell lines specifically cytotoxic to tumor associated antigens present on human tumor target cells.

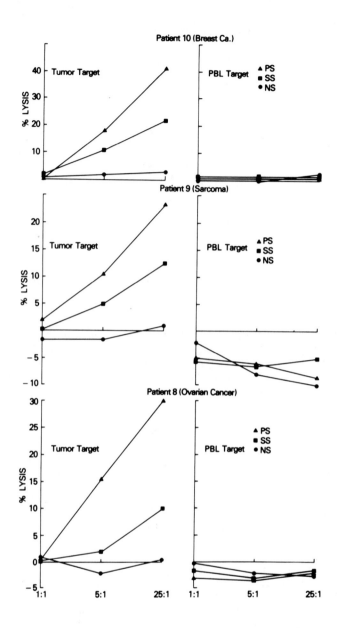

FIG. 5: Lysis of autologous fresh tumor and autologous fresh peripheral blood lymphocytes as measured in a 4-hour chromium release assay. The effector cells in these experiments resulted from incubation of the cancer patient's lymphocytes alone (NS), in a mixed leukocyte culture with a single donor stimulator cell (SS), or with a pool of multiple allogeneic donor stimulator cells (PS). In each case autologous fresh tumor was lysed by pool sensitized cells and less well by single sensitized cells. Incubation of lymphocytes alone did not result in lysis of the fresh autologous tumor. In no case were fresh peripheral blood lymphocytes lysed.

It is not known whether these nonspecifically activated cells will be useful in adoptive immunotherapy though we have begun initial phase I clinical trials of the adoptive transfer of lectin activated cells in humans with disseminated cancer.

IN VIVO TRAFFIC PATTERN OF AUTOLOGOUS HUMAN CELLS EXPANDED IN

T-CELL GROWTH FACTOR

Because of our interest in the use of cells expanded in TCGF for the adoptive immunotherapy of human tumors, Lotze et al., in our laboratory, has studied the in vivo distribution of cells expanded in TCGF when they are reinjected into the human (4). The pattern of distribution of human cells expanded in TCGF when reinjected intravenously into the human has been described (4). Human lymphoid cells expanded in TCGF traffic initially to the lung. Approximately 50% of the cells are trapped in the lung for several hours and then slowly clear from the lungs and distribute to both the liver and the spleen. Significant numbers of cells are retained in the spleen and liver for up to 10 days following cell injection. These traffic patterns appear similar to that in the in the mouse (4).

The studies reported in this paper demonstrate that lymphoid cells expanded in TCGF are capable of mediating tissue rejection when injected in vivo and provide some encouragement for the hope that these cells may ultimately play a role in the immunotherapy of tumors in man.

REFERENCES

1. Eberlein, T., Rosenstein, M., Spiess, P., and Rosenberg, S.A. (1981): J. Immunol., submitted.

2. Fefer, A., Einstein, A.B., Jr., Cheever, M.A., and Berenson, J.R. (1976): Ann. N.Y. Acad. Sci. 276:573.

3. Gillis, S. and Smith, K.A. (1977): Nature 268:154.

4. Lotze, M.T.,Line, B.R., Mathisen, D.J., and Rosenberg, S.A. (1980): J. Immunol. 125:1487.

5. Lotze, M.T., Strausser, J.L. and Rosenberg, S.A. (1980): J. Immunol. 124:2972.

6. Lotze, M.T., Grimm, E.A., Mazumder, A.M., Strausser, J.L. and Rosenberg, S.A. (1981): Cancer Res. (accepted for publication).

7. Mazumder, A.M., Grimm, E.A., Zhang, H.Z. and Rosenberg, S.A. (1980): J. Immunol., submitted.

8. Morgan, D.A., Ruscetti, F.W., and Gallo, R. (1976): Science 193:1007.

9. Rosenberg, S.A., Schwarz, S., and Spiess, P.J. (1978): J. Immunol. 121:1951.

10. Rosenberg, S.A., Schwarz, S., Spiess, P.J. and Brown, J.M. (1980): J. Immunol. 33:337.

11. Rosenberg, S.A., Spiess, P.J. and Schwarz, S. (1978): J. Immunol. 121:1946.

12. Rosenberg, S.A., Spiess, P.J. and Schwarz, S. (1980): Cell. Immunol. 54:293.

13. Rosenberg, S.A. and Terry, W. (1977): In: Adv. in Cancer Res., pp. 323-388. Academic Press, Inc., New York, N.Y.

14. Strausser, J.L., Mazumder, A.M., Grimm, E.A., Lotze, M.T. and Rosenberg, S.A. (1981): J. Immunol. 127:266.

15. Strausser, J.L. and Rosenberg,S.A. (1978): J. Immunol. 121: 1491.

16. Rosenstein, M., Eberlein, T., Kemeny, M.M., Sugarbaker, P.H. and Rosenberg, S.A. (1981): J. Immunol., in press.

17. Sugarbaker,P.H. and Chang, A.E. (1979): J. Immunol. Meth. 31:167.

18. Yron, I., Wood, T.A., Spiess, P. and Rosenberg, S.A. (1980): J. Immunol. 125:238.

19. Zarling, J.M., Robins, H.I., Raich, P.C., Bach, F.H., and Bach, M.L. (1978): Nature 274:269.

AUDIENCE DISCUSSION

Dr. Gillis: I missed the point of Con A or PHA activation to generate CTL against autologous fresh tumor. You showed that PBL from tumor-bearing patients when grown in lectin-free TCGF gave rise to these cells.

Dr. Rosenberg: There are three techniques to generate cytotoxic cells in the human that will kill fresh tumor cells. These are growth of PBL in T cell growth factor, pool sensitization and lectin activation. Thus, if one exposes lymphoid cells to lectin for two days, a cell is generated that is cytotoxic against autologous tumor. In our first clinical trial, we're using lectin-activated cells.

Dr. Gillis: Is there T cell growth factor produced during lectin activation?

Dr. Rosenberg: Yes. The conditions for activation are very similar to those we use to generate T cell growth factor.

Dr. Bach: Regarding reactivation with the TCGF, I suggest that perhaps this is what has been seen with memory cells generated both in vitro and in vivo; once they have been exposed to the antigen, what the cytotoxic cells really need for reactivation is signal II or "help". Help will reactivate them much better than exposure to antigen. This is true even at the clonal level. Do you have experiments where you have "cloned" the cloid? Have you subcloned or is there a possibility you are dealing with both types? Have you checked whether those are NK cells?

Dr. Rosenberg: I think your invention of the word "cloid" is ideal; it has already achieved common usage.

Dr. Bach: Please credit Miriam Segall with it.

Dr. Rosenberg: These are cloids. The cells have been recloned but have not yet been used in vivo. Our cloids have about 80% likelihood of having been derived from a single cell, but it's conceivable that there were two cells in those original cultures. The cells do not appear to be NK. They are Lyt 1^-2^+. These cells kill fresh tumor cells whereas NK cells don't kill fresh tumor cells to these levels.

Dr. Nabholz: Why do you want to derive clones for immunotherapy in humans when already you seem to have a very efficient way to enrich for the important cells without cloning?

Dr. Rosenberg: In the human I described the generation of cells that lyse 40-50 percent at effector-to-target ratio of 20 to 1. We can generate cells that are 100% cytotoxic at ratios of 0.1 to 1.0 by cloning reactive cells in the FBL-3 tumor system. I hope that by cloning we can find far more efficient lytic cells in the human.

Dr. Truitt: Can you or anyone tell me whether the killing efficiency of cells is increased following culture with IL 2? Is there an increase in the number of target cells that can be killed per individual cytotoxic cell?

Dr. Rosenberg: We have not done those experiments. We have demonstrated that under equivalent culture conditions one can enhance the number of cytotoxic cells generated by performing those sensitizations in lectin-free TCGF.

Dr. Greenberg: I'd like to first clarify some of the data we presented yesterday. Our results do not necessarily imply that an Lyt-1 cell is the effector cell responsible for eradicating established tumor, but rather that the host is relatively deficient in this cell population, and adoptive transfer of Lyt 1 cells promotes and/or mediates eventual tumor lysis. However, McKenzie has demonstrated that Lyt 1 cells are responsible for rejection of allogeneic skin grafts, presumably by DTH. Can you show that cloning alloreactive CTL can change the mechanism by which skin grafts are rejected? Have you looked at cloned alloreactive cells in that setting?

Dr. Rosenberg: Those experiments are in progress in both the allograft rejection assay and the FBL-3 tumor model.

Dr. Herberman: Regarding the Con A stimulated cells, do you perform the assay in the presence of Con A also or isn't that needed?

Dr. Rosenberg: Con A is thoroughly washed from the culture and all the assays are done in the absence of Con A. In fact, adding Con A to the culture does not add to the lysis. With respect to the identification of these cells as NK, although we don't know what cells are mediating the lysis, the cells lyse autologous normal cultured cells and fresh autologous tumors -- two functions which have not been ascribed to NK cells.

Dr. Mitchell: Have you tested cells activated by either TCGF or by Con A against other fresh tumors? It wasn't one of your controls; you had autologous normal cells but not other tumors. Was it tumor specific?

Dr. Rosenberg: The cells grown in TCGF kill tumors from other individuals. Normal lymphoid cells from a nontumor-bearing individual will kill fresh tumors from cancer patients. However, as soon as one moves out of the autologous setting, polyclonal activation might lead to the generation of cytotoxic cells capable of recognizing alloantigen. But the answer to your question is yes, allogeneic tumors are killed.

[Unidentified]: What about histologically dissimilar tumors?

Dr. Rosenberg: They are killed.

The Potential Role of T Cells in Cancer Therapy,
edited by A. Fefer and A. Goldstein,
Raven Press, New York © 1982.

Antitumor Reactivity *In Vitro* and *In Vivo* of Mouse and Human Lymphoid Cells Cultured with T Cell Growth Factor

*†Eli Kedar, *Ronald B. Herberman, *Eliezer Gorelik,
**Benjamin Sredni, *Guy D. Bonnard, and *Nicanor Navarro

*Laboratory of Immunodiagnosis, National Cancer Institute, and **Laboratory of Immunology, National Institute of Allergy and Infectious Diseases, National Institutes of Health, Bethesda, Maryland 20205; †Hadassah Medical School, Jerusalem, Israel*

The discovery of T cell growth factor (TCGF, or interleukin-2) and its use for in vitro cultivation of T cells (30) have provided the opportunity to produce large numbers of lymphoid cells with selected immunological reactivity. Over the past 4 years several groups have been successful in establishing lines and monoclonal cultures of specifically sensitized cytotoxic T lymphoid cells of mouse and human origin (10,26,27,32,39,42, 52). Such cells can be propagated in continuous cultures for periods ranging from several weeks up to several years, with some retention of the original cytotoxic capacity.

Since response to TCGF appeared dependent on T cell activation with consequent expression of cell surface receptors for the growth factor (3,43), it seemed likely that addition of TCGF to cultures of sensitized T cells plus the specific antigen would select for the immune T cells and promote their expansion. This has raised the obvious possibility of using TCGF for the selective growth in vitro of T cells sensitized to tumor associated antigens. Indeed, addition of TCGF to cocultures of tumor-immune T cells with tumor cells has led to the propagation of T cells with cytotoxic reactivity against tumor antigens (6,11,28) and such cultured cells have been shown to be capable, under some conditions, to retard or completely inhibit the in vivo growth of mouse tumors bearing the appropriate antigens. Since tumor-bearing individuals might be expected to have T cells sensitized in vivo to tumor associated antigens, it was expected that such cells could be selectively expanded with TCGF, without the need for further in vitro stimulation. In this respect, it has been reported recently that murine and human lymphocytes harvested from tumor-bearing hosts and propagated in TCGF frequently display a high level of cytotoxic reactivity against various fresh and cultured tumor cells (2, 37,51) including freshly harvested autochthonous tumor cells (24,50,52).

However, it has also been found that in vitro incubation of lymphoid cells from normal individuals with TCGF could also lead to the propagation of cultured lymphoid cells (CLC) with substantial cytotoxic reactivity against various tumor cells (7,31,36) and that such CLC may possess characteristics of NK cells rather than specifically immune T cells. Such observations indicate the need to carefully analyze the characteristics of CLC with anti-tumor reactivity and to determine the specificity of their cytotoxicity.

In the present study, we have initiated CLC from both tumor-bearing and normal mice and humans. Their characteristics have been examined and their cytotoxic reactivity assessed against a variety of lymphoid and solid tumor cells and also against various normal target cells. The results indicate that CLC derived from tumor-bearing and normal individuals have very similar features and that the cytotoxic cells appear to be mainly NK cells, and possibly other natural effector cells or in vitro activated lymphoid cells. Although the cytotoxicity of these CLC has not been restricted to a particular type of tumor cell, the ability to grow large numbers of cells with potent in vitro reactivity suggests that such an approach might in the future be applied for immunotherapy of experimental and human tumors. In support of this possibility, we have found that mouse and human CLC have some in vivo anti-tumor activity.

MATERIALS AND METHODS

Preparation of TCGF-Containing Medium (TCGF-M)

The method described by Gillis et al (9) and by Rosenberg et al (40) was employed with some modifications for preparation of TCGF-M for culturing of mouse lymphoid cells. Spleen cells were obtained from 3-6-month-old W/Fu rats, or from BALB/c mice, and single cell suspensions (4-7 x 10^6/ml) were incubated with 5 µg/ml concanavalin A (Con A) for 36-48 h at 37°C. The culture fluid was designated C-TCGF-M. In some experiments, Con A was depleted from the C-TCGF-M by fractional $(NH_4)_2SO_4$ precipitation or by two absorptions with Sephadex G-100. With both preparations, residual mitogen was neutralized by adding 5-10 mg/ml of α-methyl-D-mannoside. These preparations were designated mitogen-depleted TCGF-M (MD-TCGF-M).

Human TCGF-containing medium was obtained from Associated Biomedics System Inc., Buffalo, NY. It was prepared by stimulating pooled human PBL (1 x 10^6/ml) for 2-3 days with 1% PHA-M (4). Depletion of PHA from the crude TCGF (C-TCGF-M) preparations was performed by 3 consecutive absorptions with packed chicken erythrocytes and this prepartion was designated mitogen-depleted TCGF-M (MD-TCGF-M).

The TCGF preparations were tested for their ability to support growth of CLC lines, whose growth is strictly dependent on TCGF, by measuring ^{3}H-thymidine incorporation into CLC during a 48 h assay. MD-TCGF-M was shown to have 95-98% of lectin removed, as assessed by the ^{3}H-thymidine assay with fresh, normal lymphocytes, whereas at least 60-75% of the original lymphoproliferative activity for CLC was retained.

Establishment of CLC.

Cultures of mouse spleen cells were initiated with 2-5 x 10^5 cells/ml and C-TCGF or with 5-10 x 10^5/ml and MD-TCGF and then split, after a thorough pipetting (to detach adherent cells), to 1 x 10^5/ml every 3-4 days, when cell concentration reached 4-6 x 10^5/ml. Before assaying in the cytotoxicity assays, effector CLC were spun down, incubated for 30 min at 37°C with medium containing 10 mg/ml α-methyl-D-mannoside, and then washed twice with culture medium.

For culturing of human lymphoid cells, nylon-wool column nonadherent peripheral blood mononuclear leukocytes (PBL) or Percoll-fractionated

(47,48) cells were cultured for 3-6 weeks with 10-15% v/v C-TCGF-M or MD-TCGF-M. Before assaying the cytotoxic activity of the CLC, cells were washed twice, rested overnight in RPMI 1640 with 15% AB serum and washed again.

Establishment of CLC clones. Cloning of mouse CLC that were adapted to grow in C-TCGF-M for 2-3 months was performed by the limiting dilution or the soft agar techniques. In the first, cells were diluted in 25% C-TCGF-M in complete RPMI 1640 medium to 2.5, 5 and 10 cells/ml and 0.1 ml aliquots were distributed into U-shaped 96-well microtitration plates. The plates were incubated at 36°C and feeding with 50% C-TCGF-M, in 0.05 ml, was done on days 5 and 10. Clones consisting of approximately 100-1000 cells each were picked on days 10-15, transferred to 24-well Costar plates and fed with 1 ml complete PRMI 1640 medium containing 25% C-TCGF-M. Upon further growth, clones were transferred to 25 cm^2 Falcon flasks (in 10 ml) and then to larger flasks. In the second technique cells were cloned in a two-layer soft agar system in 3 cm petri dishes as described previously (45).

The human clone designated Sredni-1 was originated from a normal blood donor. T cells were isolated by rosetting with sheep erythrocytes, the cells were stimulated for 48 h with 0.0125% v/v PHA-M and seeded in PHA-containing agar (44). Colonies were picked and recloned at 200 cells per 35 mm petri dish in agar containing human TCGF. One growing clone ($i1$) was maintained for approximately 4 months using C-TCGF-M, without feeder cells. Clones Navarro-5 and Navarro-9 were derived from PBL of a normal blood donor. The cells were cloned in 96-well microplates by limiting dilutions using 1 cell per well, in the presence of irradiated (3000 rads) allogeneic PBL (1 x 10^5 per well). Clones were supplemented every 5-7 days with fresh medium and C-TCGF-M and then expanded for an additional 4 months without feeder cells.

RESULTS

Growth capacity of mouse lymphoid cells in TCGF-containing media.

Lymphoid cells obtained from the spleens of normal mice and of mice bearing the M-109 transplantable lung carcinoma were cultured in the presence of crude or mitogen-depleted TCGF of mouse and rat origin (17). Rat TCGF was superior to mouse TCGF for all types of cells, especially when cells were cultivated in large culture flasks (approximately 1000-fold increase in cell number by day 15 with rat factor, compared to about 200-fold with mouse factor). In cultures initiated and maintained with MD-TCGF-M, the majority of the cells died during the first week; subsequently the few remaining viable cells proliferated almost to the same extent as did cells maintained in C-TCGF-M. Cultures of splenocytes from nude mice and from mice with disseminated carcinoma showed a rather slow growth rate during the first 7-10 days of culture, but thereafter growth was similar to that of cultures originated from normal splenocytes. In other preliminary experiments, we compared the growth rate, in rat C-TCGF-M, of spleen, thymus, peripheral blood, peritoneal exudate, and bone marrow cells of C57BL/6 and BALB/c mice. It was found that lymphoid cells of spleen, peripheral blood, and peritoneal exudate had a similar growth rate during the period studied (2-3 months), whereas thymocytes showed a slightly lower proliferative capacity. In contrast, only a small minority of the bone marrow cells survived after the first week; the remaining cells proliferated at a much lower rate, and cultures died after 4-6 weeks.

In the course of the present studies, over 20 culture lines of splenocytes from various strains of mice were initiated and maintained for periods of 3-12 months. Under the conditions employed, cultures maintained in C-TCGF-M expanded at a rate of 10^5-10^6-fold per month with a generation time of 15-24 h.

Cytotoxic activity of mouse CLC.
The results of a large number of experiments performed with a wide range of normal and tumor target cells are summarized in Table 1. Using fresh noncultured splenocytes from normal or tumor-bearing mice, only the classical NK-sensitive lymphoma cells (YAC-1, RLδ1) were killed to an appreciable extent, whereas all the other lymphoid and solid tumor cells were resistant to lysis.

TABLE 1. Cytotoxic activity of BALB/c mouse CLC

Target Cells	% cytotoxicity (effector:target ratio usually 10:1)	
	6 h	18 h
Mouse Tumors		
YAC-1	60	88
RLδ1	36	81
M109	60	92
MT	17	41
3LL	15	31
EL4	41	80
Meth 27A	14	24
Rat Tumors		
G1	7	14
(C58NT)D	22	39
Human Tumors		
K562	10	19
SK-MES-1	6	16
Normal mouse cells		
BALB/c thymus	8	17
BALB/c peritoneal	7	14
BALB/c bone marrow	4	7
C3H lymphoblasts	14	48
BALB/c lymphoblasts	7	14
BALB/c spleen	1	5
ADCC		
Antibody-coated G1	16	31

All the cultures from either tumor-bearing or normal mice, maintained by the periodic addition of TCGF, showed strong cytotoxic activity against most of the tumor target cells tested: fresh and cultured, syngeneic and allogeneic, lymphoid and solid, NK-sensitive and NK-resistant. Cultured M109 and MT (mammary tumor) were slightly more sensitive to killing, in general, than freshly harvested transplanted M109 or primary spontaneous MT. With most of the CLC, maximum cytotoxic activity was observed after 2-3 weeks in culture. The magnitude of the cytotoxicity against various targets thereafter did not change appreciably during the first 3-4 months of culture, and a strong cytotoxic effect was noticed even at an effector/target ratio of 1/1 (data not shown). Later on, however, some lines showed a gradual diminution in cytotoxicity, particularly against the NK-insensitive solid tumor cells. CLC maintained with MD-TCGF-M and with C-TCGF-M, and those obtained from either normal or tumor-bearing mice showed a similar pattern and magnitude of cytotoxicity against most targets tested. Preliminary experiments have indicated that CLC originating from spleen, peripheral blood, and peritoneal exudate all killed a wide range of lymphoid and solid tumor targets. In contrast, TCGF-cultured bone marrow cells were mainly effective against NK-sensitive lymphoma target cells and cultured thymocytes were more cytolytic to NK-resistant solid tumor cells.

Low but significant cytotoxicity by CLC was demonstrated with xenogeneic rat and human cultured tumor cells, which are rather resistant to lysis by fresh NK effector cells. A considerable level of cytotoxicity was also found against some normal murine lymphoid target cells, especially when the ^{51}Cr assay was extended to 16-18 h. Con A-induced allogeneic lymphoblasts were more susceptible than syngeneic lymphoblasts, and among the freshly harvested normal lymphoid cells, thymus cells and adherent peritoneal exudate cells were generally more sensitive than the other cell types and spleen cells were quite resistant.

Another function associated with NK cells is ADCC activity (23,34,47). As part of the characterization of the CLC, it was therefore of interest to evaluate their ADCC activity. The data at the bottom of Table 1 show that CLC can function as effector cells in an ADCC system, against antibody-coated target cells, in addition to their ability to lyse target cells directly. The ADCC activity, but not the direct cytotoxicity, could be blocked almost completely when protein A [previously shown to selectively inhibit ADCC (15)] was added to the assay.

Surface markers of the mouse CLC. To further characterize our cultured cells, we assessed several surface markers which have been associated with either cytotoxic T lymphocytes or NK cells. Virtually all BALB/c CLC were Thy 1.2$^+$ and asialo GM1$^+$, as indicated by cell killing with specific antisera and complement and by the parallel loss in cytotoxic activity. A considerable portion of the cells expressed Lyt 2, a smaller proportion expressed Lyt 1, and a portion of the effector cells appeared to possess neither of these markers. Killing of CLC with anti-Thy 1.2 and complement required higher amounts of these reagents than those needed to lyse fresh T cells from the spleen and thymus. Whereas 1/2000 and 1/12 dilutions of the antiserum and complement, respectively, were effective with the fresh T cells, 1/200 and 1/6 dilutions, respectively, were needed to lyse $\geq$ 80% of the CLC.

Clones of mouse CLC. The cytotoxicity of the CLC against a wide array of target cells could have been due to the maintenance in culture of a very broadly reactive effector cell or to the presence of multiple types of effector cells, each with more selective reactivity. To distinguish between these possibilities, a series of clones of CLC were obtained and tested for their cytotoxic reactivity (18). Most of the clones had cytotoxic reactivity and Table 2 summarizes the results obtained with some of the cytotoxic clones. The patterns of cytotoxicity could be categorized into two main types. Several clones (e.g. clones 11, 18, 39) had strong reactivity only against the highly NK-sensitive lymphoma target cells (YAC-1 and RLδ1) and relatively low reactivity against solid tumor targets. In contrast, other clones (e.g. clones 1, 8, and 22) had a broader range of reactivity, having strong effects against NK-resistant lymphomas (e.g. EL4) and solid tumor cells (e.g. MT and M109) as well as against YAC-1 and RL♂1. The two categories of clones were therefore designated CNK-L (cultured NK cells, lymphoma targets) and CNK-SL (solid as well as lymphoma targets). The CNK-SL clones also tended to have higher reactivity against xenogeneic tumor target cells, which are relatively resistant to mouse NK activity.

TABLE 2. Cytotoxic activity of clones of BALB/c mouse CLC

Targets	% cytotoxicity (E:T, 10:1; 18 h assay)					
	Cl 1[a]	Cl 8	Cl 22	Cl 11	Cl 18	Cl 39
YAC-1	86[b]	85	92	77	85	94
RL♂1	NT[b]	92	93	90	87	95
M109	53	74	76	33	23	22
MT	31	46	39	25	21	12
EL4	92	53	90	NT	29	28
G1	46	36	47	12	18	11
(C58NT)D	31	33	42	NT	27	23
K562	22	15	13	4	5	6
SK-MES-1	12	6	12	NT	8	4
BALB/c thymus	7	24	20	9	21	13
BALB/c peritoneal	22	28	20	10	21	23
BALB/c bone marrow	7	8	15	NT	10	16
C3H lymphoblasts	29	NT	15	NT	NT	NT
BALB/c lymphoblasts	14	NT	15	NT	NT	NT
BALB/c spleen	3	3	2	NT	8	7
ab-coated G-1	95	62	79	36	52	36

[a]Cloned by soft agar technique; others cloned by limiting dilution.
[b]Not tested.

In addition to their strong anti-tumor reactivity, the BALB/c clones also reacted against some normal syngeneic target cells. This anti-normal cytotoxic effect was more evident with 18 h cytotoxicity assays and when adherent peritoneal cells or thymocytes were employed as targets. Some of the clones (e.g. clones 22 and 39) also had appreciable reactivity against syngeneic bone marrow cells. In general, both types of clones had similar reactivity against these normal targets. In contrast, normal spleen cells were resistant to lysis by the cytotoxic clones. This pattern of reactivity against normal target cells is quite similar to that found with fresh NK cells (33). Two soft agar-derived clones (e.g. clone 1) also had substantial reactivity against Con A-induced lymphoblasts, preferentially against alloblasts. In contrast, some CNK-SL clones obtained by limiting dilution (e.g. clone 22) had similar reactivity against syngeneic and allogeneic lymphoblasts.

The above results of direct testing of the clones against a variety of target cells indicated a limited degree of heterogeneity among the clones, with some reacting strongly against a relatively narrow range of targets and others showing considerably broader reactivity against most transformed cell lines of mouse, rat and human origin and against several types of normal cells. It was of interest to determine whether the reactivity of a given clone against various target cells was due to common recognition structures or whether there might be discrete recognition sites. For this purpose, we used the cold target inhibition assay (14, 22), which has been generally shown to accurately reflect either sharing , or lack of identity, of specificities between labeled targets and inhibitor cells. The results strongly suggested that most of the clones had a heterogeneity of receptors for interaction with the various targets. This was particularly well indicated by the patterns obtained with YAC-1 and M109 target cells. In most cases, and regardless of the level of susceptibility of each target to lysis, the homologous target inhibited cytotoxicity substantially more than the other target.   In contrast, in tests with clone 1, it appeared that YAC-1, EL4 and P815 shared a common specificity, with generally good cross-inhibition as well as homologous inhibition.

One concern was whether some of the observed cytotoxicity might be lectin-induced, from residual Con A on the cells. However, the cytotoxic activity of the clones maintained in MD-TCGF-M was the same as that of clones carried in lectin-containing C-TCGF-M.   In addition, reactivity remained unchanged after extensive washings of the cells followed by a 16 h incubation at either 4° or $37^\circ C$ in TCGF-free medium, before testing in the ^{51}Cr assay.

The above experiments demonstrated that the clones of CLC have spontaneous cytotoxic activity and in some ways resemble NK, natural cytotoxic (NC) (5,46), or culture-activated killer (AK) cells (19). We therefore undertook experiments to examine the clones for some of the other functions associated with such effector cells. We found that all of the BALB/c clones examined could also function as effector cells in ADCC (Table 2) and that pretreatment of the cloned cells with mouse fibroblast interferon boosted the cytotoxic activity against all targets tested, especially against the G-11 human target cell, where the spontaneous cytotoxicity was low.   These data supported the possibility that the cytotoxic clones of CLC were NK cells. Furthermore, some clones could produce relatively high levels of interferon, as has been associated with NK cells (8,41,49).

The cloned CLC have also been extensively studied in regard to their phenotype and morphology (18). All of the clones studied were Thy 1.2^+, asialo $GM1^+$, surface Ig^-, nonadherent, nonphagocytic and had no detectable histamine. In addition, it appeared that the clones were $H-2^d+$, $NK2^+$, Qa $2,3^+$, $T200^+$ and possessed the receptor for peanut agglutinin. With regard to their Lyt phenotypes, the clones were more heterogeneous. Clone 1 was Lyt $1^-,2^-$ but most of the others were Lyt 2^+ and some appeared to express low amounts of Lyt 1 as well.   Some of the clones (e.g. clone 1) contained many large cytoplasmic vacuoles and lightly-staining azurophilic granules, whereas others (e.g. clone 39) were loaded with large, densely-staining azurophilic granules.   The presence of cytoplasmic azurophilic granules in the CLC provide another analogy to NK cells, which in the human and rat have been shown to be large granular lymphocytes (47).   There was no apparent correlation between surface phenotype or morphology and the pattern of cytotoxic reactivity by the clones.

Anti-tumor activity in vivo of mouse CLC. In light of the potent antitumor activity demonstrated by the CLC in vitro, it was interesting to determine whether they could also affect tumor growth in vivo.

In Winn neutralization assays, BALB/c CLC afforded partial protection against a syngeneic lymphoma (RL♂1) and carcinoma (M109) in BALB/c mice and against an allogeneic lymphoma (MBL-2) in C57BL/6 mice (Table 3). When sufficient CLC were given (i.e., at a ratio of CLC/tumor $\geq$ 30/1) a number of mice in the experimental groups remained tumor-free and, more

over, the remaining mice developed the tumor later and showed a longer
survival time than did the control mice.   C3H CLC at a ratio of 70/1
completely inhibited mammary tumor growth and mice remained tumor-free
for more than 4 months.   In contrast to CLC, fresh BALB/c splenocytes were
totally ineffective against M109.

TABLE 3.   Tumor neutralization (Winn) assays in vivo with mouse CLC

Tumor[a]	Source of CLC[b]	CLC/tumor ratio in inoculum	Median survival time (days)	Tumor-free survivors/total (day 120)
M109	none	-	36	0/8
	N. fresh	100/1	39	0/8
	T.B. MD-TCGF-M	100/1	>120	6/8
MBL-2	none	-	24	0/8
	T.B. C-TCGF-M	100/1	68	5/8
C3H mammary tumor	none	-	77	0/10
	T.B. C3H, C-TCGF-M	70/1	>120	10/10

[a] 1×10^5 tumor cells were injected s.c. in the corresponding syngeneic
normal mice.
[b] CLC were derived from normal (N) BALB/c mice, from M109 tumor-bearing
(T.B.) BALB/c mice and from mammary tumor-bearing C3H mice, using crude
(CTGF-M) or Con A-depleted (MD-TCGF-M) conditioned medium.

Systemic administration of CLC to mice with established disseminated
tumors showed at most a limited therapeutic effect, with the survival time
of mice that died of tumor approximately 20% greater after treatment of
mammary tumor-bearing mice treated with cyclophosphamide (day 7) plus CLC
(day 8, 1.5×10^7 cells i.v.) than that of mice treated with chemotherapy
alone.
To further assess the in vivo effects of CLC, we have performed some
studies of local adoptive transfer with a radioisotopic assay (12), which
allows serial measurement of elimination of radiolabeled tumor cells from
the local site of their transplantation.   Normal spleen cells of BALB/c
mice or CLC from M109-bearing mice were admixed with 2×10^5 of [^{125}I]-
iododeoxyuridine-labelled M109 tumor cells at a ratio of 30:1 and inoculated into the footpad of BALB/c mice (13).   One day following tumor cell
inoculation, the level of the radioactivity decreased by 44% in mice
inoculated with a mixture of tumor and normal spleen cells and by 31% in
the mice transplanted with tumor cells alone.   At the same time, 81-84% of
initial radioactivity was eliminated when M109 tumor cells were transplanted in association with cells cultured with either C-TCGF-M or MD-
TCGF-M.   Subsequently, the rate of tumor cell elimination from the footpads of these mice dramatically decreased and from the second to 14th day
following tumor cell transplantation, the slope of elimination of radioactivity from the footpads was similar in all experimental and control
BALB/c mice.   In parallel with the results in the radioactivity assay, a
significant retardation in tumor appearance was observed in BALB/c mice
inoculated into the footpad with M109 tumor cells admixed with CLC.
However, once visible tumors appeared, their rate of growth in these mice
was similar to that in control mice.   As a result of the delay in tumor

appearance, at 33 days following tumor transplantation, the mean size of tumors in control mice was 12.3 mm in comparison with 7.1 and 7.2 mm in the mice transplanted with tumor cells mixed with cells cultured in C-TCGF-M or MD-TCGF-M respectively.

These data suggested that the cytotoxic effects of cultured lymphoid cells against tumor cells were transient, lasting only approximately one day. The surviving tumor cells may then proliferate and develop into visible tumors, with the latent period inversely related to the number of tumor cells remaining after the phase of elimination. To obtain a more direct indication as to whether the more rapid loss of in vivo cytotoxic activity by cultured lymphoid cells was due to their limited survival in the footpad, we inoculated $[^{125}I]$-deoxyuridine-labelled CLC into the footpads of mice. By serially measuring the level of radioactivity in the inoculated footpads, it was found that more than 95% of radioactivity disappeared by 40 h. This rapid elimination could not be attributed to the labelling, since in the presence of TCGF, the labelled cells multiplied in vitro like nonradiolabelled cultured lymphoid cells. It seemed possible that the high rate of elimination of radiolabelled cultured cells from the footpad of mice was mediated by NK cells or other natural effector cells. However, the rate of radioisotope clearance was identical in mice with either high or low NK activity. Furthermore, using ^{51}Cr-labelled CLC as targets in the in vitro cytotoxic assay, we did not find any cytotoxic effect by normal spleen cells of BALB/c nude or CBA/J mice, even at an effector:target ratio of 200:1. In another experiment, 0.5 x 10^6 radiolabelled CLC were inoculated into the footpads of BALB/c mice in 15% C-TCGF-M. This group of mice received additional injections i.p. of 0.5 ml medium with 30% C-TCGF-M at 16 and 24 h following CLC transplantation. The rate of elimination from the footpads of mice inoculated with cultured lymphoid cells in the presence or absence of TCGF was identical. The dramatic decrease of radioactivity in the footpads of mice inocualted with radiolabelled CLC could be attributed mostly to their elimination rather than to their redistribution into different parts of the body.

Because of their cytotoxic activity in vitro against some normal target cells, experiments were also carried out to evaluate the effect of inoculation of large numbers of CLC into immunodepressed recipients. In those experiments, mice pretreated with 200 mg/kg of cyclophosphamide were injected intravenously with 15 x 10^6 syngeneic CLC once, or with 10 x 10^6 CLC twice 7 days apart. The treated mice did not show any clinical symptoms of graft-versus-host disease.

Human CLC growth characteristics. About 80% of cultures originated from normal PBL expanded 200-2500-fold (mean for all normal donors, 638), whereas only 37% of the cultures from advanced cancer patients' PBL showed similar growth capacity (mean for all patients, 322-fold increase), using C-TCGF-M and AB serum over a period of 21 days (16). Five out of 38 (13%) of the cultures from normal donors and 7/27 (26%) of the cultures from patients (5 with lung carcinoma and 2 with breast carcinoma) failed to expand > 20-fold. There was no direct correlation between the growth capacity of the individual cultures and their cytotoxic activity. The growth rate in cultures supplemented with FBS and those supplemented with pooled AB serum was similar. However, with both normals and patients, a greater increase in cell number was observed in most cultures fed with medium containing autologous serum or plasma than in AB serum-containing cultures. The majority of the cultures, regardless of the type of medium used, died when they reached 5-6 weeks.

The rate of growth in cultures in MD-TCGF-M was considerably lower, especially in the first week, than in cultures supplemented with C-TCGF. In fact, apparent cell proliferation in MD-TCGF-M was observed only after 5-8 days of culture.

Unfractionated PBL and nylon wool column-enriched T cells showed similar growth kinetics in C-TCGF and AB serum, with a generation time of about 30 h. In contrast, Percoll gradient-enriched large granular lymphocytes (LGL) (47) had a lower growth rate (generation time 50-60 h) than had Percoll-enriched T cells (generation time 30-40 h).

Cytotoxic activity of CLC derived from unseparated peripheral PBL. PBL from normal donors and cancer patients were maintained in culture with either C-TCGF-M or MD-TCGF-M in AB serum, autologous serum or FBS. Cytotoxic activity of all these cultures was tested in 6 h and 18 h ^{51}Cr release assays against various tumor and normal target cells (16). When cultured cells were tested repeatedly, maximum reactivity was reached by 1-2 weeks after culture initiation, and thereafter the pattern and magnitude of reactivity against various targets were quite stable. Similar levels of cytotoxicity were seen in assays performed in the presence of FBS or AB serum.

TABLE 4. Cytotoxic activity of human CLC

Targets	% cytotoxicity (effector:target ratio, 20:1)[a]	
	6 h	18 h
Human tumors		
K562[b]	47	68
G-11[b]	38	63
9812	20	44
HT-29	18	43
MCF-7	20	52
fresh autol. lung CA	14	32
fresh allog. lung CA	15	28
Normal human cells		
autol. lymphoblasts	5	20
allog. lymphoblasts	7	25
Mouse tumors		
YAC-1	4	9
RL♂1	6	15
M109	0	1

[a] Values represent means of results from C-TCGF-M-propagated CLC of 4-28 donors, with each tested 2-4 times.
[b] Target cells highly sensitive to fresh NK cells.

The levels of cytotoxic activity varied among the individual cultures and against various targets. However, similar patterns of results were obtained with all CLC, derived from either tumor patients or normal donors. Table 4 summarizes these results. Most sensitive to killing were K562 (myeloid leukemia) and the adherent tumor lines MCF7 and G-11 (derived from breast cancer). Fresh lung tumors of autologous or allogeneic origin were also susceptible to lysis by most of the CLC but they were less sensitive than the adherent tumor lines. Moreover in the 18 h assay, autologous and allogeneic Con A-stimulated PBL were considerably susceptible to lysis.

Despite the lower growth rate of CLC in MD-TCGF, most of these CLC tested demonstrated a stronger cytotoxic activity towards most of the targets than did CLC cultured in C-TCGF. The cytotoxic activity of CLC from normal donors or patients could be potentiated by pretreating them with human leukocyte interferon. A marked increase in cytotoxicity was observed against most of the tumor targets including fresh autologous and allogeneic lung tumor cells. In contrast, treatment of CLC with interferon resulted in unchanged or lower levels (in 3 out of 5 CLC tested) of cytotoxicity against Con A-induced lymphoblasts.

Cytotoxic activity of clonal populations and of CLC derived from PBL enriched or depleted of NK cells. Because of the broad range of target cell killing seen with the CLC, we were interested in analyzing more selected cell populations. In the first series of experiments, we tested 3 lymphoid cell clones that had been propagated with C-TCGF for 4 months. The results, shown in Table 5, indicated that 2 of the clones (Navarro 5 and 9) were highly cytotoxic against SK-MES-1 and G-11 targets but had low reactivity against HT-29 and K562. In contrast, Sredni clone 1 exhibited very strong cytotoxicity against all targets tested. Thus cloned CLC showed some heterogeneity in their patterns of cytotoxicity, but even a clone of effector cells could react against a variety of tumor target cells.

TABLE 5. Cytotoxic activity of clones of human CLC and of CLC from NK-enriched and depleted mononuclear cells

CLC	% cytotoxicity (E:T, 30:1, 18 h)					
	K562	SK-MES-1	HT-29	MCF-7	G-11	Fresh lung tumors
Clones						
Sredni 1	79	93	82	64	80	20
Navarro 5	9	55	6	NT[a]	62	NT
Navarro 5	26	48	16	NT	85	NT
From Percoll fractions						
LGL	74	64	65	66	72	32
small T cell	15	53	44	58	59	23

[a] Not tested.

In the next series of experiments we obtained CLC from PBL populations enriched for, or depleted of, LGL which have been shown to mediate NK activity (47), using Percoll gradient centrifugation (Table 5). When tested fresh on day 0, the LGL population possessed higher reactivity than the unseparated cells towards all the targets, whereas the NK-depleted, T-cell fraction expressed only low cytotoxicity against either NK-sensitive (K562 and G-11) or NK-resistant target cells. After culturing for 2-4 weeks with C-TCGF, the LGL fraction displayed a similar pattern of strong reactivity against all of the cultured tumor targets, substantially increased reactivity against fresh lung tumor cells, and low, but significant, activity against allogeneic lymphoblasts. In contrast, the cultured T cell fraction showed a remarkably heightened cytotoxic activity (compared with their lack of reactivity on day 0) against all the adherent solid tumor lines as well as against fresh allogeneic lung tumor cells, and also reacted against allogeneic blasts, yet only low levels of cytotoxicity were detected against the NK-sensitive lymphoid tumor K562.

In vivo reactivity of human CLC. A local (s.c.) Winn neutralization assay was employed to assess the ability of three human CLC lines to retard the growth of tumor cells in athymic nude mice. Admixing of CLC and G-11 tumor cells at a 10/1 or 15/1 ratio completely inhibited tumor growth and all mice survived, in contrast to the death with tumor by day 65 of 8 out of 10 control mice inoculated with tumor alone. With the HT-29 cell line, which showed less susceptibility to lysis in vitro than G-11 (see Table 4), CLC delayed tumor appearance in all mice and 2 out of 5 mice did not develop tumors by day 70; in contrast, all control mice had tumors by day 15. These findings indicate that tumor cell killing by CLC can also take place in vivo.

The radioisotopic assay also was used to assess the in vivo cytotoxic activity of human CLC against human tumor-derived cell lines (13). CLC were inoculated into the footpads of BALB/c nude mice, together with 1 x 10^5 labelled G-11 cells at a 20:1 effector:target ratio. Acceleration of the radioisotope clearance was observed in mice transplanted with G-11 human tumor cells and CLC in comparison with mice inoculated with G-11 tumor cells alone. Similarly, 2 x 10^5 radiolabelled HT-29 tumor cells were inoculated into the footpad of BALB/c mice, mixed with human cultured lymphoid cells at an effector:target ratio of 30:1. At 3 days following transplantation, all tumor cells were eliminated, whereas in BALB/c nude mice inoculated only with radiolabelled HT-29 cells, a relatively high level of radioactivity remained. The cultured lymphoid cells obtained from two different donors exerted virtually the same cytotoxic effects in vivo.

DISCUSSION

The main findings of the present studies are: (a) lymphoid cells from normal or tumor-bearing mice and from normal human donors or cancer patients could be expanded in culture to very large numbers within a short period of time, using crude or mitogen-depleted TCGF preparations; (b) although no specific tumor stimulation was employed, the propagated lymphoid cells expressed a wide spectrum of cytotoxic reactivity against NK-sensitive and NK-resistant lymphoid and solid tumor cells, both fresh and cultured and of autologous, syngeneic, or allogeneic origin; and (c) under the conditions employed, the cultured cells were capable of inhibiting tumor growth in a local Winn neutralization assay but were relatively ineffective when administered systemically into hosts with established disease.

Of primary interest is the nature of the cytotoxic effector cells among the CLC. It has previously been demonstrated, in studies of CLC initiated from peripheral blood mononuclear leukocytes of normal human donors, that several types of cytotoxicity could be detected (1,36): NK-like activity, ADCC, lectin-induced cytotoxicity, and polyclonally activated cytotoxicity against allogeneic target cells. The present results indicate a similar pattern. The relatively strong reactivity of CLC against allogeneic normal blast cells is suggestive of polyclonally activated cytotoxic T cells. However, the observations of cytotoxicity also against syngeneic lymphoblasts and tumor cell lines, and of the mouse CLC against a xenogeneic target cell like K562 which has been shown to lack expression of major histocompatibility antigens (20), indicate that other types of cytotoxic effector cells exist in the cultures. It seems likely that a major contribution to the cytotoxicity was by cells with the characteristics of NK cells. The cytotoxic reactivity of CLC against a wide array of syngeneic, allogeneic, and xenogeneic target cells is reminiscent of a similar broad reactivity by NK cells. YAC-1 and RLδ1, which are widely used as sensitive target cells for murine NK cells, were both highly susceptible to lysis by the mouse CLC. The reactivity against some normal thymus cells, bone marrow cells and peritoneal exudate cells, but not against normal spleen cells, has also been observed for fresh NK cells (33). However, in addition to cytotoxicity against NK-susceptible targets, the CLC were also found to have considerable reactivity against several solid tumor cell lines, both transplantable and spontaneous, and other targets that are usually found to be resistant to NK cells. It is possible that the NK cells in the cultures are more highly activated than those found normally in the spleen and that such high reactivity, particularly in a long-term assay, can result in lysis of relatively insensitive targets. This possibility is supported by previous findings that M109, which is entirely resistant to NK activity in a 4 h *in vitro* assay, could be shown to be susceptible in longer term *in vitro* assays and in an *in vivo* assay of NK activity (38). Alternatively, or in addition, other types of natural effector cells, e.g., NC cells (5,46) which have been shown to have a predilection for reactivity against NK-resistant solid tumor target cells, might be involved. The clones of mouse CLC, designated CNK-SL, seem more likely to represent either more activated NK cells or NC cells. The human CLC initiated from LGL had a pattern of cytotoxicity quite compatible with NK cells. The CLC from LGL-depleted PBL were mainly reactive against solid tumor cells and alloblasts and may represent a mixture of activated T cells and a subpopulation of natural effector cells. The heterogeneity of the human CLC was supported by the demonstration of different cytotoxic patterns among the 3 human clones.

The findings that the cytotoxic reactivity of CLC could be appreciably augmented by pretreatment with interferon is most compatible with an involvement of NK cells and possibly NC cells, since such effector cells, but not cytotoxic immune T cells (36,46,47), have been found to be consistently augmented by interferon. Furthermore, the finding of ADCC activity by the CLC is highly indicative of the presence of NK cells, since NK cells have been shown to be the main type of nonadherent lymphoid cells mediating ADCC (23,34,47). In regard to the surface markers on the mouse CLC, and particularly on the cytotoxic cells, the findings of reactivity with anti-Thy 1 and anti-asialo GM1, and lower activity with anti-Lyt 1, are quite compatible with involvement of NK cells. Such reactivity would be unusual for freshly harvested NC cells, since they have been found to be quite resistant to complement-dependent lysis by these antibodies. The observations that monoclonal antibodies to Lyt 2 reacted with a considerable portion of the CLC and reduced their cytotoxicity activity are quite surprising since this antigen has usually not been detected on fresh NK cells (21). However, Minato *et al* (29) recently reported that Lyt 2 was present in a subpopulation of NK cells. In addition, it is quite possible that the phenotype of NK cells changes considerably in culture, acquiring more markers typical of T cells. Such observations have been made when purified populations of human NK cells have been cultured in the presence of TCGF (35). Of interest was the observation that some clones of both types of mouse CLC were Lyt 2$^+$ as well as positive for Thy 1, asialo GM1 and the NK2 alloantigen.

The ability of the CLC to kill in vitro fresh syngeneic tumor cells and to affect tumor growth in vivo without any previous intentional tumor stimulation may have practical implications. By this approach, lymphoid cells from cancer patients could be expanded directly with TCGF and subsequently administered in large quantities to the autologous donors. Our studies with TCGF-cultured lymphocytes from patients with various carcinomas have shown an appreciable cytotoxic reactivity in vitro toward autochthonous and allogeneic fresh tumor cells and such cells have also been shown to inhibit human tumor growth in athymic nude mice. However, the relative inefficiency in vivo of cultured cytotoxic cells (whether NK or cytotoxic immune T cells) undoubtedly stresses the limitations under-lying systemic employment of such cells at present. These difficulties are probably attributable to: (a) complete dependence of the cells on a continuous supply of TCGF, and (b) limited or even abnormal circulation patterns in vivo. We have shown that over 90% of radiolabeled CLC were eliminated (and probably disintegrated) within 48 h after inoculation, and the transient survival of the inoculated cells was not improved significantly by two inoculations of 0.5 ml of MD-TCGF-M. With regard to circulation, Lotze et al (25) have recently demonstrated that the vast majority of TCGF-cultured human or mouse lymphocytes are entrapped in the lungs and liver shortly following i.v. administration. While it is possible that the entrapped cells may be effective against lung and liver tumors, only a small percentage of the infused cells may be able to migrate to other tumor sites.

Despite the many difficulties foreseen in using this approach, the great potential for successful clinical application of TCGF-propagated anti-tumor effector cells should encourage further investigations aimed at a better understanding of the in vivo behavior of such cells.

References

1. Alvarez, J.M., de Landazuri, M.O., Bonnard, G.D., and Herberman, R.B. (1978): J. Immunol., 121:1270-1275.

2. Bonnard, G.D., Fagnani, R., Navarro, N., Alvarez, J.M., Kedar, E., Ortaldo, J.R., and Strong, D.M. (1980): In: International Symposium on New Trends in Human Immunology and Cancer Immunotherapy, edited by B. Serrou and C. Rosenfeld, pp. 332-244. Doin Editeurs, Paris.

3. Bonnard, G.D., Yasaka, K., and Jacobson, D. (1979): J. Immunol., 123:2704-2708.

4. Bonnard, G.D., Yasaka, K., and Maca, R.D. (1980): Cell. Immunol, 51:390-401.

5. Burton, R.C. (1980): In: Natural Cell-Mediated Immunity against Tumors, edited by R.B. Herberman, pp. 19-35. Academic Press, New York.

6. Cheever, M.A., Greenberg, P.D., and Fefer, A. (1981): J. Immunol., 126:1318-1322.

7. Dennert, G., Yogeeswaran, G., and Yamagata, S. (1981): J. Exp. Med., 153:545-556.

8. Djeu, J.Y., Timonen, T., and Herberman, R.B. (1981): In: Role of Natural Killer Cells, Macrophages and Antibody Dependent Cellular Cytotoxicity in Tumor Rejection and as Mediators in Biological Response Modifiers Activity, edited by M. Chirigos. Raven Press, New York, in press.

9. Gillis, S., Ferm, M.M., Ou, W., and Smith, KA. (1978): J. Immunol., 120:2027-2031.

10. Gillis, S. and Smith, K.A. (1977): Nature (Lond.), 268:154-156.

11. Giorgi, J.V. and Warner, N.L. (1981): J. Immunol., 126:322-330.

12. Gorelik, E. and Herberman, R.B. (1981): Int. J. Cancer, 27:709-720.

13. Gorelik, E., Kedar, E., Sredni, B., and Herberman, R. Int. J. Cancer, in press.

14. Herberman, R.B., Nunn, M.E., and Holden, H.T. (1976): In: In Vitro Methods in Cell Mediated and Tumor Immunity, edited by B.R. Bloom and J.R. David, pp. 621-628. Academic Press, New York.

15. Kay, H.D., Bonnard, G.D., and Herberman, R.B. (1979): J. Immunol., 122:675-685.

16. Kedar, E., Ikejiri, B.L., Bonnard, G.D., Reid, J., and Herberman, R.B. Submitted for publication.

17. Kedar, E., Ikejiri, B.L., Gorelik, E., and Herberman, R.B. Submitted for publication.

18. Kedar, E., Ikejiri, B.L., Sredni, B., Bonavida, B., and Herberman, R.B. Submitted for publication.

19. Klein, E., Masucci, M.G., Masucci, G., and Vanky, F. (1980): In: Natural Cell-Mediated Immunity Against Tumors, edited by R.B. Herberman, pp. 909-920. Academic Press, New York.

20. Klein, G., Zeuthren, J., Eriksson, I., Terasaki, P., Bernocco, M., Rosen, A., Masucci, G., Povey, S., and Ber, R. (1980): J. Natl. Cancer Inst., 64:725-733.

21. Koo, G.C. and Hatzfeld, A. (1980): In: Natural Cell-Mediated Immunity Against Tumors, edited by R.B. Herberman, pp. 105-116. Academic Press, New York.

22. Landazuri, M.O. and Herberman, R.B. (1972): Nature New Biol., 238:18-19.

23. Landazuri, M.O., Silva, A., Alvarez, J., and Herberman, R.B. (1979): J. Immunol., 123:252-258.

24. Lotze, M.T., Grimm, E.A., Mazumder, A., Strausser, J.L., and Rosenberg, S.A. Submitted for publication.

25. Lotze, M., Line, B., Mathieson, B., and Rosenberg, S.A. (1980): J. Immunol., 125:1487-1493.

26. Lotze, M.T., Strausser, J.L., and Rosenberg, S.A. (1980): Cell. Immunol., 124:2972-2980.

27. MacDonald, H.R., Cerottini, J.C., Ryser, J.E., Maryanski, J.L., Taswell, C., Widmer, M.B., and Brunner, K.T. (1980): Immunol. Rev., 51:93-123.

28. Mills, G.B., Carlson, G., and Paetkau, V. (1980): J. Immunol., 125: 1904-1909.

29. Minato, M., Reid, L., and Bloom, B. (1981): J. Exp. Med., in press.

30. Moller, G., editor (1980): Immunological Reviews, Volume 51.

31. Nabel, G., Bucalo, L.R., Allard, J., Wigzell, H., and Cantor, H. (1981): J. Exp. Med., 152:1582-1591.

32. Nabholz, M., Conzelmann, A., Acuto, O., North, M., Haas, W., Pohlit, H., Van Boehmer, H., Hengartner, H., Mach, J.P., Engers, H., and Johnson, J.P. (1980): Immunol. Rev., 51:125-156.

33. Nunn, M.E., Herberman, R.B., and Holden, H.T. (1977): Int. J. Cancer, 20:381-187.

34. Ojo, E. and Wigzell, H. (1978): Scand. J. Immunol., 7:297-306.

35. Ortaldo, J.R. and Timonen, T.T. (1981): In: Proceedings of the 14th International Leucocyte Culture Conference, 1981, in press.

36. Ortaldo, J.R., Timonen, T.T., and Bonnard, G.D. (1980): Behring Inst. Mitt., 67:258-264.

37. Price, G.B., Teh, H.S., and Miller, R.G. (1980): J. Immunol., 124: 2352-2355.

38. Riccardi, C., Santoni, A., Barlozzari, T., Puccetti, P., and Herberman, R.B. (1980): Int. J. Cancer, 25:475-486.

39. Rosenberg, S.A., Spiess, P.J., and Schwarz, S. (1980): Cell. Immunol., 54:293-306.

40. Rosenberg, S.A., Spiess, P.J., and Schwarz, S. (1978): J. Immunol., 121:1946-1950.

41. Saksela, E., Timonen, T., Virtanen, I., and Cantell, K. (1980): In: Natural Cell-Mediated Immunity Against Tumors, edited by R.B. Herberman, pp. 645-653. Academic Press, New York.

42. Schreier, M.H., Iscove, N.N., Tees, R., Aarden, L., and Von Boehmer, H. (1980): Immunol. Rev., 51:315-336.

43. Smith, K.A., Gillis, S., Ruscetti, F.W., Baker, P.E., and McKenzie, D. (1979): NY Acad. Sci., 332:423-429.

44. Sredni, B., Kalechman, Y., Michlin, H., and Rozenszajn, L.A. (1976): Nature (Lond.), 259:130-131.

45. Sredni, B., Tse, H.Y., Chen, C., and Schwartz, R.H. (1981): J. Immunol., 126:341-347.

46. Stutman, O., Figarella, E.F., Paige, C.J., and Lattime, E.C. (1980): In: Natural Cell-Mediated Immunity Against Tumors, edited by R.B. Herberman, pp. 187-229. Academic Press, New York.

47. Timonen, T., Ortaldo, J.R., and Herberman, R.B. (1981): J. Exp. Med., 153:569-582.

48. Timonen, T. and Saksela, E. (1980): J. Immunol. Methods, 36:285-291.

49. Trinchieri, G., Santoli, D., Dee, R.R., and Knowles, B.B. (1978): J. Exp. Med., 147:1299-1313.

50. Vose, B.M. (1981): Cancer Lett., in press.

51. Yron, I., Wood, T.A., Spiess, P.J., and Rosenberg, S.A. (1980): J. Immunol., 238-245.

52. Zarling, J.M. and Bach, F.H. (1979): Nature (Lond.), 280:685-686.

The Potential Role of T Cells in Cancer Therapy,
edited by A. Fefer and A. Goldstein,
Raven Press, New York © 1982.

Human Natural Killer Cells as Well as T Cells Maintained in Continuous Cultures with IL-2

J. R. Ortaldo, T. T. Timonen, B. M. Vose, and J. A. Alvarez

Laboratory of Immunodiagnosis, National Cancer Institute, National Institutes of Health, Bethesda, Maryland 20205

Cultured lymphoid cells (CLC) maintained with T cell growth factor or interleukin-2 (IL-2) have been cytotoxic for a wide variety of target cells. These cultures have been derived from a) mitogen-stimulated cells, b) in vitro primed cells, selected for alloreactivity and c) mixed lymphocyte tumor interactions (MLTI) in vitro (1-3, 9-12, 14). Several mechanisms for the cytotoxicity have been considered: a) human peripheral blood mononuclear leukocytes (PBL) grown on IL-2 have been very effective in lectin-induced cell-mediated cytotoxicity (1). b) PBL grown on IL-2 have been highly cytotoxic for allogeneic blasts (2, 4-7), while autologous and histocompatible blasts were not killed. This was consistant with polyclonal activation of lymphocytes against major histocompatibility determinants (10, 12). c) Some PBL grown in IL-2 mediated high levels of killing against the K562 cell line (1), which is deficient in MHC determinents, but highly susceptible to lysis by natural killer (NK) cells. This raised the possibility of the presence of NK cells in IL-2 maintained cultures (1, 2).

We present here direct evidence that human NK cells as well as typical T cells can be cultured in the presence of IL-2. In the last few years there has been considerable progress in understanding of NK cells. In fresh PBL these cells have appeared to be the major subpopulation of nonadherent cells with Fc receptors for IgG (FcγR). Recently NK and K cells, which mediate antibody-dependent cell-mediated cytotoxicity (ADCC) were found to have a characteristic morphology of large granular lymphocytes (LGL) with indented nucleus, high cytoplasmic-nuclear ratio, and azurophilic granules in the cytoplasm (15, 17). A major limitation for the detailed analysis and characterization of NK cells has been that they represent a small proportion of lymphoid cells in the peripheral lymphoid organs. The recent development of procedures to highly enrich for, or deplete, LGL by discontinuous Percoll gradient centrifugation, and the ability to morphologically identify this small subpopulation of lymphoid cells, has greatly advanced our understanding of these cells (16).

We show here that LGL can be grown in the presence of IL-2 and these cultured cells possess distinct cytotoxic capabilities. We have isolated highly enriched populations of LGL, which are virtually devoid of mature typical lymphocytes (as enumerated by morphological and surface antigen analysis using monoclonal antibodies, e.g. OKT3) and of T cells (greater than 95% sheep erythrocyte-forming and devoid of LGL and NK/K activities), and propagated both types of cells in the presence of crude or partially purified IL-2. Cultures of LGL could be initiated consistently even in the absence of lectins and the cultured LGL retained their characteristic morphology and cytotoxic activity. However, within 7-10 days after initiation, the cultured LGL changed in surface phenotype to become indistinguishable from cultured T cells.

RESULTS

When cells of actively growing cultures of peripheral blood lymphocytes were harvested and immediately tested after washing, they demonstrated indiscriminant killing of all targets tested, including low but significant levels of cytotoxicity against RLo1 (mouse target cells) (Table 1) and considerable reactivity also against a variety of other xenogeneic and human cell lines (data not shown). The possibility of lectin-induced cytotoxicity (LICC) was especially of concern since this represents a major cytotoxic activity of PBL and since PHA is a contaminant of crude IL-2 and is probably transferred to the cytotoxicity assay. To evaluate this possibility, we tested whether a 24 hr culture period in medium without IL-2 (resting) would eliminate this type of cytotoxicity. Indeed, cultures which had been rested for 24 hr had a more restricted range of reactivity, with no killing of the xenogeneic targets (RLo1). However, cytotoxicity against allogenic lymphoid target cell (particularly PHA blasts), as previously reported by several investigators (3, 10, 12, 14), was observed in rested as well as unrested cultures. Thus, polyclonal activation of T cells, rather than LICC, appeared responsible for this remaining reactivity and it seemed important to regularly monitor our cultures for such reactivity against cryopreserved allogeneic PHA blasts. As shown in the subsequent tables, rested cultures of PBL consistently demonstrated low levels of cytotoxicity against lymphoblasts.

TABLE 1. Effect of resting of CLC effectors on LICC

Experiment	Cytotoxicity (E/T = 25/1)					
	RLo1		Blasts		K562	
	Unrested	Rested*	Unrested	Rested	Unrested	Rested
1	25**	1	14	21	40	30
2	26	1	16	18	43	25
3	30	1	18	18	50	41
Mean	27	1	16	19	44	32
% Control	(-)	4	(-)	118	(-)	72

*Cells were washed and held 24 hr prior to testing in complete medium without growth factor.
**% cytotoxicity in a 4 hr ^{51}Cr release assay.

The detection of high levels of cytotoxicity against K562, by rested as well as unrested CLC suggested that NK cells also were present in the cultures. If so, one might anticipate the concomitant presence of ADCC

TABLE 2. Cytotoxicity of rested CLC*

Experiment	Cytotoxicity to			
	K562	RL♂1	RL♂1 + Antibody	Alloblast
1	16**	<0.1	21	34
2	17	<0.1	9	2.3
3	17	<0.1	5	20
4	10	<0.1	-	19
5	115	0.5	25	6
6	16	<0.1	5	8
Mean	32	0.2	13	15

*Cells were washed and held 24 hr prior to testing in complete medium
  without growth factor.
**Lytic units 30% in a 4 hr release assay.

activity since most NK cells have been shown to also mediate ADCC (15).
Because of the inability of rested culture cells to lyse xenogeneic target
cells, we were able, with great sensitivity, to test for levels of ADCC
within CLC. As shown in Table 2, rested CLC mediated high levels of
cytotoxicity against antibody-coated RL♂1 as well as K562, but were
unreactive against the mouse target in the absence of antibody. These
data indicated the probable presence of NK and K cells, in addition to
polyclonal-activated T cells in IL-2 maintained cultures. One of the most
consistent surface markers on NK and K cells from fresh PBL has been the
FcγR (5). Because of the inability to deplete cytotoxicity from cultured
cells by standard rosetting and monolayer procedures for depletion of
FcγR bearing cells (7), it was important to confirm that the apparent ADCC
was indeed mediated by FcγR-bearing cells. As shown in Table 3, Staph.
Protein A treatment abrogated the cytotoxicity against antibody-coated
RL♂1, whereas similar treatment had no effect on the cytotoxicity of K562
or allogenic blasts. This demonstrated that the FcγR was involved in the
cytotoxicity against antibody-coated RL♂1 and thus the effector cells
appeared to be K cells. As further support of the presence of NK and K

TABLE 3. Effects of Protein A on cytotoxicity by CLC

Experiment	Cytotoxicity against:					
	K562		RL♂1 + Antibody		Alloblast	
	NT*	Prot-A	NT	Prot-A	NT	Prot-A
1	809**	775	384	2.1	10.1	9.9
2	132	130	315	46.1	14.1	8.7
3	109	124	121	3.1	55.4	59.0
4	250	261	370	12.2	31.6	27.3
Mean	325	323	298	15.9	27.8	25.2
% Inhibition		1		95		6

*NT = not treated; Prot-A = Protein A, 50 µg/ml in assay medium.
**Lytic units 30% in a 4 hr release assay.

cells among the CLC, we observed that pretreatment of the cells with interferon, which is known to augment both NK and ADCC activities of PBL and LGL (4, 6), boosted the cytotoxicity by CLC (see later tables).   In contrast, it appeared that polyclonally-activated cytotoxicity against PHA blasts was not boosted.

TABLE 4.   Summary of competitive inhibition experiments

	Inhibitors		
Target	K562	Ab/RLo1	Alloblasts
K562	+++	++	-
Ab/RLo1	+	+++	-
Alloblasts	-	-	+++

To obtain further evidence for the possible presence of different effector cells among the CLC, cold target inhibition experiments with K562, antibody-coated RLo1 and alloblasts were performed (Table 4).   The cytotoxicity against PHA blasts was not inhibited by K562 inhibitors and conversely the cytotoxicity against K562 was not inhibited by alloblasts.

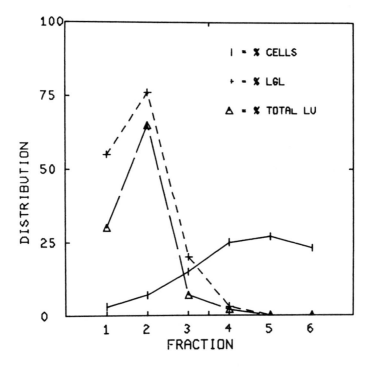

Figure 1. Percoll fractionation of nonadherent peripheral blood mono-nuclear cells by discontinuous gradient centrifugation. The distribution of LGL (+), total cell numbers (∤) and total lytic units of NK activity (△) is shown.

As seen in studies with fresh PBL, K562 and the antibody-coated target cells showed considerable cross-inhibition. These results suggest that at least two cytotoxic effector types are present when mononuclear peripheral blood lymphocytes are grown on IL-2. Similar reactivities have been seen when PBL were stimulated in mixed cultures with tumor cells or with allogenic antigens, with the concomitant presence of both allo-reactive cells as well as NK and ADCC activities.

Since it appeared that both NK and T cells could be present in IL-2 dependent cultures, we attempted to initiate cultures from highly purified LGL and T populations. Peripheral blood mononuclear cells were depleted of monocytes by adherence to plastic and of B cells by nylon wool column passage. The nonadherent lymphoid cells were then separated on a discontinuous Percoll gradient (Figure 1), with the low density fractions 1 and 2 (LGL-rich) being further depleted of contaminating T cells by 29°C rosette formation. [Previous results have demonstrated that NK cells do not form rosettes (15) at 29°C.] The resulting populations contained > 90% LGL, and $\leq$ 1% OKT3 positive cells. A detailed analysis of the pheno-type of LGL is shown in Figure 2. Most LGL showed strong reactivity with OKT10, OKM1, LYT3, and a small portion were reactive with OKT8 or anti-IA (8). There was also a high frequency of cells with FcγR, detectable by rosetting with ox-EA. The T cell population from the high density fractions 5 and 6 (Figure 1) of the Percoll gradient contained generally greater than 90% OKT3 positive cells (Figure 2) and greater than 95% formed rosettes with sheep erythrocytes at 4°C.

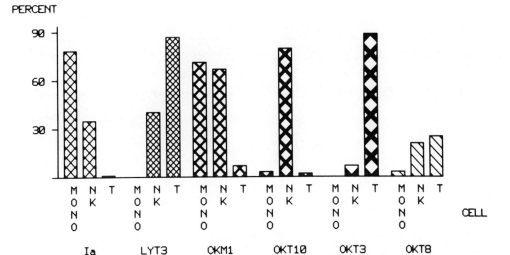

Figure 2. Purified populations of monocytes (mono), T cells (T) and LGL (NK) are summarized for reactivity with monoclonal antibodies. The percent positive cells are shown by fluorescent-activated cell-sorter analysis with 6 monoclonal reagents.

As shown in Figure 3, both highly enriched LGL cultures, as well as T cultures, underwent rapid and sustained growth in the presence of IL-2. The culture of the LGL and T populations generally resulted in an increase in the number of LGL (20-40 fold) and T cells (50-80 fold) over a four week culture period.   The analysis of the phenotype of these cells, at various times in cultures, is shown and Figure 3 (b-d).   The markers on T cultures remained relatively stable, with 1) some increase in proportion of high affinity rosettes with sheep erythrocytes , 2) a slight increase in OKT3 positive cells and 3) the appearance of Ia antigens on a high proportion of the cells.   OKT10 and OKM1 did not react with either fresh

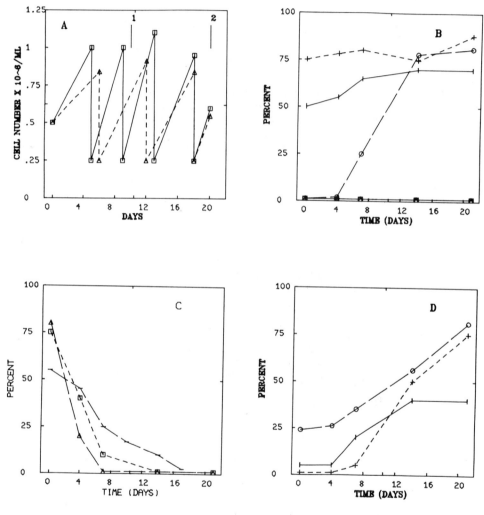

Figure 3 Cultured LGL and T cells (panel a) shows the growth of LGL (△) and T (□) cultures.   Cultures were sampled at points 1 and 2 (10 and 20 days) for cytolytic capacity (see figure 7).   T cells (panel b) and LGL (panel c and d) were examined for reactivity with OKT3 (+), OKT10 (△), OKM1 (□), anti-Ia (○), and for E-rosette-formation at 29 C (I) and for FcγR (−).

or cultured T cells. After culture of LGL, there was a dramatic loss of several characteristic markers (reactivity with OKT10, OKM1 and OX-EA) with undetectable levels being seen by 7 to 10 days (Figure 3, panel c). Conversely, there was a major increase in the proportion of LGL expressing Ia, and OKT3 antigens and high affinity receptors for sheep erythrocytes became quite apparent at approximately 7 to 10 days in culture (Figure 3, panel d).

In ten consecutive cultures, the cultured LGL retained their typical weakly basophilic cytoplasm, kidney shaped nucleus (Figure 4, panel b) in greater than 90% of the cells and the characteristic azurophilic cytoplasmic granules in 78% of the cells. In contract, cultured T cells exhibited typical blast morphology with strongly basophilic cytoplasm, and < 10% of the cells had cytoplastic granules (see Figure 4, panel d).

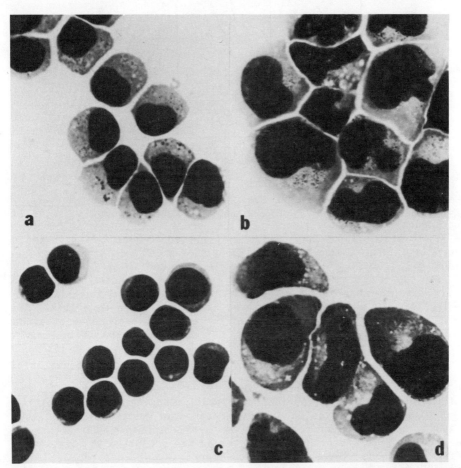

Figure 4. Morphology of fresh and cultured subpopulations of lymphoid cells (X1040). A. Fresh LGL, B. Cultured LGL at day 20, C. Fresh T cells, D. Cultured T cells at day 20. Similar morphology was seen at day 10 and as late as day 30 consistently, when the cultures were routinely discontinued.

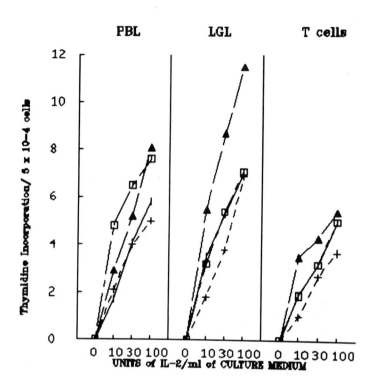

<u>Figure 5.</u> ^{3}H-thymidine incorporations of cultured PBL, LGL, and T cells in the presence of various amounts of IL-2 crude conditioned medium (CM) (---), or various species of partially purified IL-2 differing in their isoelectric points: IL-2-α (pH 6.5) (□), IL-2-β (pH 7.2) (+), and IL-2-γ (pH 8.2) (▲). Ten units of IL-2 correspond to an IL-2 activity needed for the long term growth of human and murine dependent cell lines. Data are expressed as incorporation of thymidine (c.p.m x 10^{-4}) after pulse labelling of 5 x 10^4 cells for 6 hr with 1 μCi of ^{3}H-thymidine. The cells had been previously cultured for 10 days in the presence of crude CM, and were then further cultured for 2 days in the presence of growth factors or medium alone (background).

To verify that IL-2 was responsible for the growth of the LGL, the proliferative capacities of peripheral blood lymphocytes, and of isolated LGL and T cells, were tested in the presence of human IL-2 partially purified by sequential chromatography of phenyl-Sepharose, DEAE Sephacel and AcA 54 gel filtration (13). The material was subjected to isoelectric focusing and yielded three peaks of IL-2 activity at PI's of 6.5 (IL-2 alpha), 7.2 (IL-2 beta), and 8.2 (IL-2 gamma). In Figure 5, using the IL-2 adjusted for biological activity on a IL-2 dependent murine cell line, cultures initiated from PBL, LGL, and T cells were examined for the thymidine incorporation in the presence of the various purified factors. Thymidine incorporation of cultured LGL in the presence of purified preparations was similar or higher than obtained in the presence of crude IL-2, indicating that the growth factor needed for proliferation of LGL was indeed IL-2 and that lectins and other factors in crude conditioned medium were not required after initiation of the cultures that initially responded to IL-2. In addition, the thymidine incorporation of LGL with the various preparations was similar or higher than the proliferative response obtained with T cells, indicating that once initiated, LGL cultures can proliferate at a rate equal to T lymphocytes.

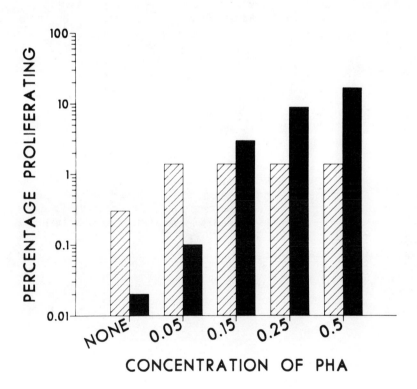

Figure 6.   Limiting dilution analysis of LGL and T cells.   Cells were grown for 7 days in IL-2 in the presence of x-irradiated feeder cells (PBL). The percent responding wells were plotted against a titration of plated cell populations at various PHA concentrations.

The frequency of cells in the purified subpopulations which prolifer-ated in different conditioned media was determined in limiting dilutions assays (Figure 6). The frequency of proliferation (f) was critically dependent upon the concentration of PHA used in culture initiation. In the presence of 0.5 µg/ml PHA, T cell expansion predominated (T cells, f = 1/11; LGL, 1/72). However, in lectin-depleted IL-2, growth of LGL was the greater (T cells, 1/5000; LGL, 1/400). These data suggest that at least a proportion of NK cells spontaneously express the IL-2 receptor as has been suggested for some mouse cells. Thus, under lectin-free conditions, LGL growth is favored, since most T cells require activation (by mitogen or antigen) before cultures can be initiated. In addition, T cells growth required the continuous presence of irradiated feeder cells, while frequency determinations showed that LGL proliferation was independent of feeders.

The cells from cultures of LGL and of T cells were tested for cytotoxic activity at days 10 and 20 after initiation and this was compared with the reactivity prior to culture. As usual, the cultured cells were rested for 24 hr prior to testing. Figure 7 shows the mean of results of 3 experiments. Cultured LGL exerted spontaneous and interferon-augmentable NK activity similar to that of fresh LGL against the susceptible target cell lines K562, MOLT 4, and G-11. They also exhibited antibody-dependent and lectin-induced cellular cytotoxicities against RLo1. They did not, however, significantly lyse NK insensitive allogeneic lymphoblasts (Figure 7, top). As previously reported (15), fresh T cells were cytotoxic only in LICC. In contrast, cultured T cells were reactive mainly in LICC, but also against allogeneic blasts, and against the monolayer target cell, G-11. However, they did not lyse the NK-sensitive target cells K563 and MOLT 4. Furthermore, cultured T cells did not demonstrate ADCC activity, indicating the lack of detectable Fc receptors on these cells.

The frequency of cytotoxic precursors was also investigated. Cultures of LGL under limiting dilution conditions showed a frequency of NK activity (K562 lysis) closely similar to the proliferative frequency (f = 1/76 - 1/350), with reactivity against alloblast or mouse target RLo1 at least 20 fold less frequent (f = 1/5000 - > 1/20,000). T cell cultures did not lyse K562 (f > 1/20,000). Taken together these data exclude the possibility that cultures from enriched LGL populations could arise by expansion of a small number of contaminating T cells.

SUMMARY

We have demonstrated that human NK cells as well as T cells can be cultured in the presence of IL-2. The cultures of highly purified NK cells were morphologically and functionally different from those of T cells, and they proliferated as rapidly as T cells cultured in the presence of IL-2. These results seemed to rule out the possibilities that either small numbers of conventional T cells among the LGL-enriched were responsible for the observed growth of NK fractions, or that minor contamination of T cells by LGL accounted for the detected cytotoxic activities of the cultured T cells. The proliferation of both NK and T cells was also supported by the reproducible presence of both NK and allo-like cytotoxic activities in PBL cultures maintained with IL-2. Although some nonselective cytotoxicity appeared in cultured T cells, several lines of evidence a) the lack of killing against K562 and other NK-susceptible targets; b) the lack of ADCC activity in these cultures; and c) the lack of LGL morphology, indicate that this was not due to classical NK cells.

ACTIVITY OF LGL

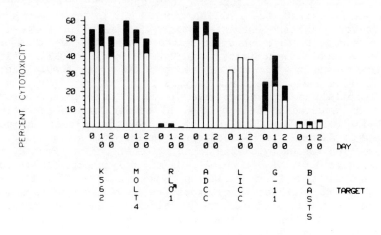

ACTIVITY OF T CELLS

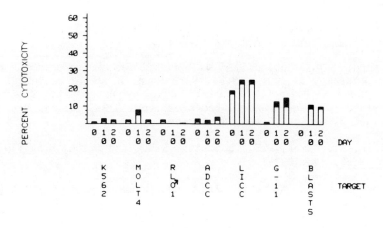

Figure 7   Cytotoxic activities of fresh and cultured LGL and T cells in a 4 hr [51]chromium-release assay (effector:target cell ratio 20:1). K562, target cell derived from a patient with chronic myelogenous leukemia; MOLT4, a T cell leukemia line; RLσ1, a murine T cell lymphoma; LICC, cytotoxicity against RLol in the presence of 1 μg/ml of PHA; ADCC, cytotoxicity against RLol coated with rabbit anti-mouse T cell serum; G-11, a cell line derived from a patient with breast carcinoma; blasts, allogenic PHA-induced blasts derived from PBL.   Solid bars: 3 hr pretreatment of effector cells with 800 IU of IFN-β (specific activity 2 x 10^7 IU/mg protein, HEM Research, Rockville, MD.).

Our demonstration of the lack of stability of surface antigens during culture and the present lack of NK-specific antigenic marker makes the analysis of the presence of NK cells in culture from a mixed population very difficult. This problem has been solved by using purified NK and T cells for initiation of cultures. This approach is of interest for several reasons. First, the proliferation of LGL in the presence of IL-2 suggests that they share characteristics with cells in the T lineage. This contention is further supported by the obervations that a majority of cultured LGL acquire reactivity with T cell specific OKT3 antibodies. Second, the technology for the expansion of NK cells should facilitate characterization and biochemical analysis of NK cells. Third, the cloning of NK cells should become feasible so that several controversial issues can be studied in detail e.g. a) specificity of sensitivity of target cells to lysis by NK cells, b) the relationship of and possible overlapping of NK cells with K cells responsible for ADCC, and c) interferon production versus cytolytic capacity of NK cells. Fourth, the use of T cells, devoid of LGL, in autologous mixed lymphocyte-tumor cultures or allogeneic MLR's, and then expansion of the stimulated T cells with IL-2, would yield more selective cytotoxic cells than those obtained from cultures of unfractionated peripheral blood mononuclear cells. This would help to determine the frequency of human T cells with specific immune cytotoxic reactivities.

References

1. Alvarez, J.M., de Landazuri, M.O., Bonnard, G.D. and Herberman, R.B. (1978): J. Immunol., 121:1270-1275.

2. Bonnard, G.D., Schendel, D.J., West, W.H., Alvarez, J.J., Maca, R.D., Yasaka, K., Fine, R.L., Herberman, R.B., De Landazuri, M.O., and Morgan, D.A. (1978): In: Human Lymphocyte Differentiation, edited by G. Serrou and D. Rosenfeld, pp. 319-326. Elsevier/North-Holland Biomedical Press, Amsterdam.

3. Gillis, S., Baker, P.E., Ruscetti, F.W., and Smith, K.A. (1978): J. Exp. Med., 148:1093-1097.

4. Herberman, R.B., Ortaldo, J.R., and Bonnard, G.D. (1979): Nature, 277:221-223.

5. Kay, H.D., Bonnard, G.D., West, W.H., and Herberman, R.B. (1977): J. Immunol., 118:2058-2066.

6. Ortaldo, J.R., Pestka, S., Slease, R.B., Rubinstein, M., and Herberman, R.B. (1980): Scand. J. Immunol., 12:365-369.

7. Ortaldo, J.R., Timonen, T., and Bonnard, G.D. (1980): Behring Inst. Mitt., 67:258-264.

8. Ortaldo, J.R., Sharrow, S.A., Timonen, T., and Herberman, R.B. (1980): J. Immunol., in press.

9. Ruscetti, F.W., Morgan, D.A., and Gallo, R.C. (1977): J. Immunol., 119:131-138.

10. Schendel, D.J., Bonnard, G.D., and Dupont, B. (1978): Transplant. Proc., 10:933-935.

11. Schendel, D.J., Wank, R., and Bonnard, G.D. (1980): Scand. J. Immunol., 11:99-107.

12. Schendel, D.J., Wank, R., and Bonnard, G.D. (1980): Behring. Inst. Mitt., 67:252-257.

13. Stadler, B.M., Dougherty, S.F., Farrar, J.J., and Oppenheim, J.J. (1981): submitted for publication.

14. Strausser, J.L. and Rosenberg, S.A. (1978): J. Immunol., 121:1491-1495.

15. Timonen, T., Ortaldo, J.R., and Herberman, R.B. (1981): J. Exp. Med., 153:569-582.

16. Timonen, T. and Saksela, E. (1980): J. Immunol. Methods, 36:285-292.

17. Timonen, T., Saksela, E., Rnaki, A., and Hayry, P. (1979): Cell. Immunol., 48:133-148.

AUDIENCE DISCUSSION

Dr. Dennert: Have you looked at the banding pattern and chromosome outfit of these cells?

Dr. Ortaldo: No.

Dr. Dennert: Can you use lectin-resistant mutants?

Dr. Ortaldo: We grow our cells in TCGF, which has been depleted of PHA, but the depletion is not 100%.

Dr. Dennert: Is the 2-week and onward LGL predominantly OKT_3 positive? Are those cells completely devoid of OKT_4, OKT_5 and OKT_8?

Dr. Ortaldo: About 60-70% are OKT_3 positive. About 10 or 15% are OKT_8 positive, but do not appear to be functional because if we deplete those we don't remove NK activity. However, the cells do express very low amounts of OKT_{10} detectable only on the FACS.

Dr. Dennert: Is the Ia detected only by the monomorphic monoclonals or does it express the polymorphic determinants?

Dr. Ortaldo: I don't know.

Dr. Bonavida: Are the various cytotoxic activities (LDCC, NK, ADCC) mediated by separate subpopulations of cells or by the same effector cells?

Dr. Ortaldo: We can't answer it without clones.

Dr. Bonavida: Data from our laboratory by Tom Bradley show that NK and LDCC cytotoxic activities are mediated by different cells. A single cell assay was used to which two targets (NK and LDCC) were bound. With unfractionated PBL, these cytotoxic activiites are separable.

Dr. Ortaldo: With the single cell assay, we have examined the frequency of these populations that bind and do kill. Fifty percent or more of the cells bind K562 and antibody targets and a very high percentage kill them. We have not done the double target binders. We do find two populations of cells which can mediate LDCC, one of which is the NK population and one of which is the small lymphocyte which is the T population. That population cannot kill antibody-coated targets or T cells. To answer your question, unless we did the same study with the same cells, we can't be sure.

[Unidentified]: How long-lasting are these cultures?

Dr. Ortaldo: In the human system, that is a technical problem. General-ly, they grow to 45-60 days and then go through a crisis period -- a problem most laboratories face in the human system and some (very few) cultures will continue to grow. Most die out. We have not attempted to look at cells more than 60 days in culture.

Ellis Reinherz: How can you rule out the possibility that there is a small number of OKT_3 cells within the LGL population that you start to expand with IL 2 and which is responsive to IL 2? Have you tried lysing the LGL population with OKT_3 and complement and then repeating the experiment?

Dr. Ortaldo: Your objection is true no matter what we do. We start with populations less than 1% of which has detectable OKT_3. The growth curve is very rapid -- not what one would expect with a population that had less than 1% OKT_3 positive. The cells do maintain the killing capability, morphology and all the other characteristics, but we cannot rule out that we have a contaminant since the frequency of responders is 1 in 70. We are concerned that we have no NK cell marker stable in culture. The best way is by cloning.

Noel Warner: Don't your specificity data make that highly unlikely because then this would have to be by chance a random contaminant T cell subset that had a totally different target cell pattern of killing.

Dr. Ortaldo: I agree.

Dr. Green: The question really is whether all these functions are due to one type of cell.

Dr. Ortaldo: To determine whether one cell has all the functions would take a single cell assay with 5 targets. But we have populations which are highly purified. For the morphology, if we take out the OKT_{10} positive cells, we lose all of the cytotoxicities, the ADCC and the NK. All the NK and K cells appear to be LGL.

Dr. Bach: Did you say that resting NK cells are OKT_8 positive and, if so, for what percentage do you have evidence that they are NK cells?

<u>Dr. Ortaldo</u>: Resting LGL are between 20 and 30% OKT_8 positive. However, if we remove the OKT_8 positive LGL, we do not remove any cytotoxicity so they appear to be nonlytic LGL. Perhaps they were once NK and have differentiated or they are pre-NK. Most of the LGL that are functional are OKT_{10} positive with a subset being Lyt 3 or OKT_{11} positive and a very small percentage Ia posiitive. OKT_8 and OKT_3 have no functional bearing on the NK.

<u>Dr. Bach</u>: They are OKT_3 negative and OKT_8 positive?

<u>Dr. Ortaldo</u>: Yes.

The Potential Role of T Cells in Cancer Therapy,
edited by A. Fefer and A. Goldstein.
Raven Press. New York © 1982.

Preliminary Characterization of a Series of Tumor Reactive Continuous Cell Lines

Lee K. Roberts, Craig W. Spellman, *Janis V. Giorgi, Anna Tai, and **Noel L. Warner

*Department of Pathology, Immunobiology Laboratories, University of New Mexico, School of Medicine, Albuquerque, New Mexico 87131; *Transplantation Unit, Department of Surgery, Massachusetts General Hospital, Boston, Massachusetts 02114; **Monoclonal Antibody Laboratory, Becton Dickinson and Company, Mountain View, California 94043*

Recently developed methods now provide a means for the long-term maintenance of T-lymphocytes in tissue culture (30). It was first reported that normal human T-lymphocytes could be maintained in continuous exponential growth cultures when supplied with T-cell growth factor (now termed Interleukin-2, IL2) derived from lectin-stimulated mononuclear cells (24, 28). These original human T-cell lines, however, appeared to be polyclonally activated and did not possess antigen-specific immunologic functions attributed to known T-cell subsets. Subsequently, numerous reports have followed describing the generation, selection, and maintenance of cloned antigen-specific murine cytotoxic T-cell lines (CTLL) (1, 13, 14, 27). In addition, antigen-specific murine helper (29, 35) and suppressor (11) T-cell lines, as well as human CTLL (17, 33), have been described. With the availability of detailed descriptions for the production and use of IL2 (30), continuous T-cell lines are now widely used to study a variety of cellular immune responses.

Continuous cell lines are currently being developed in our laboratory to investigate tumor antigens and the tumor-immune response toward a number of different tumors, as well as T-cell immunoregulatory circuits, the cellular mechanisms associated with the spontaneous development of autoimmunity, and various aspects of natural killer cell mediated cytotoxicity. In conjunction with testing each line for its antigenic specificity and immunologic functions, all the continuous lines within our laboratory are evaluated using flow cytometry analysis (FACS) to establish their expression of various cell surface markers. Combined, these data provide information that can be used to correlate immunologic function with cell surface phenotype.

EXPERIMENT APPROACH

Since we are interested in studying "normal" immune responses with continuous cell lines, our approach has been to establish lines with as few in vitro manipulations as possible. Basically, lymphocyte preparations that would be used directly in a functional assay are placed in tissue culture supplimented with IL2. The continuous cell lines that develop from these cultures are maintained by continual feeding and passing with IL2 containing media. Two to six weeks after the crisis phase, which usually occurs between two and three weeks after the culture was initiated, the now established cell line is evaluated in funcional assays and with FACS analysis. Aside from the cytotoxic T-lymphocyte lines (CTLL), none of the other continuous lines that have been developed in our laboratory receive any in vitro antigen stimulation.

To generate CTLL, cytotoxic T-lymphocytes (CTL) were first induced by coincubating normal BALB/c or (BALB/c x C57BL/6)F_1 splenocytes with 5000 rad irradiated MPC-11 cells (a syngeneic, BALB/c plasmacytoma), at responder to stimulator ratios of 100:1 (13). After 14 days in tissue culture the CTL were restimulated with irradiated MPC-11 cells at responder to stimulator ratios of 50:1. Ten days after the secondary in vitro stimulation, the CTL were resuspended in media supplemented with IL2 derived from Con A stimulated rat spleen cells. The resulting CTLL have been maintained in exponential growth cultures for approximately one year with continued addition of IL2. To establish their antigenic specificities and lytic activities, these lines have been tested, in vitro, in chromium-release assays and, in vivo, in Winn assays, for their ability to lyse various tumor targets.

Suppressor T-cell lines, as well as NK-cell lines, have been developed from spleen and/or lymph node cells that were removed from the appropriate animals and placed in tissue culture supplemented with IL2. For these particular lines, no in vitro antigen stimulation was employed during the induction period. The resulting T-cell lines have been tested in both in vitro and in vivo functional assays. The resulting suppressor T-cell lines have been evaluated for in vivo suppressor activity within the ultraviolet light tumor system (8), and the NK lines were defined by their cytotoxic activity against NK susceptible targets. Using conventional limiting dilution techniques (14, 15), many of these lines have now been cloned.

Although a number of IL2 sources are currently being evaluated for their effectiveness in maintaining our various continuous T-cell lines, two sources are routinely used. The most common source of IL2 used in our laboratory is that derived from Con A stimulated rat spleen cells (30). Briefly, spleen cells from Sprague Dawley rats, suspended at 10^6 cells/ml, are incubated in 100 ml cultures for 46 hours in Dulbecco's MEM containing 5% FCS, antibiotics, and 5 μg/ml of Con A. Our second source of IL2 is from the Con A stimulation of the T-T hybridoma FS6 (an IL2 producing cell line) (18). The tissue culture conditions are the same as those described for the rat splenocytes except that serum-free media is used and the incubation period is only 24 hours. At the end of the incubation period, the cell suspensions are centrifuged at 2000 xg for 10 minutes, and the supernatants are tested for their ability to stimulate the growth of CTLL-2 (13) and HT2 (a helper-cell line generated by J. A. Watson).

Flow cytometry analysis was used to determine the cell surface phenotypes of our different continuous T-cell lines. Characterizations

were made using either the Los Alamos National Laboratories (LANL)
multiparameter cell sorter or a FACS III cell sorter (Becton Dickinson).
When it was necessary to correlate cell volume with degrees of
fluorescence intensity after staining with different reagents, the
LANL equipment was used. Monoclonal antibodies against Thy 1.2, Lyt-1,
Lyt-2, Lyt-3, ThB, T30, and Fl (a reagent that detects T and B cell
subpopulations) were provided by Drs. J. Ledbetter and L. A. Herzenberg
(19, 22). FITC-goat anti-rat Ig was used as the second step reagent
with these particular monoclonal antibodies. The continuous lines were
also tested for the presence of membrane Ig by FITC-sheep anti-mouse
kappa; Ia antigens by ATH anti-ATL serum followed by FITC-goat anti-mouse
IgG1; and Fc receptors with a complex of FITC-BSA complexed to rabbit
IgG anti-BSA.

CONTINUOUS CELL LINES

Cytotoxic T-Cells

For some time emphasis in our laboratory has been placed on identifying the various tumor associated antigens (TAA) expressed by
plasmacytomas (PCT), in an attempt to determine their potential for the
in vitro induction of cytotoxic T-lymphocytes (CTL) that could then be
used in adoptive immunotherapy programs. The TAA that have been
identified, using conventional in vitro sensitization schemes and
assaying for lysis of various tumor targets, include: unique antigens
found on individual PCT (23), several common TAA such as oncofetal
antigens (7), common antigens shared by all PCT that are either H-2
restricted (5) or non-restricted (3), and common antigens shared by
PCT and T-lymphomas (4). While in vitro cytotoxicity by CTL against
these TAA is easily demonstrated, in vivo activity is not. For example,
anti-MPC-11 CLT are capable of in vitro function, as shown by their
ability to lyse chromium-labeled targets. Furthermore, these CTL
exhibit in vivo function when used in Winn type assays. However,
attempts to adoptively transfer immunity with anti-MPC-11 CTL indicates
that these cells do not mediate rejection of a MPC-11 tumor challenge
(2). Thus, to further analyze the CTL response to various PCT-TAA, and
possibly facilitate the use of these cells in immunotherapy procedures,
continuous T-lymphocyte lines were established and cloned so that
specific populations of cells directed against single antigenic determinants could be studied. The induction procedure for the generation of
continuous CTLL was similar to that which was used to generate PCT
specific CTL and is outlined in the experimental approach section.
Three separate anti-MPC-11 CTLL have been established in our laboratory
and are designated CTLL-1, 2 and 3 (13). CTLL-1 and 2 are syngeneic to
MPC-11, being generated from BALB/c.By splenocytes, while CTLL-3 is
semi-sygeneic, arising from (BALB/c x C56BL/6)F$_1$ spleen cells.

A consistant finding with these three CTLL is increased lytic
activity against MPC-11 compared to that of primary CTL (13). This
relationship was constant over a range of effector to target ratios
(Table 1). It is possible that the discrepancy in lytic activity between
the CTLL and primary CTL may reflect the differences between primary and
secondary in vitro tumor immune responses. A second difference we have
observed is in the range of antigen specificities recognized by the
various CTLL compared to primary CTL populations (Table 2). Although
the primary CTL response toward PCT-TAA appears to be heterogeneous in

TABLE 1

LYTIC ACTIVITY OF CTLL AND CTL POPULATIONS AGAINST MPC-11

Cytotoxic T-Cell Population[a]	CTL:Target Ratio[b]			
	1.25	2.5	5	10
1 CTLL-1	8	15	20	N.D.
CTLL-2	11	17	30	60
CTL (BALB/c)	0	2	6	10
2 CTLL-3	78	85	90	95
CTL (BALB/c x C57BL/6)F_1	5	10	20	40

[a]CTLL lines 1, 2, and 3 are compared to their appropriate CTL control. All CTLL and primary CTL were induced *in vitro* against MPC-11.
[b]Data is presented as percent specific lysis of MPC-11.

nature, i.e., directed toward numerous specificities, a limited number of antigenic determinants are recognized by the CTLL. The MPC-11 unique or H-2 restricted PCT antigens appear to be the only determinants recognized by CTLL-1. In contrast, CTLL-2 and 3 possess functional specificities for both the H-2 restricted and non-restricted PCT-TAA. CTLL-2 was the only continuous cell line that recognized antigenic determinants shared by PCT and T-lymphomas.

To correlate CTLL function with the expression of known T-cell surface markers, CTLL-2 and 3 were phenotyped using monoclonal antibodies and FACS analysis (13). A summary of these analyses is presented in Table 3. Both cell lines were positive for all the T-cell markers and negative for all B-cell markers tested. Although very low levels of Lyt-1 expression by CTLL 2 were occasionally noted over time, both CTLL-2 and CTLL-3 are now considered to be Thy-1.2$^+$, Lyt-1$^-$, Lyt-2$^+$, and Lyt-3$^+$. In addition to its variable expression of Lyt-1, the cell densities of Thy-1.2 and Lyt-2 expressed by CTLL-2 also fluctuated. With this marked variation in surface marker expression by CTLL-2, an attempt was made, using this line, to determine if the expression of Lyt-2 correlated with cytotoxic activity against MPC-11 (12). When Lyt-2 bright and dim subpopulations of CTLL-2 were sorted by FACS and then tested for their ability to lyse MPC-11, it became apparent that Lyt-2 expression and lytic activity may be unrelated (Table 4). The CTLL-2 Lyt-2 dim cells possessed the same degree of lytic activity as the Lyt-2 bright and parental CTLL-2 cell lines. Clearly, these data suggest that the expression of Lyt-2 by CTLL-2 does not necessarily correlate with its ability to either recognize or lyse tumor cells.

To determine if the CTLL were capable of *in vivo* function, a Winn assay was performed using our CTLL and MPC-11 tumor cells (13). When CTLL-2 or CTLL-3 clone 3G10 cells were mixed at a ratio of 1:1 with MPC-11·cells and injected subcutaneously into syngenic mice, the animals were protected against tumor growth. In contrast, when MPC-11 tumor cells and CTLL-3 cells were injected separately, no protection occurs and the tumor grew at the same rate as in normal, untreated control animals. Combined with earlier results, showing a marked difference in the ability of primary CTL to function in Winn assays versus tests involving the intravenous adoptive transfer of immunity, it appears that a defect in the homing mechanism may be associated with *in vitro* induced CTL and CTLL. Earlier experiments to address this point have been performed using chromium-labeled normal splenocytes and CTL to determine their tissue distribution following I.V. injection (2).

TABLE 2. ANTIGENIC SPECIFICITIES OF CTL

CTL Population[a]	Inducing Tumor[b]	Antigen Specificity[c]	Targets[d]	Blockers[e]	Reference[f]
Primary CTL	C1.18	PCT unique TAA	C1.18	C1.18	23
	HPC-10	H-2 restricted PCT-Taa	HPC-6, HPC-10	HPC-6, HPC-10	3
	MPC-11	H-2 non-restricted PCT-TAA	HPC-108, C1.18	HPC-108, HPC-6, C1.18	3
	HPC-6	PCT/T-lymphoma shared TAA	WEHI 22	WEHI 22, WEHI 7*	4
CTLL-1	MPC-11	PCT unique or H-2 restricted PCT-TAA	MPC-11	N.D.	13
CTLL-2	MPC-11	H-2 restricted PCT-TAA H-2 non-restricted PCT-TAA PCT/T-lymphoma shared TAA	MPC-11, MOPC-315 C1.18, PHC-209 WEHI 7	N.D.	13
CTLL-3	MPC-11	H-2 restricted PCT-TAA H-2 non-restricted PCT-TAA	MPC-11, MOPC-315 HPC-209	MPC-11, MOPC-315 C1.18	13

[a]The in vitro induction of primary CTL and CTLL against plasmacytomas (PCT) is described in the experimental approach section.

[b]Tumors used for induction of CTL. These tumors also served as targets in blocking experiments.

[c]Antigen specificities were determined by titering the lytic activities of CTL against chromium labeled tumor targets.

[d]Tumor targets that are lysed by a particular CTL population. MPC-11 and MOPC-315, BALB/c $H-2^d$ plasmacytoma; HPC-209, BALB/c $H2^g$ plasmacytoma; C1.18, C3H $H-2^k$ plasmacytoma; WEHI 7 and WEHI 22, BALB/c $H-2^d$ T-lymphomas; HPC-6 and HPC-10, NZB $H-2^b$ plasmacytomas.

[e]Tumors listed as blockers were capable of inhibiting the lysis of ^{51}Cr-labeled target cells by the CTL, evidence suggesting shared antigenic determinants. (*) These tumors blocked the lysis of WEHI 112, an NZB T-lymphoma, by (NZB x C57BL)F_1 anti-HPC-10 CTL. N.D. indicates the blocking experiment was not done.

[f]Data presented in the Table was compiled from published reports listed in the reference section.

(*) Burton, R.C. and Warner, N.L., 1980, J. Natl. Cancer Inst. 65:431.

TABLE 3

CELL SURFACE PHENOTYPES OF CTLL LINES

Cell Surface Marker[a]	CTLL-2	CTLL-3
Thy-1.2		+
Lyt-1	+[b]/-	-
Lyt-2	+	+
Lyt-3.2	+	+
ThB	-	-
T30	+	+
F1	-	-
M.Ig	-	-
Fc receptor	-	-
Ia	-	-

[a]FACS analysis was used to determine the expression of a surface marker. The monoclonal antibodies and antisera used are described in the experimental approach section.
[b]The symbol (+) indicates that the CTLL expresses the particular marker; (-), the marker is not expressed; and (+/-), with reanalysis over a period of time the expression of the marker is variable.

TABLE 4

CORRELATION BETWEEN LYTIC ACTIVITY AND Lyt-2 EXPRESSION BY CTLL-2

CTLL Population[a]	Percent Lyt-2 Positive Cells[b]	Lytic Activity[c]
Parental CTLL-2	94	10.8 ± 1.1
Left sort	5	21.2 ± 2.9
Right sort	98	17.7 ± 0.6

[a]Parental CTLL-2 was sorted by FACS into Lyt-2 dim (left sort: channels 128-148) and Lyt-2 bright (right sort: channels 203-255) populations.
[b]The sorted populations were reanalyzed immediately following the sort to determine the percentage of Lyt-2 positive cells in each population.
[c]Percent specific lysis ± standard deviation of chromium-labeled MPC-11 target cells at a CTLL:target ratio of 4:1 run in triplicate.

While 70% of the normal splenocytes were found in the blood and spleen with 30% in the lung and liver two hours after injection, only 30% of the CTL could be recovered from the blood and spleen with 70% being trapped in the lung and liver. An alternative explanation, however, could be that normal animals may lack the appropriate "activated" cell subsets to provide the necessary cell-interactions with CTLL that result in an effective in vivo response. Glasebrook et al. (16) have shown that by providing the appropriate "help" with non-cytotoxic cloned continuous helper cell lines or T-cell growth factor, alloantigen reactive CTLL are induced to proliferate and express cytolytic activity. Furthermore, this "help" can not be provided by antigen alone.

Suppressor T-Cells
    It has been suggested that immunoregulatory mechanisms may provide a means for tumors to escape elimination by the host's immune system (25). The use of syngeneic tumors induced by ultraviolet light (UV) has become a major experimental system for studying these types of host-tumor interactions. It is well established that the majority of UV-tumors are

rejected when transplanted into normal syngeneic mice (9, 20). These UV-regressor (UV^r) tumors will grow progressively, however, when implanted into syngeneic animals exposed to subcarcinogenic doses of UV (9). This UV-induced tumor-susceptible state has been shown to be mediated by tumor antigen-specific (Roberts, et al., manuscript in preparation; 32), Ia^+, radiosensitive, suppressor T-lymphocytes (T_s- cells) (10). Thus, the standard method used to assay for UV-induced T_s-cell activity has been to adoptively transfer the UV tumor susceptible state to normal syngeneic mice with spleen cells from UV-treated animals (8). As a result, the normal recipients of UV-induced T_s-cells are no longer capable of mounting a rejection response directed toward a UV^r-tumor implant. This type of suppression appears to be tumor-specific, since UV-treated mice are not panimmunosuppressed as established by a number of immunologic criteria (21, 31).

In an attempt to generate a continuous UV-induced T_s-cell line, spleen cells from UV-treated BALB/c.WEHI mice were passed over a nylon wool column and the nonadherent cell fraction was placed in tissue culture media containing IL2 derived from the T-T hybridoma cell line FS6. The resulting cell line (UV1) received no antigen stimulation in vitro and has been maintained by continual feedings and passages with FS6 derived IL2. FACS analysis revealed that UV1 expresses a Thy-1.2 positive, Lyt-1, 2 and 3 negative phenotype (Table 7). None of the B-cell or macrophage markers that have been tested are expressed by UV1. Of most interest was our finding that UV1 is capable of functioning in vivo. Following an injection of UV1 cells, normal syngeneic mice were rendered susceptible to the growth of a UV^r-tumor, CS-11 (Table 5). To our knowledge this is the first report of a continuous T-cell line that is capable of in vivo function. Studies are currently underway to determine if UV1 is indeed representative of the UV-induced T_s-cell population.

TABLE 5

ADOPTIVE TRANSFER OF UV-TUMOR SUSCEPTIBILITY WITH UV1

Animals[a]	Adoptive Transfer[b]	Tumor Challenge[c]	Number of TBA/ Number of Mice Challenged[d]
Normal	3×10^7 UV1 cells	CS-11	3/5
Normal	-	CS-11	0/5
UV-treated	-	CS-11	5/5

[a]Normal = normal BALB/c.WEHI. UV-treated = normal BALB/c WEHI exposed to ultraviolet light for 30 mins/day, 5 days/week, for 8 weeks prior to tumor challenge.
[b]Adoptive transfer was made by injecting 3×10^7 UV1 cells suspended in 0.3 ml serum-free PBS into the lateral tail vein of each animal prior to tumor challenge.
[c]Subcutaneous, trocar implants of 1 mm^3 tumor fragments were made with the syngeneic UV-regressor tumor CS-11.
[d]Number of tumor bearing mice/total number of animals challenged at 30 days after the tumor implant.

Natural Killer Cells

A major interest in our laboratory has been concerned with identifying the differentiation lineage and subtypes of natural killer (NK) cells (34). To assist with these studies, attempts have been made to

TABLE 6

NATURAL KILLER ACTIVITY OF NK1 AND UV1

Experiment	Continuous Cell Line[a]	E:T[b]	Target Cells[c]			
			YAC-1	HTX	WEHI-22	WEHI-164
1	NK1	100:1	34.7 ± 1.1	48.3 ± 9.2	24.6 ± 9.5	39.3 ± 7.3[d]
		50:1	0 ± 1.6	26.3 ± 4.1	0 ± 1.4	1.0 ± 1.3
2	UV1	100:1	29.9 ± 2.4	24.4 ± 2.4	24.3 ± 2.4	4.2 ± 2.4
		50:1	17.8 ± 2.1	11.5 ± 2.6	20.7 ± 1.7	0 ± 1.9
		25:1	9.1 ± 0.6	3.3 ± 0.5	13.0 ± 1.7	0 ± 1.3
3	NK1	100:1	13.3 ± 1.4	15.5 ± 0.9	15.5 ± 2.7	0.1 ± 0.3
		50:1	10.6 ± 0.2	17.4 ± 0.7	13.0 ± 0.1	0.7 ± 0.9
		25:1	8.8 ± 1.0	15.6 ± 0.5	6.0 ± 0	1.0 ± 2.3
	UV1	100:1	20.3 ± 1.7	15.5 ± 0.6	29.5 ± 1.8	0 ± 2.3
		50:1	7.8 ± 1.2	7.1 ± 1.2	19.9 ± 0.1	0 ± 0.9
		25:1	5.3 ± 0.1	1.1 ± 0	12.9 ± 0.2	0 ± 0.5

[a] The origin of these two continuous cell lines is described in the text. NK1 is the natural killer cell line derived from BALB/c nude spleen cells. UV1 was established from the nylon wool non-adherent spleen cell population of a UV-treated BALB/c.

[b] Effector to target cell ratios of 100:1, 50:1 and 25:1 were run in a 6-hour NK assay.

[c] Data is presented as the percent specific lysis of ^{51}Cr-labeled target cells.

[d] In subsequent repeats WEHI-164 has not been susceptible to lysis by NK1 or UV1.

generate continuous NK-cell lines. An example of this type of continuous cell line is NK1. This particular line was established by culturing normal splenocytes from BALB/c nudes in the presence of IL2. The resulting NK1 line possesses lytic activity against a number of known NK-susceptible targets (Table 6). In addition to its apparent suppressor T-cell function, UV1 was also found to have NK-activity. Although the levels of lysis are somewhat different, the target specificities of NK1 and UV1 are similar (Table 6). Like UV1, NK1 was shown to be Thy-1.2$^+$, Lyt-1$^-$, 2$^-$ and 3$^-$ (Table 7). At present the continuous NK lines are being compared to determine differences in target specificities and lytic activities as correlated with the expression of various surface markers.

TABLE 7

ABILITY OF DIFFERENT IL2 SOURCES TO SUPPORT GROWTH OF T-CELL LINES

Cell Lines	Surface Markers[a]				Functional Type[b]	Growth Requirements[c]		
	Thy-1.2	Lyt-1	Lyt-2	Lyt-3		RTCGF	FS6	PBL-PMA/Con A
CTLL-2	+	+/-	+	+	T_c	+++	+++	+++
HT2	+	N.D.	N.D.	N.D.	(T_b)	+++	+++	+++
NK1	+	-	-	-	NK	++	N.S.	N.S.
UV1	+	-	-	-	T_s/NK	+	+	N.T.

[a]Surface markers determined by FACS analysis. A +, indicates expression of the marker; -, the marker is not expressed; +/-, marker expression is variable; and N.D., not determined.
[b]Functional T-cell subsets were established by various *in vitro* and *in vivo* assays.
[c]IL2 growth requirements for the different lines were determined by maintaining a particular line in titrated amounts of the various IL2 sources to determine its maximum rate of growth and cell viability. A +++, indicates the cell line requires 40-50% of the particular IL2 source to maintain growth; ++, indicates a requirement of 20-30%; and +, indicates that a 10% IL2 supplement is required. N.S. signifies that the cell line could not be maintained with that IL2 source; and N.T. was not tested. The sources of IL2 tested were: RTCGF, the tissue culture supernatant from Con A stimulated rat splenocytes; FS6, supernatant from Con A stimulation of the FS6 cell line; and PBL-PMA/Con A, a IL2 containing supernatant produced by human peripheral blood leukocytes at 10^6/ml stimulated with 7 µg/ml Con A and 4 ng/ml PMA in media containing 5% human plasma for 48 hours.

CONCLUSIONS

Induction protocols were followed to develop continuous cell lines from normal spleen and lymph node cell populations. Although CTLL were established using *in vitro* antigen stimulation, suppressor T-cell and NK cell lines were developed from lymphocyte populations taken directly from the animal and placed in tissue culture supplemented with IL2, without *in vitro* antigen stimulation. Thus, the eventual cell lines that emerged appear to represent those subpopulations of cells that were activated within the animal at the time of removal, as determined by conventional immunologic assays.

Attempts to correlate cell surface phenotypes, using available monoclonal antibodies and antisera, with specific immunologic function have not provided sufficient information to establish a reference catalog that can be used to separate different T-cell subpopulations from the normal lymphoid population. One example is the variation in Lyt-2 expression by different CTLL. Although Lyt-2 has been ascribed to a surface marker on cytotoxic T-cells (6), for our particular CTLL there appears to be no correlation between Lyt-2 expression and lytic activity. This finding is consistant with data reported earlier (16) which indicate that neither Lyt-2 nor Lyt-3 are required for the lethal hit in T-cell mediated cytolysis, although they may contribute to the functional antigen receptor for alloantigen recognition by CTLL. In the case of CTLL-2, which has functional specificity for syngeneic tumor antigens, Lyt-2 is not required for either antigen recognition or cytolysis. Thus, using a single marker such as Lyt-2 as the sole criterion to define all CTL subsets may be inappropriate.

One aspect regarding the continued development of continuous T-cell lines centers around their potential usefulness in immunotherapy procedures. Aside from some assays using CTLL, continuous T-cell lines appear to be incapable of mediating an in vivo effect (2, 13). This could be due to either a defect in homing mechanisms, associated with T-cells held in tissue culture that are fully differentiated, or the inability of these cells to cooperate with other cell populations required in mediating an immunologic effect. Using UV1, the continuous suppressor T-cell line, these questions might now be addressed. Although UV1 may be mediating its in vivo effect through the production of suppressor factors, a mechanism shown for T_s-cells in other tumor systems (26), it may be possible, by comparing it to other continuous lines, to identify differences in cell surface properties that would account for its ability to function in vivo. Experiments have been initiated to evaluate these differences, and possibly provide a mechanism to modulate the surface properties of continuous T-cell lines that would restore their in vivo functional capabilities.

In addition to the development and evaluation of new continuous T-cell lines, we are presently engaged in testing different sources of IL2 for their abilities to provide the appropriate "growth factors" to the different lines. It appears that various cell lines may not only require different sources of IL2, but the amounts that are necessary to maintain growth is widely variable among the different lines (Table 7). By using numerous T-cell lines and different IL2 sources, an experimental model system might be developed to identify a wider range of IL2 like molecules. Combined with antigenic specificities, phenotypic characteristics, and functional properties of different continuous lines, these data may provide insight into the various cellular interactions and immunoregulatory mechanisms involved in different immunologic responses against cancer.

Acknowledgment

This work was supported by Grants CA22268, CA05921, CA06804 and CA27115, awarded by the National Cancer Institute, DHHS.

REFERENCES

1. Baker, P.E., Gillis, S., and Smith, K.A. (1979): J.Exp.Med., 149: 273-278.
2. Burton, R.C., and Warner, N.L. (1977): Cancer Immunol. Immunother., 2:91-99.
3. Burton, R.C., Chism, S.E., and Warner, N.L. (1977): J.Immunol., 118:971-980.
4. Burton, R.C., and Warner, N.L. (1978): Aust.J.Exp.Biol.Med.Sci., 56:587-595.
5. Burton, R.C., and Warner, N.L. (1978): Fed.Proc., 37:1569.
6. Cantor, H., and Boyse, E.A. (1975): J.Exp.Med., 141:1390-1399.
7. Chism, S.E., Burton, R.C., and Warner, N.L. (1976): J.Natl.Cancer Inst., 57:377-387.
8. Daynes, R.A., and Spellman, C.W. (1977): Cell.Immunol., 31:182-187.
9. Daynes, R.A., Spellman, C.W., Woodward, J.G., and Stewart, D.A. (1977): Transplantation, 23:343-348.
10. Daynes, R.A., Schmitt, M.K., Roberts, L.K., and Spellman, C.W. (1979): J.Immunol., 122:2458-2464.
11. Fresno, M., Nabel, G., McVay-Boudreau, L., Furthmayer, H., and Cantor, H. (1981): J.Exp.Med., 153:1246-1259.
12. Giorgi, J.V., and Warner, N.L. (1981): Fed.Proc., 40:956.
13. Giorgi, J.V., and Warner, N.L. (1981): J.Immunol., 126:322-330.
14. Glasebrook, A.L., and Fitch, F.W. (1979): Nature, 278:171-173.
15. Glasebrook, A.L., and Fitch, F.W. (1980): J.Exp.Med., 151:876-895.
16. Glasebrook, A.L., Sarmiento, M., Loken, M.R., Dialynes, D.P., Quintans, J., Eisenberg, L., Lutz, C.T., Wilde, D., and Fitch, F.W. (1980): Immunol.Rev., 54:219-266.
17. Gouling, E., Blokland, E., van Rood, J., Charmot, D., Malissen, B., and Mawas, C. (1980): J.Exp.Med., 152:182-190.
18. Harwell, L., Skidmord, B., Marrack, P., and Kappler, J.W. (1980): J.Exp.Med., 152:893-904.
19. Herzenberg, L.A., Herzenberg, L.A., Black, S.J., Loken, M.R., Okumura, K., Van der Loo, W., Osborne, B.A., Hewgill, D., Goding, J.W., Gutman, G., and Warner, N.L. (1976): Cold Spring Harbor Symp.Quant.Biol., XLI:33-45.
20. Kripke, M.L. (1974): J.Natl.Cancer Inst., 53:1333-1336.
21. Kripke, M.L., Lofgreen, J.S., Bread, J., Jessup, J.M., and Fisher, M.S. (1977): J.Natl. Cancer Inst., 59:1227-1230.
22. Ledbetter, J.A., and Herzenberg, L.A. (1979): Immunol.Rev., 47: 63-90.
23. MacKenzie, M.R., Burton, R.C., and Warner, N.L. (1978): Int.J. Cancer, 21:789-795.
24. Morgan, D.A., Ruscetti, F.W., and Gallo, R.C. (1976): Science, 193: 1007-1008.
25. Naor, D. (1979): Adv.Cancer Res., 29:45-125.
26. Perry, L.L., Benacerraf, B., and Greene, M.I. (1978): J.Immunol., 121:2144-2147.
27. Rosenberg, S.A., Schwarz, S., and Spiess, P.J. (1978): J.Immunol., 121:1951-1955.
28. Ruscetti, F.W., Morgan, D.A., and Gallo, R.C. (1977): J.Immunol., 119:131-138.
29. Schreier, M.H., and Tees, R. (1980): Int.Arch.Allergy Appl.Immunol., 61:227-237.
30. Smith, K.A. (1980): Contemp.Topics Immunobiol., 11:139-155.

31. Spellman, C.W., Woodward, J.G., and Daynes, R.A. (1977):
     Transplantation, 24:112-119.
32. Spellman, C.W., and Daynes, R.A. (1978): Cell.Immunol., 38:25-34.
33. Strausser, J.L., and Rosenberg, S.A. (1978): J.Immunol., 121:
     1491-1495.
34. Tai, A., and Warner, N.L. (1980): In: Natural Cell-Mediated
     Immunity Against Tumors, edited by R. Herberman, pp. 241-264.
     Academic Press, Inc.
35. Watson, J.D. (1979): J.Exp.Med., 150:1510-1519.

AUDIENCE DISCUSSION

Dr. Bach: I'm worried that some antisyngeneic tumor cells can kill allogeneic normal targets perhaps based on cross-reactivity which has been demonstrated. Could that be the reason?

Dr. Warner: No. We have used the C3H plasmacytoma and other H2K-bearing tumors (not myelomas) and they are not killed.

Dr. Bach: Have you shown that cultured cells will be effective in immunotherapy?

Dr. Warner: Not with our myeloma tumors.

Dr. Bach: What about cells immunized in vivo and not cultured?

Dr. Warner: All our work has been with cultured cells.

Dr. Bach: You also don't know whether the tumors are susceptible to therapy.

Dr. Warner: All our tumors are very susceptible to an in vivo induced state of tumor-specific immunity.

Dr. Nabholz: We have made hybrids between BW5147 which does not express Ly-2 or Ly-3 and two types of H-2 restricted cloned CTL lines, one of which is hapten-specific; the other is MSV-specific. We have obtained a series of hybrids which kill specifically and show the same H-2 restriction pattern as the CTL parent. None of these hybrids express any Ly-2. We could conclude that your suggestion that Ly-2 has something to do with H-2 restriction is wrong. One of the problems with all of these studies (yours, mine, and maybe Fitch's) is that we don't know what it means when a monoclonal antibody no longer reacts with the cells -- the molecules could still be there but be undetected. One should speak not about presence or absence of Ly-2, but of reactivity with a given antibody.

Dr. Warner: I agree.

Dr. Nabholtz: The antibody may not even bind to the cell at all, but still be there but be covered up by a change in the carbohydrate moiefy.

Dr. Warner: That is an alternative explanation.

Dr. Bonavida: The fact that some clones are Lyt 2⁻ and express cytotoxicity does not rule out a role of Lyt 2 antigens in cytotoxicity. It is possible that some of the clones may have bypassed or circumvented an essential step (i.e. involving Lyt 2 antigens) and still retained cytotoxic activity.

Dr. Warner: I agree. The molecule on the surface may not be essential.

Dr. Bonavida: Regarding the generation of clones which lack a surface marker, can one draw conclusions regarding the role of such markers and functional activity? Are clones to be considred analogous to in vivo cells or should they be considered aberrant?

Dr. Warner: That is a major point about the surface markers -- we've heard today of several which have been considered aberrant expressions.

We know little about the function of these surface markers, whether it be T8 or LY2 in a suppressor/cytotoxic function.

Dr. Greenberg: In the lysis by apparently nonrestricted CTL, it's conceivable that those cells might be recognizing a cross-reactive H-2 determinant. Have you looked at blocking with antibody to H-2 and shown that it has no effect on cytolysis?

Dr. Warner: The plasmacytoma is the only H2K tumor that is capable of being killed. Unfortunately, it's the only H2K plasmacytoma we have. It doesn't kill T lymphomas and other cells known to have H2K.

Dr. Greenberg: But if it's recognizing a tumor antigen in association with, for example, a shared public H2K determinant, it is conceivable that your activities actually represent H-2 restricted lysis.

Dr. Warner: That's a possibility. We need other H2K myelomas to look at that.

Dr. Green: Did you say that the UVI suppressor line did not kill normal thymocytes?

Dr. Warner: We haven't looked at normal thymocyte targets. The only cells it kills are tumors that we quote as being "NK sensitive type targets." In our hands, none of the UV established tumors have been susceptible to NK killing.

The Potential Role of T Cells in Cancer Therapy.
edited by A. Fefer and A. Goldstein.
Raven Press. New York © 1982.

Cloned T Cell Lines with Multiple Functions

Gunther Dennert and John F. Warner

Department of Cancer Biology, The Salk Institute for Biological Studies, San Diego, California 92138

One of the well accepted dogmas in cellular immunology is the mono-functionality of regulatory and effector T lymphocytes (3, 4, 9). This line of thinking has led to experiments aimed at delineating T cell subsets, each endowed with certain functions and cell surface markers which interact in a complicated network of regulatory lymphocytes. Recent advances in tissue culture techniques have made possible the establishment of T cell lines and clones with functional activity, which could serve as a powerful tool in characterizing the functions and cell surface markers of the many T cells which play a role in the immune system. Here we report the cloning of a T cell line established and maintained against H-2 alloantigens by antigenic selection. This cell line was cloned by limiting dilution, subsequently assayed for its functions and analyzed with regard to its Lyt phenotype.

RESULTS AND DISCUSSION

Allospecific T cell line C.C3.11.75 is a Balb/c ($H-2^d$) anti-C3H ($H-2^k$) cell line which was established in 1975 and maintained continuously by antigenic stimulation (6). The cell line recognizes a private specificity in the H-2 IA subregion in all functional assays, including cell proliferation, cell mediated cytotoxicity, delayed type hypersensitivity (DTH) and helper activity in a humoral response to sheep erythrocytes (5, 7). C.C3.11.75 was cloned by limiting dilution in the presence of 5×10^6 irradiated $H-2^k$ spleen stimulator cells in 1 ml culture tubes containing conditioned medium. This medium consisted of 30% Con A supernatant (Con A CM) prepared from normal spleen cells stimulated for 48 hr with 10 µg/ml Con A, and 70% fresh RPMI 1640 medium supplemented with fetal bovine serum (5%), antibiotics, L-glutamine, sodium pyruvate and non-essential amino acids. Initially the cell line was cultured at 100 cells per tube followed by reculturing at 10 cells and 2 cells per tube and finally at 0.5 cells per tube. Several cloned sublines were assayed for their cell surface markers by flow microfluorometry employing monoclonal antibody. The phenotype of these sublines was identical to that of the parent line (12) in that it was Thy 1.2^+, Lyt 1^+2^-, and $T200^+$. In functional assays we initially tested eight

221

individual sublines of the 2-cell per tube cloning stage. If challenged
with H-2^k stimulator cells, these sublines showed only about a three-
fold stimulation of cell proliferation compared to a thirty-fold effect
with the parent line. This rather small effect with cloned sublines is
presumably a reflection of the fact that the sublines, in contrast to
the parent line, are dependent on both Con A CM and stimulator cells for
optimal proliferation. In the cytotoxic reaction, all sublines showed
specific cytotoxicity on targets carrying the IA^k antigens, while H-2^d
or H-2^b targets showed no lysis. These results are presented in Fig. 1

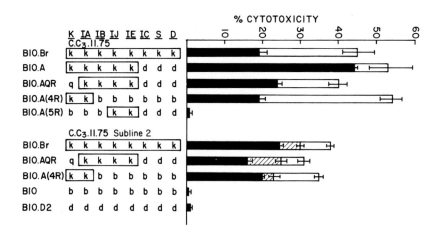

FIG. 1. Cytolytic specificity of line C.C3.11.75 and subline 2.
Cytolytic effector cells were assayed on day 3 LPS spleen blast cells
in a 3 hr ^{51}Cr release assay at a ratio of 50:1 ☐ and 15:1 ■ for
C.C3.11.75 and in a 5 hr assay in the case of subline 2 at ratios of
10:1 ☐, 5:1 ▨, and 2:1 ■ (7).

where the effects with subline 2 are compared to those of the parent
line. Interestingly, very similar results were seen when the cloned
sublines were tested for activity in the DTH reaction. Subline 2
causes a strong DTH reaction if injected with IA^k positive stimulator
cells into the footpad of Balb/c mice (Fig. 2). Hence in both cell
mediated assays, namely cytotoxicity and DTH, the cloned sublines
express different activities with similar specificity. Even more surprising was the finding that the sublines when mixed with anti-Thy 1.2
+ C'-treated spleen cells (B cells) and sheep erythrocytes, were able
to stimulate a humoral antibody response provided the B cells expressed
the IA^k antigens (Fig. 3). Obviously, the finding that cloned cell
lines may express cytotoxicity, DTH and allohelp, three functions
originally assigned to three distinct subsets of T cells, raises an
important question of whether these sublines are true clones.
Conceivably cloning at two cells per tube could result in cell lines

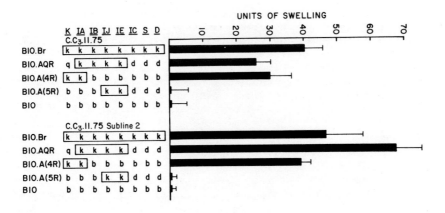

FIG. 2. Specificity of DTH reaction caused by line C.C3.11.75 and subline 2. C.C3.11.75 (10^6) or subline 2 (5×10^5) responder cells were
mixed with 2×10^7, 3000 r-irradiated spleen cells and injected into the
footpads of Balb/c mice. The differences in swelling were plotted in
units for the 24 hr timepoint (15).

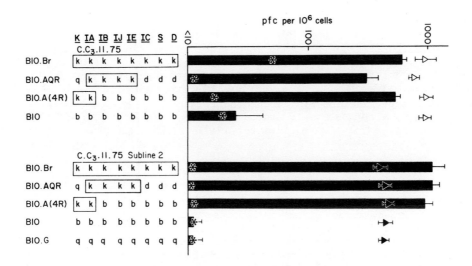

FIG. 3. Specificity of allohelp reaction of line C.C3.11.75 and subline
2. Cells were treated with mitomycin C and assayed for their ability to
give help to various B cells in the primary response to SRBC.
* = background response of B cells to SRBC. Δ = response of B cells
caused by nylon column purified allogeneic Balb/c T cells. This serves
as a control for optimal B cell responsiveness. B cells ($5-8 \times 10^5$/well,
anti Thy 1.2 + C'-treated spleen cells) were cultured with optimal
numbers of cells from the T cell line or Balb/c T cells in Falcon 3040
Microtest II plates in a 0.1 ml final volume plus SRBC (0.1%) (7).

consisting of two different cell types, although the probability of two cell types rather than one being responsible for the various activities assayed in the case of seven isolated tests is very low with P = 0.012. In order to verify this, therefore, subline 2 was recloned at 0.5 cells per tube and three individual isolates, C.C3.11.75/2 E6, C.C3.11.75/2 B10, and C.C3.11.75/2 H5 were assayed in the three functional assays (Table 1). These three sublines showed IA^k-specific activities similar to those exhibited by the parent cell line and subline 2 in all three assays using B10, B10.AQR, and B10.A(4R) spleen cells. It therefore appears that the sublines tested are in fact clones of T cells with multiple functions.

These findings raise several important questions. The first question is whether or not this multifunctionality is a general property of T cells. C.C3.11.75 has been in culture since 1975 and has retained a normal chromosome set. Yet it is possible that the cell line has become deregulated, thereby expressing several rather than one predominant functional activity. A second question is whether Lyt 2 can be the T killer cell receptor in view of the fact that this cytolytic cell line is Lyt 1^+2^- (12). Obviously the failure of detecting Lyt 2 antigen on these cells would strongly argue against Lyt 2 being the T killer cell receptor. An interesting point put forward by these results is whether there is in fact a correlation between T cell function and Lyt phenotype, since cytolytic T cells are usually of Lyt 2^+ phenotype. Recently it was reported that T killer cells sensitized to IA antigens in a primary mixed lymphocyte culture are high in Lyt 1 and low in Lyt 2 antigen (13). This demonstrates that the cell surface phenotype of our cell line is not aberrant and suggests that there is no correlation between Lyt phenotype and T cell function. Yet, as pointed out previously (12), it is possible that the Lyt phenotype of T cells correlates with antigen recognition. Thus T cells specific for H-2KD region antigens may be Lyt 2^+ and T cells specific for H-2I region antigens may be Lyt 1^+2^-. Further experiments will show whether this hypothesis is tenable or not.

A very important question regarding this cell line is whether the functions observed are representative of the functions seen with other T cells. The cytolytic reaction clearly requires cell-cell contact and lysis is not caused by lymphotoxin released into the cell culture supernatant. Therefore there is no indication that this function is different from that of the other T killer cells. The DTH reaction induced by these cells exhibits the time kinetics and histological characteristics of a DTH reaction (15). An interesting feature of this reaction is that it is H-2 unrestricted while being specific. The H-2 unrestricted nature of DTH reactions to H-2 coded antigens has previously been reported by Smith and Miller (10). The question whether the DTH reaction caused by these cells is identical to that of other T cells cannot be answered, however, since this reaction is insufficiently defined. The helper activity of the cell line clearly does not require cell-cell contact between the B and T cell. We have previously shown that the C.C3.11.75 cell line, upon antigenic stimulation, releases activities capable of stimulating B cells for antibody synthesis (14). Consequently there is no conceptual problem of a cytolytic T cell being able to also provide helper activity. Yet there is the question of whether the helper activity displayed by this cell line is similar to that of other T helper cells. Only further experiments will show whether this is the case. Recently an attempt was made to characterize the T cell replacing activity released by this cell line upon antigenic

TABLE 1

Functional activity of clones derived from C.C3.11.75 subline 2

Function	Cytotoxicity*			DTH*			Allohelp*		
Clone	E6	B10	H5	E6	B10	H5	E6	B10	H5
B10 (bbbbbbb)	3 ± 0.1	1 ± 0.5	< 1	5 ± 3	3 ± 4	7 ± 5	300	350	390
B10.(AQR) (qkkkkddd)	25 ± 0.3	31 ± 1.2	29 ± 2.1	29 ± 3	35 ± 5	38 ± 4	1800	1200	1100
B10.A(4R) (kkbbbbbb)	28 ± 0.5	32 ± 0.01	35 ± 0.3	41 ± 1	31 ± 7	33 ± 6	1100	1400	1200

*Functional assays were done as in Fig. 1, 2, 3. The a/t ratio for the cytotoxicity assay was 3:1 and the 5 hr timepoint is shown. For the DTH reaction, 3×10^5 responder cells were injected per mouse. For the allohelp reaction, 6×10^5 responder cells were titrated with varying numbers of cloned T cells and the optimal responses are given.

stimulation (11). Results showed that release of the activity is dependent on specific stimulation with IA^{k+} stimulator cells but the activity itself is not antigen specific (14). Preliminary fractionation of this activity showed that following ammoniumsulfate precipitation, gel filtration, isoelectric focusing and polyacrylamide gel electrophoresis, activities could be separated which stimulate both B cell proliferation and Ig synthesis or only Ig synthesis (M. Thoman, J. Watson, G. Dennert, unpublished results). Experiments are in progress to further purify this activity to biochemical homogeneity.

In summary, our experiments seem to point to a more flexible nature of T cells regarding their function. There are several recent reports which also support this conclusion. Bianchi et al. (2) isolated a cloned T cell line with both helper and DTH activity. Nabel et al.(8) described a Lyt 1^+2^- T cell clone which displayed the following functions: stimulation of B cells for Ig synthesis, induction of bone marrow cells to produce granulocyte and macrophage colonies and stimulation of T cell proliferation. Recently Lin and Askonas (cited in reference 1) isolated a cloned T cell line specific for influenza virus infected targets which was cytolytic and active in the DTH reaction. The usual observation, therefore, that T cells are generally monofunctional in nature, could be due to cyclic regulation of these functions, for example, via interaction with antigen or regulatory lymphocytes.

Acknowledgement. We thank Cheryl Bry for excellent technical assistance. This work was supported by U. S. Public Service Grants CA 15581 and CA 19334 (G. D.) and a grant by the American Cancer Society #IM-284 (G. D.).

REFERENCES

1. Ada, G. L., Leung, K-N., and Ertl, H. (1981): Immunological Rev., 58:5-24.

2. Bianchi, A.T.J., Hooijkaas, H., Benner, R., Tees, R., Nordin, A. A., and Schreier, M. H. (1981): Nature 290:62-63.

3. Cantor, H., and Boyse, E. A. (1977): Cold Spring Harbor Symp. Quant. Biol. 41:23-32.

4. Dennert, G. (1974): Nature (London), 249:358-360.

5. Dennert, G. (1979): Nature, 277:476-477.

6. Dennert, G., and DeRose, M. (1976): J. Immunol., 116:1601-1606.

7. Dennert, G., Swain, S. L., Waterfield, J. D., Warner, J. F., and Dutton, R. W. (1981): Euro. J. Immunol., 11:62-64.

8. Nabel, G., Greenberger, J. S., Sakakeeny, M. A., and Cantor, H. (1981): Proc. Nat. Acad. Sci., 78:1157-1161.

9. Shiku, H., Kisielow,P., Bean, M. A., Takahashi, T., Boyse, E. A., Oettgen, H. F., and Old, L. J. (1975): J. Exp. Med. 141:227-241.

10. Smith, F. I., and Miller, J.F.A.P. (1979): J. Exp. Med. 150:965-976.

11. Swain, S. L., Dennert, G., Warner, J. F., and Dutton, R. W. (1981): Proc. Nat. Acad. Sci. 78:2517-2521.

12. Swain, S. L., Dennert, G., Wormsley, S., and Dutton, R. (1981): Eur. J. Immunol. 3:175-180.

13. Vidovic, D., Juratic A., Nagy, Z., and Klein, J. (1981): Eur. J. Immunol. (in press).

14. Waterfield, J. D., Dennert, G., Swain, S. L., and Dutton, R. (1979): J. Exp. Med. 149:808-814.

15. Weiss, S., and Dennert, G. (1981): J. Immunol. 126:2031-2035.

AUDIENCE DISCUSSION

Dr. Ihle: What is the frequency with which you derive these antigen-independent cloned cells?

Dr. Dennert: It only happened once, a year ago.

Dr. Ihle: Are these independent lines cytotoxic?

Dr. Dennert: No, neither with or without lectin. The only activity which we have seen is helper activity and TRF activity in cell supernatants produced by these cell lines.

Dr. Ihle: Your cell lines are essentially identical to the LY1 positive cell lines that we established with IL 3.

Dr. Bach: Whereas I have nothing against the concept that a single cell may perform the functions of both help and cytotoxicity, your conclusion that you are dealing with a clone -- when the vast majority of your data involves plating of at least two cells per well -- should be stricken from the record. To make such an assertion, one must follow the approach of Michael Widmer, who truly has isolated an apparently helper-independent cytotoxic clone, where the probability of nonclonality is 1×10^{-7}. At the very least, you need confidence of 1×10^{-4} to know that you are dealing with a clone with dramatic dual functions. Have you characterized the populations you are growing for their normal chromosome constitution   ? How do you define DTH? I think your definition is not a classical one and should be discussed.

Dr. Dennert: Judy Johnson in Munich has looked at these lines and particularly the one which has been continuously in culture for six years and found no chromosomal abnormalities by banding.

Dr. Bach: Is that one of the lines with which you demonstrated all these things also?

Dr. Dennert: Yes. Most of the data I showed were with cell lines which were cloned at two cells per well. We examined ten different isolates of this cloning for the various functions, and all displayed all the functions. The p value for these functions being affected by more than one cell is 0.05. Recently, we recloned one of these lines, at 0.05 cells per well, and examined three clones for help, cytolytic activity,

and DTH. The isolates were positive for all three functions. The only
way to do a more conclusive cloning is by isolation of single cells by
micromanipulation. Incidentally, DTH is defined by a swelling reaction
which is maximal at 24 hours and which shows the typical histological
picture of a DTH reaction with massive infiltration by monocytes and
neutrophils, indicating recruitment of host cells into the site of the
reaction.

Dr. Rosenberg: I do not think you can equate your assay with classical
delayed hypersensitivity. There are a large number of irritants that
can cause swelling. When you combine two types of cells, they may die
and release lysozyme, or produce a large number of lymphokines which can
result in swelling.

Dr. Dennert: What would you call it?

Dr. Rosenberg: A nonspecific inflammatory process. If one injected HCl
into the skin one would get swelling but one wouldn't call it delayed-
type hypersensitivity.

Dr. Dennert: Our reaction is specific and depends on specific stimulation.

Dr. Rosenberg: Did you study the histology of the swellings? Did it
look like a delayed hypersensitivity reaction?

Dr. Dennert: Yes.

Dr. Rosenberg: While it's possible that the same clone would have both
proliferative and cytotoxic activity, have others observed this?

Dr. Bach: The clone I mentioned was derived by Dr. Michael Widmer. He
derived a clone -- with the probability of nonclonality being approximately 1×10^{-7} -- which proliferated when stimulated with its target
antigen, which incidentally is the D^d antigen. The cells of the helper-
independent cytotoxic clone produce a factor(s) into the supernatant
which the cells can utilize to grow. This clone is, thus, different
from those isolated by Glasebrook and Fitch.

Dr. Rosenberg: Will it proliferate when it meets DBA antigen?

Dr. Dennert: Yes.

Dr. Fitch: Among the 50 or so clones that we've studied, I don't think
that we found any that did not have either helper or the cytolytic
activity. None had both activities.

Dr. Shu: About 70% of the original clones were not cytolytic. Have you
looked at those clones for helper function?

Dr. Dennert: Yes. All have helper and DTH function.

The Potential Role of T Cells in Cancer Therapy,
edited by A. Fefer and A. Goldstein,
Raven Press, New York © 1982.

Murine T Cell Clones Having Defined Immunological Functions

Frank W. Fitch, John M. Ely, Michael B. Prystowsky,
Deno P. Dialynas, and *Andrew L. Glasebrook

*The Committee on Immunology and the Department of Pathology, The University of Chicago,
Chicago, Illinois 60637; *The Swiss Institute for Experimental Cancer Research,
CH-1066 Epalinges S/Lausanne, Switzerland*

With development of procedures for cloning T lymphocytes, it is now possible to obtain large numbers of homogeneous T lymphocytes having different defined immunological functions. Helper (14,26,33), cytolytic (14,23,26,33), and suppressor (10) T cell clones have been developed. Still other cloned T cells proliferate when stimulated by specific antigens (7,31). These cloned T lymphocytes are proving to be useful for defining the repertoire of antigens recognized by T cells, for characterizing the role of particular cell surface structures for given immunological functions, and for determining the molecular basis for interactions between T lymphocytes and other cells during immune responses. They also have potential usefulness for therapy of tumors and immunodeficiency states and for modulating specific immune responses.

Although T cell clones can be derived and maintained with relative ease, cloned cells obtained by different investigators have displayed rather varied characteristics. Explanations for some of these differences have become evident. The following discussion will compare several methods for deriving T cell clones and will consider the effects of culture conditions on the functional properties of cloned T cells. Some of the expected and unexpected properties of the cloned cells will be described.

CONDITIONS FOR DERIVING AND MAINTAINING T CELL CLONES INFLUENCE THE EASE OF CLONING AND THE CHARACTERISTICS OF CLONED CELLS

Two rather different strategies have been used to derive and maintain T cell clones. Both approaches utilized conditioned medium obtained from activated T lymphocytes. It had been found in 1976, that conditioned medium (CM) obtained from mitogen-stimulated human T lymphocytes could support the sustained growth of T lymphocytes in culture (20). Although the relevant biological activity in such CM usually is attributed to interleukin 2 (IL 2) (also called T cell growth factor), a variety of other biological activities are also mediated by such CM. Since crude culture supernatant fluids or partially purified materials usually have been used to derive and maintain cloned T cells, it is not possible to exclude a role for factors other than IL 2 in the long term growth of cloned cells.

Some T cell clones have been developed using only CM. Often, these clones have been obtained from antigen-stimulated cultures prepared with cells from animals sensitized in vivo. The cultured cells have been exposed repetitively to CM in vitro (1,10,15,21,22,27,34). However, the frequency of T cells capable of growing at low cell density in CM alone seems to be low since it has been necessary to passage cells in bulk cultures for weeks to months before cloning has been successful (15). Frequently, such cultured T cells have been observed to undergo a "crisis" after about two months in culture. When this occurs, they show impaired growth characteristics, and sometimes cultures cannot be maintained. If cells can be "nursed" through such a crisis, they usually demonstrate improved growth and cloning then is possible. However, the great majority of cloned cells capable of sustained growth in CM have shown gross karyotypic abnormalities (4), and some cytolytic clones have shown fluctuating levels and patterns of cytolytic activity (22).

An alternative strategy for developing T cell clones involves the use of stimulating antigen and irradiated adherent cells from lymphoid tissues in addition to CM (2,5,11,12,16,17,32,35). T cell clones have been derived from primary mixed leukocyte culture using this strategy, and cloning efficiency may approach 100% if responding cells from secondary mixed leukocyte cultures are used (12). Irradiated adherent cells from lymphoid tissues appear to serve as "antigen presenting" cells for soluble antigens (7). For alloreactive T cell clones, such adherent cells may provide the source for stimulating alloantigen (14). However, the adherent cells may serve other functions as well, since cloned alloreactive T cells derived using this strategy survive much better when cultured with syngeneic irradiated lymphoid cells and conditioned medium than they do when cultured with conditioned medium alone (12). Adherent cells may be a source of interleukin 1 (IL 1) which promotes production of IL 2 by appropriately stimulated lymphocytes (25), although other functions for adherent cells have not been excluded.

ONLY T CELLS WHICH HAVE BEEN CLONED
SHOULD BE CONSIDERED TO BE CLONED CELLS

Although cells from long term bulk cultures which are capable of sustained growth in CM may appear to be "have cloned themselves" (15), maintenance of cells in long term culture does not insure that such cells actually represent a clone. Indeed, when intentional cloning of a cytolytic mouse T cell "line" was performed after 14 months in continuous culture, at least three distinct cell types were isolated (1). The characteristics of these different cell types were stable in subclones. In other instances, repetitive cloning was necessary before cells isolated from soft agar colonies demonstrated stable and unique phenotypic characteristics (17,30). Thus, it is evident that several different T cells may be maintained simultaneously in long term cultures stimulated with CM. Cells can be assumed to be cloned only if suitable approaches have been used to obtain cloned cells.

Three approaches have been used for cloning T cells. Soft agar with an underlying feeder layer has been used commonly to derive T cell clones (5,22,32,34). However, direct contact between antigen presenting cells and cloned T cells is not possible using the soft agar technique. Also, T cells can migrate within the agar. It may be difficult to be certain that extraneous T cells have not contaminated a colony, either during the culture period or at the time colonies were collected. As noted above, colonies collected from soft agar have been found to contain a mixture of cells in some instances (17,30).

The limiting dilution technique also has been used frequently to clone T cells (12,22,35). Using this approach, it is necessary to plate at fractional cell densities per well in order to be reasonably certain that proliferating cells are clonally distributed. This method facilitates sampling of putative clones for assessment of their functional characteristics before selecting particular cells for expansion. A statistical estimate of the likelihood that a given colony or well represents a clone can be obtained using both the soft agar and limiting dilution methods (24). However, if plating efficiency is low, it may be difficult to be certain that cells having mixed characteristics or unusual phenotypes represent cloned cells.

Micromanipulation also has been used to isolate individual cells for cloning (21). This approach may be particularly useful for subcloning after putative clones that proliferate well have been identified.

VARIANT CELLS CAN AND WILL EMERGE

The growth rate of different cloned T cells varies, depending in part upon culture conditions and upon the characteristics of the particular clone. However, doubling times are usually 24 hours or less. Given this rate of proliferation, it is not unexpected that variant cells will emerge. The use of stimulating antigen together with less than maximal levels of conditioned medium may favor selection of antigen-reactive cells (12,19). Variant cells may arise spontaneously (1 and unpublished observations) or may be induced by treatment of cloned T cells with a mutagen (3). Such variant cells may be useful for particular purposes (3 and unpublished observations). For example, it has been possible to derive variant clones from a cloned cytolytic T cell by selection with antibody and complement after treatment of the cells with the mutagen ethyl methanesulfonate. A clone of variant cells lacking Thy-1.2 expressed the same levels and specificity of cytolytic activity as the parent clone from which it was derived indicating that Thy-1, a convenient cell surface marker for T cells, is not required for expression of cytolytic activity by cytolytic T cells (3). Cloned variant cells lacking Lyt-2 had markedly reduced cytolytic activity for specific target cells in conventional cytolytic assays; however, in the presence of appropriate lectins, the level of cytolytic activity wss indistinguishable from that of the parent cloned cytolytic T cell from which it was derived. These observations indicated that Lyt-2 is not required for cytolytic activity but appears to be necessary for establishment of effective interactions between effector and target cells (3).

If cloned T cells having particular characteristics are to be maintained in continuous culture, it is necessary to adopt suitable approaches for avoiding the overgrowth of variant cells. It is desirable to reclone every few months and to select those cells which have retained the phenotypic characteristics of particular interest.

THE "IMAGINATION" OF CLONED T CELLS
MAY EXCEED THAT OF THE INVESTIGATORS STUDYING THEM

Antigen-recognition Repertoire of Cytolytic T cells

Some T cell clones have demonstrated a number of unexpected characteristics. Although many cytolytic cloned T cells react with target cells as anticipated, unexpected reactivity patterns have been observed rather frequently. Such unusual patterns of reactivity are observed more frequently as the panel of target cells is expanded. For example, at least 7 different patterns of lysis were observed when 9 separate clones of cytolytic T cells derived from secondary C57BL/6 anti-DBA/2 MLC were tested on a panel of 11 different target cells (12). Sherman studied the fine specificity of lysis by short-term T cell clones derived from $H-2^d$ spleen cells selected for lytic activity on $H-2K^b$ target cells (28). Since numerous $H-2K^b$ mutant mice which express different antigenic determinants were available, it was possible to discriminate fine patterns of reactivity. When assayed on a panel of target cells from 7 distinct $H-2K^b$ mutant mouse strains, 43 individual clones demonstrated 23 out of the possible 128 reactivity patterns (28). These different reactivity patterns would not have been differentiated in assays employing conventional $H-2^b$ target cells.

Virus and hapten determinants appear to be recognized by cytolytic T cells concomitantly with cell surface antigens specified by the major histocompatibility complex (MHC) of antigen-presenting cells (37). Analysis of the cytolytic activity of virus- and hapten-reactive cloned cytolytic T cells also have indicated multiple patterns of reactivity. Cloned cells reactive with Moloney leukemia virus (MoLV) -associated cell surface antigens displayed at least 3 different reactivity patterns: some clones reacted with syngeneic MoLV-derived tumor cells only, some were cross-reactive with allogeneic MoLV-derived tumor cells, and some were cross-reactive with normal allogeneic cells (35). The clones reactive with MoLV-infected syngeneic tumor cells showed further heterogeneity since the lytic activity of some clones was inhibited by anti-$H-2D^b$ monoclonal antibodies while the reactivity of other clones was not (36). Some hapten-reactive clones reacted with haptenated cells of a single haplotype while others reacted with hapten-coupled cells from several different haplotypes (15,33).

Collectively, these results indicate that the antigen-recognition repertoire of cytolytic T cells has a considerable degree of heterogeneity. The MHC-restriction which often appears stringent in bulk cell populations may show lesser degrees of restriction at the clonal level.

Antigen-recognition Repertoire of Non-Cytolytic T cells

Non-cytolytic alloreactive T cell clones and T cell clones reactive with "conventional" antigens have helped clarify the relationships among I-region encoded MLC-stimulating determinants, Ia antigens, and immune response genes. Proof for the existence of unique stimulating determinants on F_1 hybrid cells, previously suggested by results obtained with whole lymph node cells, was provided by clones of non-cytolytic T lymphocytes which could be stimulated to proliferate only by F_1 alloantigens (5). The stimulating determinant appeared to be derived from trans-complementation between the I-A-region gene products of the two parents (6,7).

I-A-region genes also appear to be of major importance in the MHC-restriction of antigen-specific mouse T cell clones. All possible combinations of gene products of the I-A region can provide the restriction elements (8,17,18). In addition, trans-complementation I-A and I-E subregion gene products may serve as restriction elements since T cell clones reacting to antigen only in the presence of β_{AE}-α_E Ia molecules have been identified (29). Thus, antigen-reactive cloned T lymphocytes which proliferate when stimulated by soluble antigen appear to require antigen-presenting cells bearing appropriate gene products encoded by the I-A region. A given clone appears to recognize only a single combination, but clones have been identified which react with antigen in association with each of the possible combinations of I-A gene products including complementation of an α-chain encoded by the I-E subregion and a β-chain encoded for by the I-A subregion.

Non-cytolytic cloned T cells may have dual antigen reactivity. Cloned T cells, reactive with DNP-ovalbumin in the presence of cells bearing syngeneic I-A^k antigens, also proliferated when cultured with cells bearing I-A^s alone; other haplotypes did not induce proliferation (30,31).

Multiple Biologically Active Factors
Can be Produced by a Single Non-Cytolytic T Cell Clone

Non-cytolytic cloned T cells may secrete biologically active "factors" into the culture medium upon stimulation with appropriate antigens. "Helper" activity for both T cells (11,12,14,19,21,26) and B cells (13,26,27) has been described. With cloned helper cells reactive with sheep erythrocytes, the antibody response to a separate unrelated erythrocyte was "helped" in vitro if the second erythrocyte was included in culture; only antigen-specific help was observed with such cells in vivo (27).

Culture fluid from a single antigen-stimulated helper T cell clone may produce a wide variety of biological activities. IL-2, factor(s) which stimulate B cells (BCSF), granulocyte/macrophage colony stimulating factor (CSF), interferon, macrophage migration inhibitory factor (MIF), factors causing the recruitment of Ia$^+$ macrophages into the peritoneal cavity and the induction of Ia-antigen expression by macrophages in vitro, and factors which stimulate the production of complement components by guinea pig macrophages have been found in the supernatant of a non-cytolytic T cell clone reactive with Mls alloantigen (11,13, and unpublished observations). Multiple biological activities also have been found in culture supernatants of cloned T cells reactive with heterologous erythrocytes (26) and with cloned T cells maintained only with CM (21). Although it is not known with certainty how many chemically distinct lymphokines are responsible for these various activities, biological criteria suggest that some differences exist. There must be at least two physically distinct molecules since the time course of the production of IL-2 differs from that of BCSF and CSF. Also, a variant clone derived from a parent clone which produces IL-2, BCSF, and CSF has lost the ability to produce IL-2 while retaining the ability to secrete the other two activities (unpublished obsertations).

Antigen-specific suppressor T cell clones have been reported recently. These suppressor cells which have been maintained in CM alone secreted a soluble antigen-binding glycoprotein (10). Suppression of primary antibody responses appeared to be due to direct inhibition of T helper cell activity (9).

SUMMARY

T cell clones are proving to be useful for studying a number of immunological phenomena. Rigorous approaches must be used to derive T cell clones, since it is possible to maintain mixed populations of T cells in long term culture by repetitive stimulation with conditioned medium. The conditions used for deriving and maintaining T cell clones may influence the ease with which T cell clones can be derived and may have profound effects on the characteristics of the cloned T cells. Although some T cell clones will grow well in IL 2-containing conditioned medium alone, the combination of antigen, "filler" cells, and conditioned medium results in better cloning efficiency and appears to favor the growth of stable clones which express a "normal" phenotype. Variant cells may develop spontaneously in culture, and the yield of variant cells may be increased by treatment with mutagenic agents. Frequent recloning is necessary to insure that unwanted variant clones do not contaminate the culture to a significant extent. A considerable heterogeneity has been observed in antigen-reactivity patterns for both cytolytic and non-cytolytic cloned T cells. "Factors" mediating a wide variety of biological activities may be produced by a single clone of antigen-stimulated non-cytolytic T cells. T cell clones will be useful for further characterization of the molecular and cellular events that occur during immune responses.

REFERENCES

1. Baker, P.E., Gillis, S., and Smith, K.A.(1979): J. Exp. Med. 149:273.
2. Braciale, T.J., Andrew, M.E., and Braciale, V.L.(1981): J. Exp. Med. 153:910.
3. Dialynas, D.P., Loken, M.R., Glasebrook, A.L., and Fitch, F.W.(1981): J. Exp. Med. 153:595.
4. Engers, H.D., Collavo, D., North, M., von Boehmer, H., Haas, W., Hengartner, H., and Nabholz, M.(1980): J. Immunol. 125:1481.
5. Fathman, C.G., and Hengartner, H.(1978): Nature 272:617.
6. Fathman, C.G., and Hengartner, H.(1979): Proc. Natl. Acad. Sci. (USA) 76:5863.
7. Fathman, C.G., and Kimoto, M.(1981): Immunological Rev. 54:57.
8. Fathman, C.G., Kimoto, M., Melvold, R., and David, C.S.(1981): Proc. Nat. Acad. Sci. (USA) 78:1853.
9. Fresno, M., McVay-Boudreau, L., Nabel, G., and Cantor, H.(1981): J. Exp. Med. 153:1260.
10. Fresno, M., Nabel, G., McVay-Boudreau, L., Furthmayer, H., and Cantor, H.(1981): J. Exp. Med. 153:1246.
11. Glasebrook, A.L., and Fitch, F.W.(1979): Nature 278:171.
12. Glasebrook, A.L., and Fitch, F.W.(1980): J. Exp. Med. 151:876.

13. Glasebrook, A.L., Quintans, J., Eisenberg, L., and Fitch, F.W.(1981): J. Immunol. 126:240.
14. Glasebrook, A.L., Sarmiento, M., Loken, M.R., Dialynas, D.P., Quintans, J., Eisenberg, L., Lutz, C.T., Wilde, D., and Fitch, F.W.(1981): Immunological Rev. 54:225.
15. Haas, W., Mathur-Rochat, J., Pohlit, H., Nabholz, M., and von Boehmer, H.(1980): Eur. J. Immunol. 10:828.
16. Hengartner, H., and Fathman, C.G.(1980): Immunogenetics 10:175.
17. Kimoto, M., and Fathman, C.G.(1980): J. Exp. Med. 152:759.
18. Kimoto, M., and Fathman, C.G.(1981): J. Exp. Med. 153:375.
19. Lutz, C.T., Glasebrook, A.L., and Fitch, F.W.(1981): J. Immunol. 127: (in press).
20. Morgan, D.A., Ruscetti, F.W., and Gallo, R.(1976): Science 193:1007.
21. Nabel, G., Greenberger, J.S., Sakakeeny, M.A., and Cantor, H.(1981): Proc. Natl. Acad. Sci. (USA) 78:1157.
22. Nabholz, M., Engers, H.D., Collavo, D., and North, M.(1978): Curr. Top. Microbiol. Immunol. 81:176.
23. Nabholz, M., Conzelmann, A., Acuto, O., North, M., Haas, W., Pohlit, H., von Boehmer, H., Hengartner, H., Mach, J.-P., Engers, H., and Johnson, J.P.(1980): Immunological Rev. 51:125.
24. Quintans, J., and Lefkovits, I.(1973): Eur. J. Immunol. 3:392.
25. Smith, K.A., Lachman, L.B., Oppenheim, J.J., and Favata, M.F.(1980): J. Exp. Med. 151:1551.
26. Schreier, M.H., Iscove, N.N., Tees, R., Aarden, L., and von Boehmer, H.(1980): Immunological Rev. 51:315.
27. Schreier, M.H., and Tees R.(1980): Int. Arch. Allergy Appl. Immunol. 61:227.
28. Sherman, L.A.(1980): J. Exp. Med. 151:1386.
29. Sredni, B., Matis, L.A., Lerner, E.A., Paul, W.E., and Schwartz, R.H.(1981): J. Exp. Med. 153:677.
30. Sredni, B., and Schwartz, R.H.(1980): Nature 287:855.
31. Sredni, B., and Schwartz, R.H.(1981): Immunological Rev. 54:186.
32. Sredni, B., Tse, H.Y., and Schwartz, R.H.(1980): Nature 283:581.
33. von Boehmer, H., and Haas, W.(1981): Immunological Rev. 54:27.
34. von Boehmer, H., Hengartner, H., Nabholz, M., Lernhardt, W., Schreier, M.H., and Haas, W.(1979): Eur. J. Immunol. 9:592.
35. Weiss, A., Brunner, K.T., MacDonald, H.R., and Cerottini, J.-C.(1980): J. Exp. Med. 152:1210.
36. Weiss, A., MacDonald, H.R., Cerottini, J.-C, and Brunner K.T.(1981): J. Immunol. 126:482.
37. Zinkernagel, R.M., and Doherty, P.C.(1979): Adv. Immunol. 27:51.

AUDIENCE DISCUSSION

Dr. Paetkau: Is the L2 variant which doesn't produce IL 2 a suitable continued source for L3? Do you ever in the presence of Con A see killing against syngeneic targets in the clones that you've analyzed? Our brief experience suggests they don't show up.

Dr. Fitch: The cytolytic clone will kill syngeneic target cells in the presence of Con A; the L3 clone of C57BL/6 origin lyses EL4 as well as C57BL/6 LPS blasts in the presence of Con A. The L2 variant does not support the growth of L3. The variant is antigen responsive, and both the variant and the parent cell line are responsive to Con A stimulation as well as to alloantigen stimulation for release of factors.
Dr. Greenberg: Is your helper line seeing MLS in the context of an H2 antigen or is it seeing MLS independently?
Dr. Fitch: It sees MLS in the context of any haplotype that we've been able to find.
Dr. Kedar: Do any of your clones function as specific or nonspecific suppressor cells?
Dr. Fitch: Yes, the cytolytic clones can function as specific suppressor cells by destroying the stimulating alloantigen. But this is a rather trivial mechanism for suppression. We have become discouraged by inability to derive suppressor clones after 18 months. The only suppressor clones I know of are those of Harvey Cantor; they are not now antigen reactive. He maintains them with conditioned medium only.
Dr. Greenberg: How would you look for them?
Dr. Fitch: Suppression of a primary MLC and suppression of antibody responses. The particular culture system we've used gives very brisk responses.
Dr. Bonavida: Do any of the factors generated by the clones have immunologic function? Are any of the factors cytotoxic?
Dr. Fitch: We have not tested the cytolytic clones specifically for production of lymphotoxin. We have not tested to see if the clones or their products will mediate reactions in vivo. We intend to do that.
Dr. Grimm: Your data suggest that perhaps we're not really able yet to clone terminally differentiated CTL, that perhaps we're really cloning something just prior to that step and that by constantly adding the antigen, the cytolytic activity can be turned on or off and that if we leave out the alloantigen we lose the cytotoxic activity.
Dr. Fitch: That's not true. Our L3 clone will retain full cytolytic activity on syngeneic filler cells with supernatant containing maximal amounts of an IL 2. Alloantigen is not required for the growth of those cells. When we have tried to maintain these clones with a Con A supernatant, they begin to get "funny." They may display bizarre cytolytic activities. I suggest that for both cytolytic and noncytolytic clones in the presence of a not-too-strong source of IL 2 and stimulating alloantigen, you exert a strong selective pressure to keep the antigen reactive cells around. If you want to look at long-term cloned antigen-reactive cells, I urge you to consider the Glasebrook culture conditions. Everyone else who has tried it (Tom Braeiole with the influenza viral specific CTL clones and Art Weiss with his Moloney leukemia virus-specific cells) has been able to get cloned cells within a few months using this technique. These results are quite different than those obtained with the kind of long-term culturing of cells before cloning. The characteristics of the cloned cells are quite different. For one purpose you may want to use one procedure, for another purpose, another. The culture conditions clearly influence the properties of the cloned cells you get.

The Potential Role of T Cells in Cancer Therapy,
edited by A. Fefer and A. Goldstein.
Raven Press, New York © 1982.

T-Cell Clones Reactive with Soluble Antigen

C. G. Fathman

Department of Medicine, Division of Immunology, Stanford University School of Medicine, Stanford, California 94305

Recent technological advances in cellular immunology have allowed us as well as others to maintain murine T-cells in culture which proliferate in response to soluble antigen in the context of MHC restriction (1, 2,6,7,9,10,12,13,15). From such long-term antigen reactive T-cell lines, we have been able to isolate clones of murine T-cells which exhibit antigen recognition in the context of I-region restricted recognition (2,6,7). Initial studies in our laboratory were performed with the synthetic amino acid polymer (L-Glu^{60}, L-Ala^{30}, L-Tyr^{10})n (GAT). It was possible to obtain antigen specific proliferating T-cells from mice immunized with GAT which could be maintained in vitro by repeated antigen stimulation in the presence of syngeneic irradiated spleen cells. The antigen specific proliferation could be maintained in vitro only by antigen stimulation in the context of I-A compatible presenting cells. The reactivities of such GAT reactive T-cells (recognition of antigen on a panel of antigen presenting cells) derived from hybrid (B6A)F$_1$ mice could be classified into three categories. One group of T-cell clones exemplified by clone 12.5.a.24 (Table 1) recognized antigen in the context of parental A and syngeneic F$_1$ cells. The second group exemplified by clone 17.2 recognized antigen in association with the products present on clone B6 and syngeneic (B6A)F$_1$ cells, whereas the third group exemplified by clone 12.5.a.1 recognized antigen only in the context of hybrid antigen restricting determinants on (B6A)F$_1$ cells which were not present on cells from either parental A or B6 mice. These data suggest two important points; first that there exist unique antigen restriction sites or antigen presenting determinants on F$_1$ cells which are not present on cells from either parent; and secondly, there exist clones of T cells from F$_1$ mice which uniquely recognize antigen in the context of such hybrid antigen presenting determinants. Genetic mapping studies were performed using antigen-presenting spleen cells derived from various congenic recombinant and F$_1$ mice. These studies showed that the expression of F$_1$ specific antigen presenting determinants for GAT reactive T-cells was controlled by the I-A subregion (Table 2). The most likely interpretation of these results is that the F$_1$ specific antigen presenting determinants are hybrid I-A molecules derived by free combinatorial association of alpha and beta chains which result in combinatorial I-A antigens $A_\alpha^k A_\beta^b$ or $A_\alpha^b A_\beta^k$ (Figure 1). Antibody blocking experiments using monoclonal anti-I-A antibodies as well as studies using (bm12 x B10.A)F$_1$ mice as a source of antigen presenting cells further support this concept as described below. In addition to transcomplement-

Table 1

GAT Reactive T Cell Clones From (B6A)F$_1$ Mice

Antigen Presenting Cells	12.5.a.24 GAT	17.2	12.5.a.1 GAT
		^{3}HTdR uptake (Δcpm)	
A	15,831	15	315
B6	904	6,787	236
A + B6	16,798	4,730	418
(B6A)F$_1$	10,428	5,807	14,908

Data in Tables 1, 2, 3 and 5 are expressed as (mean) Δcpm (experimental – control) of an overnight pulse of 2μCi of ^{3}HTdR of triplicate culture of 1 x 10^4 cloned T cells in the presence of 1 x 10^6 (3300R irradiated) splenic filler cells (as a source of antigen presenting cells) and 100μg/ml antigen in 200μl medium (6).

Table 2

Genetic Mapping of F_1 Specific Antigen Presenting Determinants

Antigen Presenting Cells	H-2 Haplotype K A E D				Clone 12.5.a.2 MED	GAT
					^{3}HTdR uptake (Δcpm)	
A	k	k	k	d		162
B6	b	b	b	b		458
A + B6	k	k	k	d		519
	b	b	b	b		
(B6A)F_1	k	k	k	d		10,517
	b	b	b	b		
B10.A(4R)	k	k	b	b		519
[B10.A(4R) x B6]F_1	k	k	b	b		12,876
	b	b	b	b		
[B10.A(4R) x B10.A]F_1	k	k	b	b		95
	k	k	k	d		
[B10.MBR x A.AL]F_1	b	k	k	q		267
	k	k	k	d		

Data in Tables 1, 2, 3 and 5 are expressed as (mean) Δcpm (experimental - control) of an overnight pulse of 2µCi of ^{3}HTdR of triplicate culture of 1 x 10^4 cloned T cells in the presence of 1 x 10^6 (3300R irradiated) splenic filler cells (as a source of antigen presenting cells) and 100µg/ml antigen in 200µl medium (6).

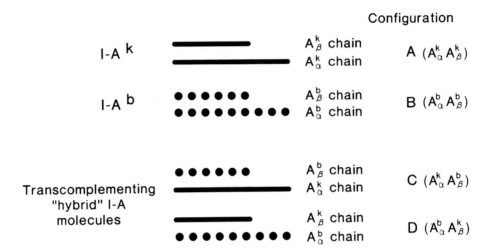

Figure 1:   An artist's representation of I-A products
from $(H-2^a \times H-2^b)F_1$ mice.

ing hybrid I-A molecules which restrict the recognition of antigen by
murine T-cell clones, there exists a second class of combinatorial I-A
molecules. These are formed by combinatorial association of the alpha
chains encoded within the I-E region and beta chains encoded within the
I-A region (Ae). Such AE molecules have been described by biochemical
technology by Pat Jones and her collaborators (5). Data obtained by
Sredni et al suggested that such AE molecules can restrict the recognition of T-cell clones which respond to GL Ø (14). Additional data
presented by Sredni et al suggested that such recognition could be
effectively blocked by a monoclonal antibody directed at the $A_e E_\alpha$ Ia
molecule.   Studies in our laboratory using keyhole limpet hemocyanin
(KLH) reactive T cell clones have yielded similar data (11). It has
been possibie for us to isolate KLH reactive T cell clones from
(B6 x C3H)F_1 mice which recognize antigen only in the context of F_1
antigen presenting cells bearing the E^k and A^k chains. These data are
presented in Table 3. In this table it can be seen that clone 1 recognizes KLH in association with antigen presenting cells which have the E
region and A region k haplotype. Although this is not conclusive evidence that such clones recognize the $A^k_e E^k_\alpha$ product, data (Table 4) utilizing monoclonal antibody blocking studies show that monoclonal antibody
Y.17, used in the studies by Sredni et al (14) will effectively block
antigen presentation to this clone (11). Thus, it has been possible to
show that in the KLH system alpha/beta complementation exists in cis
configuration for restriction of antigen recognition by certain T cell
clones.

Table 3

Genetic Restrictions Imposed Upon Recognition of KLH By T-Cell Clones

Antigen Presenting Cells	K	A	E	D	Clone 1	Clone 11	Clone 9
					^{3}HTdR Uptake (Δcpm)		
C3H	k	k	k	k	3248	26	39
B6	b	b	b	b	139	0	0
(B6 x C3H)F$_1$	k b	k b	k b	k b	5431	20807	17946
B10.A(4R)	k	k	b	b	15	0	0
B10.A(5R)	b	b	k	d	0	N.T.	N.T.
[B10.A(4R) x B10.A(5R)F$_1$	k b	k b	b k	b d	7170	12460	N.T.
B10.MBR	b	k	k	q	1793	N.T.	N.T.
[B10.A(4R) x B6]F$_1$	k b	k b	b b	b b	107	19357	24743
[B10.MBR x A.AL]F$_1$	b k	k k	k k	q d	4955	157	0

Data in Tables 1, 2, 3 and 5 are expressed as (mean) Δcpm (experimental - control) of an overnight pulse of 2μCi of ^{3}HTdR of triplicate culture of 1 x 10^4 cloned T cells in the presence of 1 x 10^6 (3300R irradiated) splenic filler cells (as a source of antigen presenting cells) and 100μg/ml antigen in 200μl medium (6).

Monoclonal Anti-Ia Antibodies Can Block Antigen
Recognition By Murine T-Cell Clones

Using a panel of monoclonal antibodies generously provided by Dr. Gunther Hammerling, Heidelberg, Germany, we were able to show that anti-Ia antibodies blocked the ability of antigen presenting cells to present

antigen to murine T cell clones reactive with KLH. Two separate monoclonal antibodies 10.2.16 and H150.13 react with the same Ia determinant
(Ia.17) present on I-A^k products. These antisera can discriminate
between clones which recognize transcomplementing hybrid I-A molecules
when compared with blocking capabilities of an αI-A^k monoclonal antibody
reactive with Ia19. These data are presented in Table 4. Additionally,
as shown in this table, using monoclonal antibody Y.17 it was possible
to block the $E_\alpha^k A_e^k$ molecule which was used to restrict the ability of KLH
reactive T-cell clone number 1 to recognize KLH in association either
with C3H or (C3H x B6)F_1 antigen presenting cells. These data show that
the transcomplementing products exist and that each is capable of presenting antigen to the appropriate antigen specific T cell clone. These
data additionally confirm our interpretation of the results obtained by
genetic mapping studies and suggest that cis complementing AE molecules
are utilized by certain KLH reactive T-cell clones. In order to more
fully document the fact that the alternative transcomplementing I-A
hybrid products can be recognized effectively as antigen-presenting
determinants, we studied antigen presentation of hybrid mice which have
as one parent, the I-A^b mutant mouse B6.C-H-2^{bm12}. The data presented
above have suggested that there exist F_1 specific determinants which can
function as restriction determinants for antigen recognition by immune
T-cell clones. We suggested that such hybrid determinants were formed

Table 4

Anti-Ia Monoclonal Antibody Inhibition of   KLH   Presentation

	Clone 14	Clone 2	Clone 9	Clone 11	Clone 1
Exp. 1	^{3}HTdR uptake (cpm)				
Media	103939	7813	18089	24284	18432
αIa17	0	6543	0	28312	15644
αIa19	4793	3894	15941	7252	19714
αIa.m.44	83600	3915	15029	22101	46
I-A configuration recognized by T cell clone	$A_\alpha^k A_\beta^k$	$A_\alpha^b A_\beta^b$	$A_\alpha^b A_\beta^k$	$A_\alpha^k A_\beta^b$	$A_e^k E_\alpha^k$

Methods are the same as in the legend to Table 2. 2μl of
purified antibody at 1mg/ml are added at the initiation of
culture and can be compared to media controls (top row).

by free combinatorial association of alpha and beta chains from the I-A subregion. In an attempt to prove this hypothesis, we studied the antigen presenting characteristics of F_1 mice derived from B10.A and the mutant B6.C-H-2^{bm12} (bm12). A variety of studies have shown that the mutation of gain and loss type was in the I-A^b product (reviewed in reference 3). By tryptic peptide analysis, Dr. David McKean at Mayo Clinic has shown that there is a defect in the A_β^{bm12} chain, but was unable to detect any differences in the A_α^{bm12} chain (8). If the mutation in bm12 results only in structural alteration of the beta chain of the I-A^{bm12} subregion product, it would suggest that of the four possible I-A determinants expressed on (B6A)F_1 cells (see Figure 1), there would be only two normal products on the cell surface of (bm12 x B10.A)F_1 cells; the two which contain the A_β^{bm12} chain would be different. Utilizing clones of murine antigen reactive T-cells, it was possible to provide evidence for this interpretation. These data were gathered in experiments aimed at testing the hypothesis that the altered form of the I-A determinant expressed on bm12 and/or (bm12 x B10.A)F_1 cells might function as an antigen restricting site for antigen reactive murine T-cell clones. Table 5 shows representative results of reactivity patterns of selected antigen reactive clones derived from KLH and (T,G)-A--L immune mice. KLH reactive T cell clone 11 cannot recognize KLH presented by [B10.A(4R) x bm12]F_1 antigen presenting cells, whereas KLH reactive T-cell clone 9 can see KLH presented equally well by (B6 x C3H)F_1 and [B10.A(4R) x bm12]F_1 antigen presenting cells. These data substantiate the hypothesis following antibody blocking studies (see Table 4) which suggested that clone 9 recognized the combinatorial product $A_\alpha^b A_\beta^k$, whereas clone 11 utilized the reciprocal combination $A_\alpha^k A_\beta^b$. Similar data are presented for two (T,G)-A--L specific clones derived from (B6A)F_1 mice. Clone 2e.SA.13 recognized (T,G)-A--L presented by (bm12 x B10.A)F_1 antigen presenting cells as well as it recognized antigen presented by (B6A)F_1 antigen presenting cells. However, clone 2e.SA.12 did not recognize antigen presented by (bm12 x B10.A)F_1 antigen presenting cells, although it recognized (T,G)-A--L presented by (B6A)F_1 cells. Again, the most likely explanation of these results is that the different (T,G)-A--L reactive clones use different transcomplementing hybrid I-A products as the restricting element for recognition of (T,G)-A--L. Thus the mutation in the A_β^{bm12} chain is in or near the site used for both KLH and (T,G)-A--L restriction. Whether this is actually a mutation within the "restriction site", or causes tertiary changes in the molecule cannot be resolved by data presented in this paper. The data presented above have documented the existence of unique hybrid Ia molecules present on cells obtained from heterozygous mice. Such molecules are formed by free combinatorial association of alpha and beta chains encoded within the I-A region, as well as by free combinatorial association of alpha chains encoded in the I-E region and with the Ae beta chains encoded within the I-A region. Studies in progress in our laboratory have suggested that such antigen specific MHC restricted T cell clones provide antigen specific MHC restricted help to B cells in their maturation to immunoglobulin producing plasma cells (4). That such hybrid determinants are present and are functionally effective for immunocompetent cellular interactions suggests that these hybrid I-A products are functional counterparts of the conventional I-A product recognized on homozygous mice. That such hybrid determinants exist and that individuals within a species must recognize such hybrid determin-

Table 5

Antigen Presentation by (bm12 x B10.A)F_1 Cells to F_1 Specific

(T,G)-A--L or KLH Reactive T Cell Clones

Antigen Presenting Cells	(T,G)-A--L		KLH	
	2e.SA.12	2e.SA.13	11	9
	^{3}HTdR uptake (Δcpm)			
A/C3H	21	42	26	39
B6	590	458	0	0
(B6A)F_1/(B6 x C3H)F_1	11,33	22,702	20,807	17,946
[B10.A(4R) x B6]F_1	12,964	22,293	19,357	24,743
[B10.MBR x A.AL]F_1	140	147	157	0
(bm12 x B10.A)F_1	460	16,241	0	18,429

Data in Tables 1, 2, 3 and 5 are expressed as (mean) Δcpm (experimental - control) of an overnight pulse of 2µCi of ^{3}HTdR of triplicate culture of 1 x 10^4 cloned T cells in the presence of 1 x 10^6 (3300R irradiated) splenic filler cells (as a source of antigen presenting cells) and 100µg/ml antigen in 200µl medium (6).

ants suggests that recognition of self I-region restricting products must be a learned phenomena. Thus, we suggest that T-cells are positively selected within that environment for recognition of expressed I-region products. Such positive selection may well take place within the thymus supporting earlier observation by Zinkernagel and his collaborators (16). Whether such hybrid I-region antigens exist in other mammalian species has not yet been determined. It is of considerable interest for successful organ transplantation and/or cellular immunotherapy to recognize whether these hybrid molecules exist in humans prior to attempted reconstitution studies with T-cell clones as has been suggested at this meeting.

References

1. Augustin, A.A., Julius, M.H., and Cosenza, H. (1979): Eur. J. Immunol., 9:665.

2. Fathman, C.G., Kimoto, M., Melvold, R., and David, C. (1981): Proc. Natl. Acad. Sci. USA, 78:1853.

3. Fathman, C.G., Kimoto, M., Melvold, R., and David, C. (1981): Proc. Natl. Acad. Sci. USA, 78:1853.

4. Hodes, R.J., Kimoto, M., Hathcock, K.F., Fathman, C.G., and Singer, A.: Proc. Natl. Acad. Sci. USA, (in press).

5. Jones, P.P., Murphy, D.B., and McDevitt, H.O. (1978): J. Exp. Med., 148:925.

6. Kimoto, M., and Fathman, C.G. (1980): J. Exp. Med., 152:759.

7. Kimoto, M., and Fathman, C.G. (1981): J. Exp. Med., 153:375.

8. McKean, D.J., Melvold, R.W., and David, C.: Immunogenetics (in press)

9. Schrier, R.D., Skidmore, B.J., Kurnick, J.T., Goldstine, S.N., and Chillu, J.M. (1979): J. Immunol., 123:2525.

10. Schreier, M.H., Tees, R. (1980): Int. Arch. Allergy Appl. Immunol., 61:227.

11. Shigeta, M., and Fathman, C.G. Immunogenetics (in press).

12. Sredni, B., Tse, H.Y., and Schwartz, R.H. (1980): Nature, 283:581.

13. Sredni, B., Tse, H.Y., Chen, C. and Schwartz, R.H. (1981): J. Immunol., 126:341.

14. Sredni, B., Matis, L.A., Lerner, E.A., Paul, W.E., and Schwartz, R.H. (1981): J. Exp. Med., 153:677.

15. Watson, J. (1979): J. Exp. Med., 150:1510.

16. Zinkernagel, R.M., Callahan, G.M., Althage, A., Cooper, J., Klein, P.A., and Klein, J.(1978): J. Exp. Med., 147:882.

Acknowledgements

This work was supported by NIH grants AI 18716 and AI 18705 and by Research Career Development Award AI 00485.

AUDIENCE DISCUSSION

<u>Dr. Bonavida</u>: Do any products from the plasmacytoma form an association with the antigen and can be presented to the T cell clones?

<u>Dr. Fathman</u>: Lonai showed that there is an antigen complex between a nominal antigen like TGAL and an Ia "antigen" from the antigen-presenting cell, the so-called IAC, which is recognized by T cells in a binding assay. His preliminary results suggest that it also can cause proliferation of a cloned helper line as well as long-term lines. So there probably is some type of a molecular association between an antigenic epitope and Ia. We haven't yet looked for it. We've had these data about a month now on David McKean's lymphoblastoid antigen-presenting cells.

<u>Dr. Greenberg</u>: Will your cloned line not bind soluble antigen alone in the absence of an antigen-presenting cell?

<u>Dr. Fathman</u>: These cloned lines will not bind soluble antigen alone in the absence of antigen-presenting cells at large excess ratios of "hot" antigen. These are helper cells as evidenced by data from Hodes and Singer. They provide antigen-specific help in the context of the appropriate I region restriction. That kind of help is somewhat dissimilar from what Rich has seen in that there is no obligate hapten carrier association. You can trigger these cells with the carrier TGAL and get a KLH-TNP hapten response. So, unlike most of the other systems, in this there is obligate hapten carrier association, the carrier need only be seen in the context of the appropriate antigen presentation to trigger help. The antigen specificity is contained in the T cell's ability to recognize the antigen.

The Potential Role of T Cells in Cancer Therapy,
edited by A. Fefer and A. Goldstein,
Raven Press, New York © 1982.

Somatic Cell Hybrids as Tools for a Genetic Analysis of Cytolytic T-Cell Functions

M. Nabholz, A. Conzelmann, and M. Cianfriglia

Genetics Units, Swiss Institute for Experimental Cancer Research, 1066 Epalinges, Switzerland

Since the discovery that cloned functionally active cell lines can be derived from cytolytic T-lymphocyte (CTL) populations (2,3,10) our work has concentrated on the use of such CTL-lines for a somatic cell genetic approach to the identification of the genes whose expression is required for the CTL-specific functions (specific target cell recognition, cytolytic capacity, dependence on T-cell growth factor (TCGF = IL-2))(9). Recently we have discovered that cytolytically active hybrids can be derived from crosses between inactive T-lymphoma-derived lines and CTL-lines when the hybrids are selected in medium (7) supplemented with TCGF containing culture supernatants. The results described below indicate that such hybrids will allow the identification of some of the chromosomes which carry genes which control the manifestation of the CTL-phenotype.

RESULTS

On the Nature of Murine CTL-Lines

All murine CTL-lines described so far have been derived from populations enriched in CTL by one or several in vitro stimulations with allogeneic, tumor, virus infected or haptencoupled stimulator cells. Almost all of them fall into one of two classes : (1) After (re)stimulation CTL-populations are maintained in medium supplemented with a source of TCGF, usually supernatant from mitogen activated spleen cells (e.g. Concanavalin A supernatant = CS) without further addition of filler or stimulator cells (2,10). Such populations grow quite vigorously for one to several months and then undergo some sort of crisis. When good growth resumes the populations often consist of a single clone of cells, which morphologically are different from normal CTL and carry abnormal chromosomes (5,9). After the crisis many such lines can be cloned with high efficiency (100%) when plated at limiting dilutions in TCGF-containing medium without filler cells. (2) Normal CTL can be cloned immediately after stimulation in a mixed leukocyte culture (MLC) system in TCGF-containing medium in the presence of irradiated spleen cells (3,4). CTL-clones isolated in this way can also be maintained for apparently indefinite periods but they continue to depend not only on TCGF but also on co-cultivation with filler cells. The nature of the requirement provided for by the addition of filler cells is not clear. Such lines appear to maintain a normal karyotype and also morphologically resemble more normal CTL (M. Cianfriglia, A. Glasebrook, unpublished). We have called this latter type of lines CTL-A line (8), as we believe that the former type called CTL-B line is derived from CTL-A cells by a transformation event of unknown nature which renders CTL-B cells independent of the filler cell requirement. Attempts to derive TCGF-independent variants from CTL-B lines by mutagenesis have, so far, not been successful (9).

The derivation of cytolytically active hybrids between murine CTL-lines and T-lymphomas.

From crosses between CTL-A or B-lines or normal CTL from a secondary MLC with several T-lymphoma lines hybrids can be obtained with a high frequency. In our hands all of several hundred such hybrids selected in the absence of TCGF were cytolytically inactive, whereas a large proportion of the hybrids selected in TCGF-containing medium displayed lytic activity (7,8).

Hybrids derived from CTL-B can easily be cloned and maintain their activity with adequate stability. They continue to depend on TCGF (in the experiments described here in the form of CS), while TCGF-independent hybrids do not become cytolytic when cultured in CS. Hybrids derived from CTL-A lines or normal CTL are much less stable : They tend to lose rapidly CTL-activity and TCGF-requirement.

CTL-B or CTL-A hybrids express the specificity of the CTL-parents although in some cases loss of certain crossreactions has been observed. A limited search for the expression of new specificities contributed by the thymoma parents has given negative results (8).

TCGF-dependence is correlated with the expression of other CTL-specific characteristics.

TCGF-dependent (CS^+) and independent (CS^-) hybrids differ from each other not only in their cytolytic competence : Morphologically CS-hybrids resemble thymoma cells, while in some crosses CS^+ hybrids show a strong tendency to spread out and adhere to tissue culture plastic, a property which they share with some CTL-B lines (7).

When the cell surface glycoproteins (GP) are labelled with ^{3}H-borohydrid after treatment with galactose oxidase and neuraminidase and the solubilized cells are run in SDS-polyacrylamide gel electrophoresis the two types of hybrids produce very different patterns : that of CS^- hybrids resembles the one of the lymphoma parent, while CS^+ hybrids give a pattern similar to the one of the CTL-parent. This difference is probably related to the observation that Vicia Villosa lectin (VV), which inhibits the growth of CTL-but not lymphoma lines (1), has the same effect on CS^+ but not on CS^- hybrids.

CS⁻ variants can be isolated from CS⁺ hybrids.

The expression of several of the attributes of the CTL-phenotype (VV-sensitivity, GP-pattern, CTL-activity) by CS⁺ but not CS⁻ hybrids suggests that these characteristics are subject to co-ordinated control. Our working hypothesis is that the two types of hybrids differ in their chromosomal constitution. The two simplest possibilities are : a) A hybrid containing all parental chromosomes is CS⁻ due to a lymphoma gene which represses not only TCGF-dependence but also the other attributes of the CTL-phenotype. CS⁺ hybrids are the result of the loss of the lymphoma chromosome carrying this gene. b) Alternatively a hybrid containing full complements of parental chromosomes is CS⁺ because a gene active in CTL and the hybrid cells but not in lymphomas renders the cell TCGF-dependent. This or other genes on the same chromosome control the expression of the other properties that distinguish the two types of hybrids. As the homologous gene(s) of the lymphoma do not become active in the CS⁺ hybrids, loss of this CTL-chromosome results in CS⁻ hybrids.

The evidence which favours the latter alternative is (i) that the only cross in which many CS⁺ but no CS⁻ hybrids were obtained involved a tetraploid CTL-line and (ii) that it is possible to select CS⁻ variants from cloned CS⁺ hybrids. Such hybrids resemble hybrids directly isolated in TCGF-free medium in their morphology, their VV-resistance and their GP-pattern. Most of the CS⁻ variants express no detectable CTL-activity but some are still very weakly cytolytic. Preliminary results show that the difference between the chromosome numbers of CS⁺ hybrids and of their CS⁻ variants can be small.

DISCUSSION

Our results are compatible with the hypothesis that several of the properties in which CTL- and lymphoma lines differ from each other are controlled by one gene or several genes on a single chromosome. These genes are active in CTL and in TCGF-dependent hybrids, but not in lymphomas. The homologous lymphoma genes are not activated in the CS⁺ hybrids and when the CTL-chromosome carrying them is lost the hybrids revert to the CS⁻, lymphoma like phenotype.

That some of the CS⁻ variants still express weak cytolytic activity suggests that expression of the gene controlling TCGF-dependence or a closely linked CTL-gene has a strong quantitative influence on but is not absolutely required for cytolytic competence. This influence could e.g. be mediated by effects of the gene controlling TCGF-dependence on the organisation of the cytoskeleton and thus on cell motility or on the distribution of cell surface charge, etc. It is possible that the TCGF-independent CTL-hybrids described by Kaufmann et al. (6) are similar to the weakly cytolytic CS⁻ variants described here.

One of the characteristics of CTL which appears not to be controlled by genes on the same chromosome as that responsible for TCGF-dependence is the expression of receptors for TCGF. Preliminary experiments show that CS⁺ hybrids as well as their CS⁻ variants absorb per cell similar amounts of TCGF from CS, while the parental thymoma cells absorb at least 10-fold less. These results show that TCGF-dependence is not simply the consequence of the expression of receptors for this growth factor.

The identification of the CTL-chromosome which according to our hypothesis carries the gene(s) controlling the expression of TCGF-dependence
and the associated CTL-characteristics is complicated by (1) the fact
that the hybrids described here are intra-specific and (2) by the high
numbers of chromosomal abnormalities in the CTL-B parent lines. We are
trying to overcome these obstacles by producing hybrids between T-cell
lines from other species and karyotypically normal CTL-A lines.

REFERENCES

1. Conzelmann, A., Pink, R., Acuto, O., Mach, J.P., Dolivo, S., and
   Nabholz, M. (1980): Eur. J. Immunol, 10:860-868

2. Gillis, S. + Smith, K.A. (1977): Nature, 268:154-156

3. Glasebrook, A.L. + Fitch, F.W. (1979): Nature, 278:171-173

4. Glasebrook, A.L., Sarmiento, M., Loken, M.R., Dialynas, D.P.,
   Quintans, J., Eisenberg, L., Lutz, C.T., Wilde, D., and Fitch, F.W.
   (1981): Immunological Rev., 54:225-266

5. Haas, W., Mathur-Rochat, J., Pohlit, H., Nabholz, M., and v. Boehmer,
   H. (1980): Eur. J. Immunol, 10:828-834

6. Kaufmann, Y., Berke, G., and Eshhar, Z. (1981): Proc. Natl. Acad.
   Sci. USA, 78:2502-2506

7. Nabholz, M., Cianfriglia, M., Acuto, O., Conzelmann, A., Haas, W.,
   v. Boehmer, H., MacDonald, H.R., Pohlit, H., and Johnson, J.P.
   (1980): Nature, 287:437-440

8. Nabholz, M., Cianfriglia, M., Acuto, O., Conzelmann, A., Weiss, A.,
   Haas, W., and v. Boehmer, H. (1980): In: Monoclonal Antibodies and T
   cell Hybridomas, edited by G.J. Hämmerling, U. Hämmerling and J.
   Kearney, Elsevier/North Holland Publishing Company, inpress

9. Nabholz, M., Conzelmann, A., Acuto, O., North, M., Haas, W., Pohlit,
   H., v. Boehmer, H., Hengartner, H., Mach, J.P., Engers, H., and
   Johnson, J.P. (1980): Immunol. Rev.51, 125-156

10. Nabholz, M., Engers, J.D., Collavo, D., and North, M. (1978):In:
    Current Topics in Microbiology and Immunology, edited by F. Melchers,
    M. Potter, and N.L. Warner, Springer-Verlag, Vol 81, pp. 176-187

AUDIENCE DISCUSSION

Dr. Bonavida: Did you hybridize with in vivo drived CTL or do you need
a cultured line for hybridization? What's the method for hybridizing?
Dr. Nabholz: The hybrids were all derived from CTL-B lines; that is,
cell lines that were maintained from MLC cultures grown in TCGF, dependent only on TCGF, not on filler cells. We can also make hybrids from
normal CTL or CTL-A lines (which resemble more closely normal CTL than

CTL-B lines). But such hybrids are much less stable. It is difficult to clone them and maintain the CTL-positive phenotype. We assume this is because they lose CTL chromosomes more rapidly than the hybrids derived from the CTL-B lines. This is not an unreasonable assumption, given other situations where established cell lines are crossed with normal cells of the same species. One of the problems we have to deal with are the chromosomal abnormalities in the CTL-B lines. We can't hope to make chromosomal assignments if we work with cell lines where 30 to 50 percent of the chromosomes are structurally unidentified.

Dr. Wunderlich: Do any of the TCGF-independent lines derived from a TCGF-dependent cytotoxic line still show binding activity for the target cells?

Dr. Nabholz: We haven't tested that. We think that the binding tests are so frought with problems of interpretation, that unless you can do criss-cross experiments, it's not worth doing them.

Dr. Fathman: I'm intrigued by the concept that there is a dominant chromosomal CTL addition. Do you then perceive the event of a CTL precursor going to a CTL line to be switching on at this dominant gene since you now have this locked in to a new chromosomal arrangement only on one of the chromosomes; because if that were not the case, then with the loss of one chromosome you should expect in that homozygous cell that you would have a second chromosome there, still allowing the dominance in the CTL-TCGF addition. How do you envision the triggering event which allows the line to become TCGF-dependent? Why would it lose that with the single chromosomal loss?

Dr. Nabholz: I'm not talking about a single chromosomal loss. I think that both copies of the gene which makes the CTL and their hybrids TCGF-dependent are active. Thus, in order to get TCGF-independent hybrids both chromosomes must be lost. There's nothing against that. The system works well because we have a selective systems. We can select rare variants from the TCGF-dependent cloned hybrids in and the frequencies by which they arise are not inconsistent with those of chromosome losses in other systems of somatic cell hybridization. We don't know whether this explanation is correct. Moreover, if the TCGF-dependence is imposed on the cell by the activity of a single gene and if that gene would be allelically excluded (i.e. expressed only in one copy), then we should be able to get TCGF in dependent mutants from the CTL-B lines with reasonable frequencies by using a mutagenesis protocol and selecting for TCGF-independent cells. We have not been able to do that. The frequency of TCGF-independent mutants is more than a thousandfold lower than, for instance, HGPRT-deficient mutants, where we also select for the loss of a single copy of a gene.

Dr. Fernandez-Cruz: For immunotherapy it might be as important to have cloned T helper lines as cytotoxic lines.

Dr. Nabholz; We will hear more about that in Dr. Fitch's and Dr. Fathman's talks.

Dr. Paetkau: You mentioned that the variants which are CS- still retain the binding for IL 2. Have you primarily derived CS- which do not or which do? Are there some growth factor independent lines that you pick out at the first instance which do not bind?

Dr. Nabholz: We have not tested that. The problem is that we were trying to get the absorption experiments to the point where we can be reasonably sure that we look at receptors on the cell surface and we have only done preliminary experiments with the hybrids. Now we can screen many hybrids.

Dr. Bernard: To establish the value of the Vicia Villosa lectin binding as a marker on these CTL lines, do you know if this lectin will also inhibit the helper T cell lines?
Dr. Nabholz: I don't know.
Dr. Bernard: Don't you think it's important to establish if you want to have the Vicia Villusa binding as a marker for CTL?
Dr. Nabholz: I don't want to have it as a marker for CTL. All I say is that CTL lines are sensitive to Vicia Villosa, bind to Vicia Villosa and that we have the correlation in the hybrids between Vicia Villosa sensitivity, TCGF dependence and CTL activity. Maybe we can find out, using the system, whether this Vicia Villosa binding means something for the function of CTL. A mere correlation with cell types will not yield a definitive answer. We know that Vicia Villosa binding itself is not important for the CTL phenotype because we can select mutants (not hybrids), which are Vicia Villosa resistant and still are able to kill specifically -- they don't lose the CTL phenotype.
Dr. Bonavida: Can you speculate on the glycoproteins that you see on the positive lines and about any differences among the lines?
Dr. Nabholz: I would not like to speculate.
Dr. Bach: Is it the T200 you are looking at which is the same as Ly 5?
Dr. Nabholz: Yes.
Dr. Bach: I thought that had been mapped to chromosome #1. Sarmiento, working with Frank Fitch, and Widmer and Dunlap working with me have been looking at Ly 5 expression on normal cloned T lymphocytes. There are cytotoxic T lymphocyte clones that have high molecular weight markers of 222,000 and 240,000; there are other Tc that have lower Ly 5 markers (210,000 and 225,000) but still higher than the regular thymoma. The protein backbone of all the Ly 5 bands ranging form 187,000 to 240,000 seems to be very similar. Could some of what you are showing us not be loss of bands, and if it is loss have you looked at chromosome #1 or could it be regulation?
Dr. Nabholz: The changes in the glycoprotein patterns between TCGF-dependent hybrids and independent variants suggest that we're looking not at loss of structural protein backbones of certain glycoproteins but at changes in the expression of glycosyetransferases which affect a whole slew of glycoproteins. We haven't looked at Ly 5 on these hybrids directly. We suspect that they all have it.

The Potential Role of T Cells in Cancer Therapy,
edited by A. Fefer and A. Goldstein,
Raven Press, New York © 1982.

Strategies for Regulating the Human Immune Response by Selective T Cell Subset Manipulation

Ellis L. Reinherz and Stuart F. Schlossman

Division of Tumor Immunology, Sidney Farber Cancer Institute and the Department of Medicine, Harvard Medical School, Boston, Massachusetts 02115

The precise dissection of cellular mechanisms and interactions involved in the generation of human T cell responses has been facilitated in recent years by advances in four areas: first, the development of in vitro methods for characterization and identification of human T lymphocyte subsets by cell surface markers; second, the development of new techniques for the isolation of highly purified subclasses of human T lymphocytes depending on cell surface markers; third, the development of in vitro techniques to discriminate functional properties and interactions of the isolated subsets of T lymphocytes and other cells (that is, B cells, null cells and macrophages); and fourth, the capacity to correlate normal and abnormal in vitro functional properties of T lymphocyte subpopulations with in vivo disorders of the immune response. These advances have made possible the elucidation of the major T lymphocyte subsets in man and their unique functional programs.

The genetic program of the human T lymphocyte is a complex one as it includes immunoregulation as well as the capacity to recognize specific antigens and to execute unique effector functions. Thus, T lymphocytes proliferate to soluble and cell surface antigens and polyclonal activators, including the mitogens phytohemagglutinin (PHA) and Concanavallin A (Con A).[1,2] They are responsible for cytotoxic killer activity in cell-mediated lympholysis (CML)[3] and they produce a host of soluble factors[4,5] which effect a variety of cellular functions. Perhaps more importantly, T lymphocytes are involved in virtually all regulatory interactions, including helper and suppressor cell function[6,7].

In this review, we will focus upon the recent developments in understanding of the differentiative history of T lymphocytes and their functional maturation. We will also provide evidence which supports the notion that, during differentiation, T cells diverge into functionally distinct subsets programmed for their respective inducer (helper) and cytotoxic/suppressor functions which can be defined by unique cell surface glycoprotein antigens.

Differentiation of T Lymphocytes

A thymic microenvironment is necessary for the differentiation of T cells in all species. It appears that precursor bone marrow cells (pro-thymocytes) migrate to the thymus gland, where they are processed, be-come functionally competent, and are then exported into the peripheral lymphoid compartment.[8-11] Moreover, profound changes in cell surface antigens mark the stages of T cell ontogeny.[12,13]

In man the earliest lymphoid cell within the thymus lack mature T cell antigens but bear antigens shared by bone marrow cells of several lineages.[14] This population accounts for approximately 10% of thymic lymphocytes and is reactive with two monoclonal antibodies, anti-T9 and anti-T10 (Stage I)(Fig. 1). Although these two antibodies are not speci-

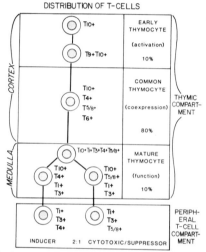

Fig 1. Stages of T Cell Differentiation in Human Beings. Three dis-crete stages of thymic differentiation can be defined on the basis of reactivity with monoclonal antibodies. The most mature thymocyte pop-ulation (Stage III) gives rise to the peripheral T cell inducer and cytotoxic/suppressor subsets. The cell surface antigens expressed during T cell ontogeny are shown.

fic for T cells[14,15] (since they are reactive with normal, activated, and malignant cells of non-T lineages), they are useful in providing an understanding of antigenic changes occurring during T cell ontogeny. With maturation, thymocytes lose T9, retain T10, and acquire a thymocyte distinct antigen defined by anti-T6. Concurrently, these cells express antigens defined by anti-T5 and anti-T5/T8 (Stage II). The $T4^+$, $T5/8^+$, $T6^+$, and $T10^+$ thymocytes account for approximately 70% of the total thy-mic population. With further maturation, thymocytes lose the T6 antigen, maximally express the T1 and T3 antigens, and then segregate into $T4^+$ and $T5^+$ subsets (Stage III). ($T5^+$ cells also express the T8 antigen. For simplification, however, these cells are referred to as $T5^+$ rather than $T5^+/8^+$.) Immunologic competence is acquired at this stage but is not fully developed until thymic lymphocytes are exported.[16] Outside the thymus the resting ($T1^+,T3^+,T4^+$) and ($T1^+,T3^+,T5^+$) subsets lack T10 and represent the circulating inducer (helper)[17,18] and cytotoxic/suppressor populations,[19-21] respectively.

Unlike the majority of the thymocytes which express little or only faint reactivity with anti-T1 and anti-T3,[22] all of the circulating peripheral T cells are strongly reactive with T1$^+$ and T3$^+$. The T4 antigen is expressed on approximately 55-65% of peripheral T cells, and the T5[18] antigen is present on 20-30%. These two subsets correspond to TH$_2$$^-$ helper and TH$_2$$^+$ cytotoxic/suppressor cells, respectively.[19,23] Moreover, unlike Stage II thymocytes, T4 and T5/T8 antigens are expressed on mutually exclusive subsets of mature T cells.[14,20,24] Table I lists the cell surface expression of antigens defined by monoclonal antibodies and indicates their preliminary biochemical characterization.[25-30] Also listed is a monoclonal antibody, anti-T11, which defines an antigen comprising or closely associated with the sheep erythrocyte receptor. Since this antigen is expressed on all thymocytes and peripheral T cells, it will not be discussed further.

Functions of Mature T Lymphocyte Subsets

Given the existence of two distinct subpopulations of peripheral T cells and the multiplicity of functional responses effected by T lymphocytes, it was important to determine whether an individual T lymphocyte possessed all of these effector and regulatory functions or, alternatively, whether T cells within a subset were unique with respect to their functional repertoire. A series of functional studies on isolated subpopulations of peripheral T lymphocytes has demonstrated that the latter hypothesis is correct and that the specific program of T cells is linked to the expression of a particular cell surface antigen.

For example, only the T1$^+$,T3$^+$,T4$^+$ population responded to soluble antigen.[17] In contrast, both subsets of cells show a maximal response to cell surface antigens (alloantigens). In additional studies, it was shown that the T1$^+$,T3$^+$,T4$^+$ population responds maximally to PHA, while the T1$^+$,T3$^+$,T5$^+$ subset shows a diminished response at all doses tested. Both populations of cells respond comparably to Con A.

As mentioned above, one of the major effector functions of human T lymphocytes is the capacity to become sensitized to HLA-A, -B and -C locus antigens and to effect specific cell-mediated killing. It was found that only the T1$^+$,T3$^+$,T5$^+$ subset [20,24] contained a cytotoxic effector population when separated after allogeneic activation in mixed lymphocyte culture. The T1$^+$,T3$^+$,T4$^+$ population, although capable of proliferating to alloantigen did not become cytotoxic when separated after sensitization.[17]

Perhaps the most important difference between these T cell subsets was evident from their differential regulatory effects on the immune response.[6,7] The T1$^+$,T3$^+$,T4$^+$ cells were shown to provide inducer (helper) function in the T-T, T-B, and T-macrophage interactions. For example, although the T1$^+$,T3$^+$,T4$^+$ cells were not cytotoxic effectors when separated after allogeneic stimulation, they were required for optimal development of cytotoxicity within the T1$^+$,T3$^+$,T5$^+$ effector population[17] This is similar to findings in previous studies which showed that the TH$_2$$^+$ population defined by heteroantisera contained the cytotoxic effector cell, while the TH$_2$$^-$ population contained the helper cell for development of cytotoxicity.[23]

Thus the T1$^+$,T3$^+$,T4$^+$ (T4$^+$) T cells provided an inducer function in T-T interactions. In addition, T4$^+$ T cells provided helper function in T-B interactions as well.[18,21] Only the T4$^+$ T cell subset provided the signals necessary to help autologous B cells to proliferate and differentiate into immunoglobulin-containing cells (Fig. 2). In contrast, the

Table 1. Monoclonal antibodies to human T cell surface antigens

Monoclonal antibodies	Approximate molecular weights of antigens 25-30		Cell surface expression (% reactivity with antibodies)			Trade designations
	Non-reduced	Reduced	Thymocytes	T cells	Non-T cells	
Anti-T1[∞]	69K	69K	10[+]	100	0	OKT1, Leu1*
Anti-T3	19K	19K	10[+]	100	0	OKT3, Leu4
Anti-T4	62K	62K	75	60	0	OKT4, Leu3a/3b
Anti-T5	76K	30K + 32K	80	25	0	OKT5
Anti-T8	-	-	80	30	0	OKT8, Leu2a/2b
Anti-T6[⊖]	49K	49K	70	0	0	NAI/34, OKT6
Anti-T9[∞]	190K	94K	10	0	0	OKT9, 5E9
Anti-T10[∞]	37K	45K	95	5	0	OKT10
Anti-T11[††]	50K	50K	100	100	≤10	OKT11, Leu5, NEI-016 SFCI 3pt2H9

*OK designations are available through Ortho Pharmaceuticals, Raritan, NJ. Leu designations are available through Becton-Dickinson, Mountain View, CA. 5E9 is available through NIAID monoclonal antibody serum bank, Bethesda, MD. NAI/34 is available through Accurate Chemical, NJ.

[∞]T9 and T10 antigens are not T lineage specific and are found on normal and malignant populations of non-T cells.[14,15] In addition, both antigens are expressed on a fraction of peripheral T cells following mitogen stimulation.[27]

[+]10% of thymocytes express a high density of T1 and T3 antigens while the remaining thymocytes express little or faint reactions with anti-T1 and anti-T3.[22]

[⊖]T6 is B2 microglobulin associated.

[††]See references 56 and 57.

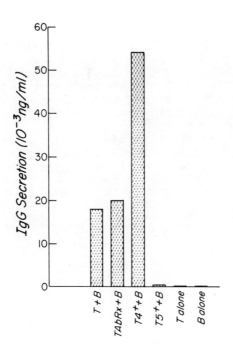

Fig. 2. Influence of Isolated T Cell Subsets on B Cell IgG Secretion. Isolated populations of T cells and T cell subsets, B cells, and autologous T-B combinations were cultured in the presence of PWM for 7 days. Subsequently, culture supernatants were harvested and IgG secretion quantitated by RIA. The TAbRx population was treated with anti-T4 or anti-T5 and G/M FITC, but not fractionated into subsets. As shown, the T4+ T cell subset helps B cells secrete IgG and its inductive effect is significantly greater than the unfractionated T cell population. In contrast, the T5+ subset provides no inducer function for IgG secretion. Results are representative of four experiments performed.

T1+,T3+,T5+ (T5+) T cells neither induced B cells to proliferate nor to differentiate. Moreover, the inducer role of the T4+ T cells for B cell immunoglobulin production was shown in both a pokeweed mitogen[18] and an antigen-stimulated system.[31]

Prior studies demonstrated that antigen triggered T cells produced helper factors, including lymphocyte mitogenic factor,[4] which induced proliferation of all major lymphocyte subclasses (T cell, B cell, null cell and macrophage) and, T cell replacing factor which initiated B cell immunoglobulin synthesis in the absence of T cells. In recent studies, it was found that only the T4+ subset made these nonspecific helper factors.[31] The T cell subset restriction of these factors in man further stresses the importance of this subset of T cells in its inductive influence on the human immune response.

The above findings helped assign an inducer role to the T4+ population in T-T, T-B and T-macrophage interactions. Moreover, they provided additional evidence that a proliferative response to soluble antigen is restricted to the inducer population. The regulatory effects of the T4+ population do not appear limited to cells of lymphoid lineage. Since it is known that antigen-stimulated T lymphocytes produce helper factors which modulate erythroid stem cell production in vitro, it is probably that the T4[+] population of lymphocytes is important in some aspect of erythroid differentiation.[32] Similarly, osteoclast-activating factor[33] and soluble factors inducing fibroblast proliferation and collagen synthesis have been shown to be derived from antigen-stimulated T lymphocytes.[34] These findings suggest a much broader biologic role for the T4[+] inducer population in man.

The T5[+] subset in contrast contains a mature population of cells with cytotoxic and suppressor function but not inducer functions.[20,21] Following activation with Con A, T5 cells suppressed autologous T cells responding in MLC. In addition, this same T5[+] population suppressed B cell immunoglobulin production (Fig. 3). It should be emphasized at this

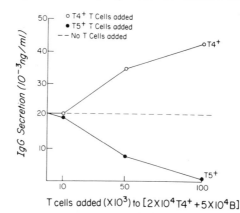

Fig. 3. Suppressive Effect of the T5[+] T Cell Subset on Autologous B Cell IgG Secretion. The capacity of T4[+] and T5[+] T cells to effect IgG secretion by a mixture of 2×10^4 T4[+] T cells and 5×10^4 B cells was determined. T cell subsets were separated as described in Materials and Methods. Subsequently, different numbers of T4[+] (o) or T5[+] (●) T cells were added to the constant T4[+] T-B mixture and supernatants harvested after 7 days in culture with PWM. As shown, T5[+] cells were capable of suppressing IgG secretion while a comparable number of T4[+] cells provided additional T cell help. Results are representative of four experiments performed.

point that although both the T4[+] and T5[+] subpopulations proliferated equally well to mitogenic stimulation by Con A, only the T5[+] population became suppressive. These results support the view that the T4[+] and T5[+] subpopulations are programmed for their respective helper and suppressor functions independent of their ability to discriminate and react to nonspecific polyclonal mitogens or antigens. Moreover, these results suggest that the programming of the specific cell function is linked to the expression of a particular cell surface phenotype and that such programming occurs before cell activation.

Further evidence substantiating this notion is the subsets' differential susceptibility to expression of Ia antigens following specific activation stimuli.[35] In several species, immunoregulatory activities are mediated by intercellular signals involving products of the I region of the major histocompatibility complex. Human Ia-like antigens were first defined by alloantisera[36] and subsequently by heteroantisera[37] and monoclonal antibodies.[35] In man, Ia antigens are expressed on the surface of B cells, most monocytes and a subset of null cells, but are not detected on resting T cells.[35,38] Activation of human T cells results in de novo biochemical synthesis and cell surface expression of Ia antigens.[39] Thus, the appearance of Ia antigen on T cell subsets serves as a marker of specific T cell activation. Following alloactivation in MLC or stimulation by PHA and Con A, both $T4^+$ and $T5^+$ T cell subsets express Ia antigens. In contrast, when the T cell population is specifically activated by soluble antigens, only the $T4^+$ subset expresses Ia. The appearance of Ia antigens on unique T cell subsets therefore depends upon the activation stimuli used and the ability of that individual subset to respond to a given stimulus.

The observation that only a fraction ($\sim$40%) of $T4^+$ T cells expressed Ia antigen upon activation suggested that the $T4^+$ population might be heterogeneous. To test this possibility, antigen activated $T4^+$ T cells were separated into $T4^+Ia^+$ and $T4^+Ia^-$ populations and characterized.[40] It was found that the $T4^+Ia^+$ population contained the majority of proliferating T cells and that most of this proliferation was nonspecific. Elimination of the $T4^+Ia^+$ T cell subset with monoclonal anti-Ia and complement treatment diminished subsequent proliferation to both the triggering antigen and to unrelated antigens. In addition, the antigen induced $T4^+Ia^+$ subset alone produce nonspecific helper factors. Although the Ia^- fraction represents 60% of the $T4^+$ population, it showed minimal proliferation to soluble antigen and did not elaborate helper factors. Nonetheless, a mixture of both $T4^+Ia^+$ and $T4^+Ia^-$ T cells was required for maximal Ig secretion by B cells since these two $T4^+$ subsets worked in a synergistic fashion.

Other studies have provided additional evidence to support the existence of heterogeneity within the $T4^+$ subset. Specifically it was shown that approximately 35% of $T4^+$ T cells and 10% of $T5^+$ cells were reactive with an antibody found in the serum of many patients with active juvenile rheumatoid arthritis.[41] These $T4^+JRA^+$ cells are required to induce the $T5^+$ subset to mediate suppression of B cell Ig secretion. Thus $T4^+JRA^+$ T cells appear to be the inducer cells of suppression while $T4^+JRA^-$ are the T inducers of help (Fig. 4). Yet to be determined is the relationship of $T4^+Ia^+$ lymphocytes to the $T4^+JRA^+$ subset.

Therefore the $T4^+$ subset is analogous to the murine Lyt^+2^- subset which provides helper function through both specific and nonspecific signals and induces suppressor cell activation as well.[42] In this regard, $T4^+JRA^+$ subset has a counterpart in the $Lyt1^+Qa1^+$ murine subpopulations[43] and the $T4^+Ia^+$ in the $Lyt1^+2^-Ia^+$ subset.[44] The $T5^+$ T subset in man appears to be analogous to the murine $Lyt2,3$ subset which mediates both cytotoxic and suppressor functions.[42] Based on the evolutionary conservation of other cell surface molecules (that is, immunoglobulins, MHC encloded antigens, etc.), it is likely that the antigens defining the phenotypes of inducer and suppressor populations in man and mouse will be biochemically similar. There is already good evidence to indicate that the T5 antigen and the Lyt2,3 antigen are homologous.[27]

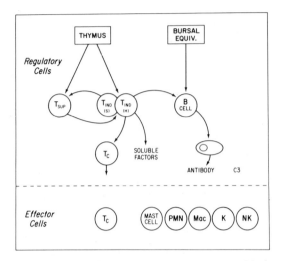

Fig. 4. The Human T Cell Circuit. Cellular and humoral responses are regulated by T4$^+$ inducer (Tind) and T5$^+$ suppressor (Tsup) T lymphocytes. One subpopulation of T4$^+$ cells (Tind$_{(S)}$), reactive with JRA autoantibodies, induces T5$^+$ suppressor cell activation while a second subpopulation of T4$^+$ cells (Tind$_{(H)}$) induces help for cytotoxic T cell (Tc) effector function, B cell differentiation and immunoglobulin production. Many of the effector cells illustrated above including NK, K, mast cells, polymorphonuclear leukocytes (PMN) and Macrophages (Mac) are under the influence of these regulatory cells and their products.

However, whether the T4 antigen and the Lyt1 antigen are similar is less certain. Nonetheless, given the observation that T4 and T5 are on reciprocal subsets in man with similar functions to the murine Lyt1$^+$2$^-$ and Lyt2$^+$ populations it is likely that an antigen equivalent to T4 exists on a murine Lyt1$^+$2$^-$ subset.

Clinical Disorders of T Lymphocytes

In the present review, we have provided evidence to support the theory that it is possible to detect T lymphocyte subpopulations with unique biologic functions on the basis of their cell surface antigenic components. The application of this technology to human immunodiagnosis is just becoming appreciated. It is now possible to define the heterogeneity of T cell malignancies; diseases of T cell maturation and/or premature release; diseases associated with loss of T cells; diseases associated with imbalances of T cell subset restricted functions; and diseases associated with activation of T cell subsets.

Since immunologic functions are acquired only at the latest stage of intrathymic ontogeny, premature release of immunologically incompetent cells or aberrations of T cell maturation resulting in blocked differentiation could lead to immunodeficiency. The development of probes that make it possible to define points along the differentiative pathway should help in the understanding of heterogeneity within congenital immunodeficiencies. In this regard, it has already become evident that patients with severe combined immunodeficiency may have thymocytes blocked in differentiation either at Stage I (T10[+] or T9[+]T10[+]) or Stage III (T3[+]T4[+]T5/8[+]T10[+]).[45] As expected, only those patients with the latter population express any T cell function (i.e. MLC proliferation).

Major immunologic abnormalities result from alterations in the mature T cell subsets. For example, some patients with acquired agammaglobulinemia lack the T4[+] population and possess a T cell population that is incapable of triggering B cell synthesis of immunoglobulin. This specialized circumstance must be discriminated from that in the majority of patients with agammaglobulinemia, who have B cell abnormalities, but possess normal T cells.[6,7]

Circulating activated T4[+] cells appear to result in different immunopathologic abnormalities including the formation of autoantibodies directed at red cells, white cells and platelets. Activated helper cells have been demonstrated in patients with active graft-versus-host disease,[46] and similar abnormalities have been seen in patients with sarcoid, scleroderma, and Sjogren's syndrome. Not only is there an increase in T4[+] cells, but these activated T lymphocytes, unlike resting lymphocytes, express Ia-like (HLA-D related) antigens. The presence of activated T lymphocytes in human disease does not appear to be uncommon.[47] Whether the activated T4[+]T cells account for hyperglobulinemia, lymphocytosis, dermal infiltration, granuloma formation, or fibrotic lesions in the diseases mentioned above is under investigation.

It is obvious that defects in immunoregulation could result from either a loss or persistent activation of the T5[+] population. Loss of the T5[+] T cells should result in unopposed inducer functions, whereas activated T5[+] cells should suppress the immune response. In patients with acute graft-versus-host disease, in which activated helper cells have been demonstrated, there is also a loss of suppressor cells.[46] A similar loss of T5[+] cells has been seen in naturally occurring autoimmune diseases including systemic lupus erythematosus,[48] hemolytic anemia,[49] multiple sclerosis,[50] severe atopic eczema, hyper IgE syndrome and inflammatory bowel disease.[7] Moreover, the loss of the T5[+] population may correlate temporally with the severity of clinical disease. The precise mechanism by which one population is lost or another activated is not clear. There is evidence from patients with lupus that autoantibodies are present in the serum and directed at the T5[+] population.[51] Autoantibodies may selectively eliminate the suppressor population or modulate its functional properties. Similarly, in studies of patients with juvenile rheumatoid arthritis, the loss of suppressor cell function correlates with increased B cell Ig secretion, the presence of autoantibodies to a T4[+] subset which induces suppressor cell function, and increased disease activity.[41]

In contrast, the presence of excessive numbers of activated suppressor cells results in severe immunodeficiency. For example, in a smaller number of patients with acquired agammaglobulinemia, activated T5[+]Ia[+] cells were responsible for suppressing autologous B cell production of immunoglobulin.[49] Increased numbers of activated suppressor cells have also been seen after viral infections including those caused by Epstein-Barr virus and cytomegalovirus.[52] In infectious mononucleosis, the self-limited increase in suppressor cells may account for transient immunologic hyporesponsiveness, but in patients with chronic graft-versus-host disease, persistent circulating suppressor cells cause prolonged immunologic incompetence.[46] Moreover, antigen-specific suppressor cells may result in human disorders. Patients with lepromatous leprosy have a $T5^+$ population that can be specifically activated by lepromin.[53] In this case, activation of $T5^+$ T cells is antigen-specific; nevertheless, these activated suppressor cells may cause generalized immunosuppression. Presumably, the anergy seen in tuberculosis, systemic fungal infections, and protozoan infections may result from similar mechanisms. Finally it should be noted that an imbalance in the inducer:suppressor cell ratio is itself sufficient to result in diminished immunoglobulin production in vitro and agammaglobulinemia in vivo. The finding of a relative increase in suppressor cells is a common finding in patients with acquired agammaglobulinemia and circulating B cells.[48]

Human T Cell Malignant Diseases

The ability to define cell surface antigens that appear at specific stages of T cell differentiation has, in addition, allowed for the orderly dissection of T cell malignant processes in human beings. In fact, these T cell diseases reflect the same degree of heterogeneity and maturation as is seen in normal T cell ontogeny.[14] For example, the tumor cells in most cases of acute T cell lymphoblastic leukemia arise from an early thymocyte or prothymocyte compartment (Stage I), whereas in only 20% of cases the cells are derived from a common thymocyte compartment (Stage II) and therefore bear the T6 antigen. To date, we have found only one T cell acute lymphoblastic leukemia tumor that arose from the most mature thymic compartment and expressed the T3 antigen (Stage III). Since normal thymocytes have not acquired mature T cell functions at either the level of the Stage I or II thymocytes, it is not surprising that the vast majority of acute lymphoblastic leukemia T cell in human beings have no demonstrable function.

The tumor populations from patients with T cell chronic lymphocytic leukemia, Sezary syndrome and mycosis fungoides are derived from the mature T cell compartment bearing the T1 or T3 antigens or both.[15,54] Therefore, it is not unexpected that some of these tumor cells display helper or suppressor functions. In this regard, all tumor populations from patients with Sezary syndrome bear the $T1^+T3^+T4^+$ phenotype and may demonstrate the functional capacity to provide help for B cell Ig synthesis. T cell CLL tumor populations are of either the mature inducer or suppressor phenotypes. Since 6 of 8 T-CLL tumor populations studied to date have been of the helper phenotype, it would appear the the frequency of subset derivation corresponds to that expected from the normal ratio of inducer:suppressor cells (i.e. 2-3:1).

Immunotherapy by Selective T Cell Subset Manipulation

The ability to dissect normal lymphoid differentiation and to define the biology of lymphocytes in health and disease will allow for an understanding of disorders of the human immune response. In addition to their immunodiagnostic utility, the reagents described in this review may be potent therapeutic tools themselves. It is also likely that certain drugs will have selective effects on individual T cell subsets such that they could be utilized to alter the ratio of T inducer and T suppressor cells.

Finally, it is important to note that these monoclonal antibody-defined cell surface antigens may themselves represent important cell surface receptors. For example, anti-T3 alone was found in earlier studies to block proliferative responses of T lymphocytes to both soluble and cell surface antigens (Fig. 5).[55] As few as 10^4 molecules of anti-T3

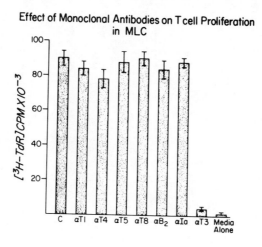

Fig. 5. Unique Capacity of Anti-T3 to Inhibit MLC Proliferation. The effect of anti-T3 and other monoclonal antibodies to inhibit MLC proliferation was determined by incubating responding T cell and mitomycin treated stimulator cell mixtures with antibodies during the in vitro culture period. Results are expressed as ^{3}H-TdR incorporation.

per cell appeared to inhibit these responses when added early in the culture period.

In addition to abrogating antigen-stimulated T cell proliferation responses, anti-T3 blocked the ability of T cells to provide help to autologous B lymphocytes in a T-dependent, PWM-driven system (Fig. 6). Thus, in the presence of anti-T3, Ig secretion by the T-B mixture was reduced to the level of Ig secretion found in B cells alone. Similar to the inhibition of T cell proliferation, anti-T3 inhibition of PWM-driven Ig secretion occurred during an early phase of cell-cell interaction. The capacity of anti-T3 to inhibit both T cell proliferation itself as well as T-B cooperation suggests that anti-T3 defines an important T cell interaction molecule. Both the failure of all other T cell specific antibodies to block these functions and the fully developed expression of the T3 antigen late in thymic differentiation at the time of acquisition of immunologic competence suggest that T3 is an important molecule.[55]

Furthermore, other T lymphocyte surface molecules may be critical for a variety of T cell effector functions. Recently, several monoclonal antibodies, anti-T5, anti-T8 and anti-T8$_A$, were found to define antigens on cytotoxic effector T cells (unpublished data).[14,20] More importantly, as shown in Table 2, anti-T8$_A$ markedly inhibited cell mediated lympholysis, anti-T8 partially effected CML, and anti-T5 had no effect. Immunoprecipitation studies and competitive binding experiments indicated that anti-T8 and anti-T8$_A$, like anti-T5, defined a related 33,000 dalton

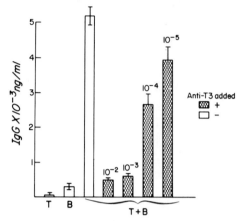

Fig. 6. Inhibition by Anti-T3 of T Cell
Help in PWM-Driven B Cell IgG Secretion.
The capacity of anti-T3 to effect IgG secretion by a mixture of T and B cells was
determined. Anti-T3 was added to cultures
in dilutions ranging from 10^{-2} to 10^{-5}.
As shown, IgG synthesis is significantly
inhibited by anti-T3 even at a dilution
of 10^{-4}.

molecular weight antigen. Taken together, these results suggest that
the single epitope marked by anti-T8$_A$ is critical for the cytolytic
mechanism.

TABLE 2.   Effect of pre-incubation of CTL with monoclonal antibodies.

		% Specific lysis		
Monoclonal antibody	E/T ratio:	40/1	20/1	10/1
Control		28 ± 2	29 ± 1	21 ± 1
Anti-T5		30 ± 2	28 ± 2	22 ± 2
Anti-T8		16 ± 2	14 ± 2	15 ± 1
Anti-T8$_A$		2 ± 1	2 ± 1	1 ± 1

Additional studies in the murine system indicate that regulatory
molecules (i.e. IJ), like effector molecules, are expressed on the cell
surface membrane of some T lymphocytes. It is likely that antibodies to
such determinants may serve to inhibit suppressor T cell function. In
this regard, abrogation of suppressor cells has been shown to markedly
alter the host immune response to autologous tumor cells (see Discussion
by M. Greene in this symposium).
Utilization of soluble regulatory products from T lymphocytes as well
as manipulation of T cells and their cell surface receptor may be of
paramount importance in controlling immune function. Given the recent
evolution of T-T hybridomas in murine systems and the possibility of developing similar hybridomas in humans, it is conceivable that homogene-

ous helper and suppressor products could be produced. These and other strategies should prove useful to the host if manipulations are based on sound principles of immunobiology.

SUMMARY

Functional T lymphocyte subpopulations can be identified in humans by antibodies which detect stable glycoprotein antigens on their surface. Thus, inducer T lymphocytes bear an antigen termed T4 while suppressor T lymphocytes bear a different antigen termed T5. Immune homeostasis results from a delicate balance between inducer and suppressor subsets within the T cell circuit. Perturbation in subset dynamics may initiate a wide variety of immunopathologic disorders. An understanding of this circuit will be important for the elucidation of the pathogenesis of a number of diseases and should permit the orderly manipulation of the human immune response through modulation of selected T cell subsets.

REFERENCES

1. Chess, L., MacDermott, R.P. and Schlossman, S.F. (1974). J. Immunol. 113:1113-1121.
2. Chess, L., MacDermott, R.P. and Schlossman, S.F. (1974). J. Immunol. 113:1122-1127.
3. Sondel, P.M., Chess, L., MacDermott, R.P. and Schlossman, S.F.(1975) J. Immunol. 114:982-987.
4. Geha, R.S., Schneeberger, E., Rosen, F.S. and Merler, E. (1973). J. Exp. Med. 138:1230-1247.
5. Rocklin, R.E., MacDermott, R.P., Chess, L., Schlossman, S.F. and David, J.R. (1974). J. Exp. Med. 140:1303-1316.
6. Reinherz, E.L. and Schlossman, S.F. (1980). Cell 19:821-827.
7. Reinherz, E.L. and Schlossman, S.F. (1980). N. Engl. J. Med. 303: 370-373.
8. Moore, M.R.S. and Owen, J.T.T. (1967). J. Exp. Med. 126:715-725.
9. Owen, J.T.T. and Ritter, M.A. (1969). J. Exp. Med. 129:431-437.
10. Owen, J.T.T. and Raff, M.C. (1970). J. Exp. Med. 132:1216-1232.
11. Stutman, O. and Good, R.A. (1971). Transplant Proc. 3:923-925.
12. Raff, M.C. (1971). Transplant. Rev. 6:52-80.
13. Konda, S., Stockert, E. and Smith, R.T. (1973). Cell. Immunol. 7: 275-289.
14. Reinherz, E.L., Kung, P.C., Goldstein, G., Levey, R.H. and Schlossman, S.F. (1980). Proc. Natl. Acad. Sci. USA 77:1588-1592
15. Reinherz, E.L. and Schlossman, S.F. Cancer Research (In press).
16. Reinherz, E.L., Kung, P.C., Goldstein, G. and Schlossman, S.F. (1979). J. Immunol. 123:1312-1317.
17. Reinherz, E.L., Kung, P.C., Goldstein, G. and Schlossman, S.F. (1979). Proc. Natl. Acad. Sci. USA 76:4061-4065.
18. Reinherz, E.L., Kung, P.C., Goldstein, G. and Schlossman, S.F. (1979). J. Immunol. 123:2894-2896.
19. Reinherz, E.L. and Schlossman, S.F. (1979). J. Immunol. 122:1335-1341.
20. Reinherz, E.L., Kung, P.C., Goldstein, G. and Schlossman, S.F. (1980). J. Immunol. 124:1301-1307.
21. Reinherz, E.L., Morimoto, C., Penta, A.C. and Schlossman, S.F. (1980). Eur. J. Immunol. 10:570-572.
22. Bhan, A.K., Reinherz, E.L., Poppema, S., McCluskey, R. and Schloss-

man, S.F. (1980). J. Exp. Med. 152:771-782.

23. Evans, R.L., Lazarus, H., Penta, A.C.and Schlossman, S.F. (1978). J. Immunol. 120:1423-1428.

24. Reinherz, E.L., Hussey, R.E. and Schlossman, S.F. (1980). Immunogen 11:421-426.

25. van Agthoven, A., Terhorst, C., Reinherz, E.L. and Schlossman, S.F. (1981). Eur. J. Immunol. 11:18-21.

26. Martin, P.J., Hanson, J.A., Nowinski, R.C. and Brown, M.A. Immunogen. (In press).

27. Terhorst, C., van Agthoven, A., Reinherz, E.L. and Schlossman,S.F. (1980). Science 209:520-521.

28. Terhorst, C., van Agthoven, A., LeClair, K., Snow, P., Reinherz, E.L. and Schlossman, S.F. Cell (In press).

29. McMichael, A.J., Pilch, J.R., Galfre, G., Mason, D.Y., Fabre, J.W. and Milstein, C. (1979). Eur. J. Immunol. 9:205-210.

30. Ledbetter, J., Evan, R.L., Lipinski, M., Cunningham-Rundles, C., Good, R.R. and Herzenberg, L.A. J. Exp. Med. (In press).

31. Reinherz, E.L., Kung, P.C., Breard, J.M., Goldstein, G. and Schlossman, S.F. (1980). J. Immunol. 124:1883-1887.

32. Lipton, J.M., Reinherz, E.L., Kudisch, M., Jackson, P.L., Schloss- man, S.F. and Nathan, D.G. (1980). J. Exp. Med. 152:350-360.

33. Horton, J.E., Raiza, L.G., Simmons, H.A., Oppenheim, J.J. and Mor- genhargen, S.E. (1972). Science 177:793-795.

34. Cohen, S., Pick, E. and Oppenheim, J.J. (1979) Academic Press

35. Reinherz, E.L., Kung, P.C., Pesando, J.M., Ritz, J., Goldstein,G. and Schlossman, S.F. (1979). J. Exp. Med. 150:1472-1482.

36. Winchester, R.J., Fu, S.M., Wernet, P., Kunkel, H.G., Dupont, B. and Jersild, C. (1975). J. Exp. Med. 141:924-929.

37. Humphreys,R.E., McCune, J.M., Chess, L., Herrman, H.D., Malenka, D.J., Mann, D.L., Parham, P., Schlossman, S.F. and Strominger,J.L. (1976). J. Exp. Med. 144:98-112.

38. Schlossman, S.F., Chess, L., Humphreys, R.E. and Strominger, J.L. (1976). Proc. Natl. Acad. Sci. USA 73:1288-1292.

39. Evans, R.L., Faldetta, T.J., Humphreys, R.E., Pratt, D.M., Yunis, E.J. and Schlossman, S.F. (1978). J. Exp. Med. 148:1440-1445.

40. Reinherz, E.L., Morimoto, C., Penta, A.C. and Schlossman, S.F. (1981). J. Immunol. 126:67.

41. Morimoto, C., Reinherz, E.L., Borel, Y., Mantzourais, E., Stein- berg, A.D. and Schlossman, S.F. J. Clin. Invest. (In press).

42. Cantor, H. and Boyse, E.H. (1977). Cold Spring Harbor Symp. Quart. Biol. 41:23-32.

43. Eardley, D.D., Hugenberger, J., McVay-Boudreau, L., Shen, F.W., Gershon, R.K. and Cantor, H. (1978). J. Exp. Med. 147:1106-1115.

44. Keller, D.M., Swierhosz, J.E., Marrock, P. and Kappler, J.W.(1980). J. Immunol. 124:1350-1359.

45. Reinherz, E.L., Schlossman, S.F. and Rosen, F.S. Elsevier/North- Holland, Amsterdam. (In press).

46. Reinherz, E.L., Parkman, R., Rappaport, J.M., Rosen, F.S. and Schlossman, S.F. (1979). N. Engl. J. Med. 300:1061-1068.

47. Yu, D.T.Y., Winchester, R.J., Fu, S.M., Gibofsky, A., Ko, H.S. and Kunkel, H.G. (1980). J. Exp. Med. 151:91-100.

48. Morimoto, C., Reinherz, E.L., Steinberg, A.D., Schur, P.H., Mills, J.A. and Schlossman, S.F. (1980). J. Clin. Invest. 66:1171-1174.

49. Reinherz, E.L., Rubinstein, A., Geha, R.S., Rosen, F.S. and Schlossman, S.F. (1979). N. Engl. J. Med. 301:1018-1022.

50. Reinherz, E.L., Weiner, H.L., Hauser, S.L., Cohen, J.A., Distaso, J.A. and Schlossman, S.F. (1980). N. Engl. J. Med. 303:125-129.
51. Morimoto, C., Reinherz, E.L., Abe, T., Homma, M. and Schlossman, S.F. (1980). Clin. Immunol. & Immunopathol. 16:474-484.
52. Reinherz, E.L., O'Brien, C., Rosenthal, P. and Schlossman, S.F. (1980). J. Immunol. 125:1269-1274.
53. Mehra, V., Mason, L.H., Rothman, W., Reinherz, E.L., Schlossman, S.F. and Bloom, R.R. (1980). J. Immunol. 125:1183-1198.
54. Boumsell, L., Bernard, A., Reinherz, E.L., Nadler, L.M., Ritz, J., Coppin, H., Richard, Y., Dubertret, L., Degos, L., Lemerle, J., Flandrin, G., Dausset, J. and Schlossman, S.F. Blood (In press).
55. Reinherz, E.L., Hussey, R.E. and Schlossman, S.F. (1980). Eur. J. Immunol. 10:758-762.
56. Kamoun, M.P., Martin, P.J., Hansen, J.A., Brown, M.R., Siadan,A.W., and Nowinski, R.C. (1981). J. Exp. Med. 153:207-213.
57. Howard, F.D., Ledbetter, J.A., Wong, J., Bieber, C.P., Stinson,E.B. and Herzenberg, L.A. (1981). J. Immunol. 126:2117-2122.

AUDIENCE DISCUSSION

Dr. Warner: In regards to infectious mononucleosis, is there a distinction in the response of the two subsets to DRW versus HLA antigens?
Dr. Reinherz: There are data which indicate that the T_4^+ population proliferates specifically to differences in DR, whereas the T_5^+ or T_8^+ does not recognize DR differences. This can be shown in recombinant family studies. The T_4^+ population from one member can proliferate to lymphocytes of another member which differs only at DR whereas the $T_{5/8}$ cannot. Moreover, the autologous MLR is a property of the T_4^+ population and not the $T_{5/8}^+$ population.
Dr. Warner: That certainly is analogous to the mouse situation. What about the infectious mono then, where it's primarily an Ia DRW bearing type B cell? Why isn't the T_4 cell then primarily stimulated?
Dr. Reinherz: I think there's something unique about lymphoblastoid cells which appears to trigger suppressor cells, whether these be LPS blasts or EBV transformed cells. If one uses lymphoblastoid cells rather than resting lymphocytes as an allogeneic stimulus, one gets a much better proliferative response by T_5 cells. I think that there is a transformation that takes place when the cell becomes a blast which is serving as a trigger for T_5 cells. Incidentally, I don't want to leave you with the impression that the T_4 population or the T_5 population in and of themselves are homogeneous. There's a lot of heterogeneity even within these two subpopulations. For example, some studies indicate that the T_4 population is divisible into at least two major subpopulations, one of which appears to induce suppressor cells and the other which does not. At present we are looking only at the major subpopulations of immunoregulatory cells.
Dr. Fernandez-Cruz: Do you have any data on the imbalance of the helper/suppressor ratio in patients with solid tumors?
Dr. Reinherz: No. It is beginning to be looked at.
Dr. Grimm: You used OKT reagents to define the cytotoxic effector cell in an allogeneic sensitization. You sorted the T_5 positive and negative populations. The T_5 negative population had some residual cytotoxic activity. Does this represent another subpopulation of cytotoxic

effector cells or could you get rid of this with OKT_8 and perhaps with the use of complement or are we faced with a hazy area where we can't get rid of all of the allocytotoxicity with these monoclonals?

Dr. Reinherz: If you perform an allosensitization and then separate cells at day 6, virtually all of the cytotoxic effector function is in the T_5 positive or T_8 positive population -- a level of specific lysis which is 10-20% in the T_5 negative population and 80% or so in the T_5 positive population. Almost the entire cytotoxic effector potential is within the T_5 population. However, when you separate T cells into subsets prior to the initiation of the MLC -- then all bets are off, because the T_4 positive population develops into a cytotoxic effector population. It appears that in the absence of regulation from T_5 cells, T_4 cells can become cytotoxic and this cytotoxicity is specific. In addition, the allogeneic stimulus also results in generation of T cells which perform NK and ADDC and those two cytotoxic functions are not restricted to either T cell subset. When one simply looks at a crude chromium release assay, some of the activity seen results from these latter cytotoxic functions.

Dr. Grimm: Was you target a fresh lympocyte target or a blast target?

Dr. Reinherz: It was a blast. When fresh lymphocytes are used, there is much less background activity.

Dr. Curtis: In trying to hypothesize on the reason for the differential course of recovery or progression to lymphoma, does the HLA type of the individual plays a role?

Dr. Reinherz: It is not known. One would guess, however, given the situation with multiple sclerosis and other autoimmune diseases in which there is a very strong DR relationship, that this may well be the case. Even if there isn't a DR correlation, one would believe that there are immune response genes in the human, and that they may act at the level of individual T cell subpopulations. For example, some individuals may have an immune constitutuon such that antigen X induces selective triggering of T4 cells and results in autoimmunity whereas the same antigen induces T8 cells to suppress yielding a selective immunodeficiency state in another person.

Dr. Fathman: In the murine system the isolation of targets which bear DR specificity equivalents, the Ia molecules, depends upon the isolation of blasts of the equivalent cell type and the Dennert-Swain suggestion is that the Ly 1 type killer is directed at the DRW equivalent, the Ia antigen. Therefore, what you might be seeing in your residual killing with allostimulation is a DR kill with your helper-inducer type of cytotoxic cell. Have you asked that question with the appropriate blasts or the appropriate immunization?

Dr. Reinherz: We have not, but that's an excellent point.

The Potential Role of T Cells in Cancer Therapy,
edited by A. Fefer and A. Goldstein.
Raven Press, New York © 1982.

Regulation of the Immune Response to Cell Surface Antigens

Jonathan S. Bromberg, Muneo Takaoki, ManSun Sy, Akira Tominaga,
Linda Perry, and Mark I. Greene

Department of Pathology, Harvard Medical School, Boston, Massachusetts 02115

If immunology is to be of consequence to the therapy of tumors, then neoplasms must bear antigens on the cell surface. This follows from the absolute necessity to accurately distinguish malignant cells from normal ones. The host must also have a receptor repertoire which is capable of recognizing these tumor specific antigens. The antigen itself can be either a de novo tumor specific transplantation antigen (TSTA) or a component which is normally present in only a restricted number of tissues or cells and/or at certain stages of differentiation as examplified by so-called oncofetal antigens. If these cell surface structures are not present, then it is doubtful that specific immune responses can make a substantial contribution to cancer therapy.

Assuming that some tumors do meet these requirements, there are two major avenues of experimentation to immunotherapy. One is the development of syngeneic effector clones in vitro which can be transferred into the tumor bearing host. Many of the participants at this meeting have begun to develop this methodology and their findings and insights are reported elsewhere in this volume. The second approach deals with the nature of the ongoing immune response to the tumor in the host. If the tumor bears antigens, then why is it not promptly rejected? Studies conducted in our laboratories over the past several years have shown that the apparent lack of an immune response is due in some cases to the effects of active suppression by thymus-derived suppressor cells (Ts). A detailed understanding of suppressor cells could therefore have a significant impact on approaches to immunotherapy: interference with suppressor cell regulatory networks may be more efficacious than attempts to induce effector cell clones or at the very least provide an adjunct which assures the success of effector mechanisms.

Much of the work reported here deals with immunity and suppression to the hapten azobenzenearsonate (ABA). One of the advantages of this system is the ease with which haptens can be manipulated. Secondly, in the A/J strain of mice, ABA protein conjugates induce an antibody response dominated by a predominant cross-reactive idiotype (CRI) (10). This idiotypic determinat has enabled us to investigate receptor structure and specificity and to manipulate cell interactions. The results of the analysis of the ABA system seem applicable to antigens not known to

be under the control of a predominant idiotype such as certain other haptens, alloantigens and TSTA.

The Suppressor Cell Network

Delayed-Type Hypersensitivity

Delayed-type hypersensitivity (DTH) or cell mediated cytotoxicity
(CMC) to ABA-cell surface structures can be induced by injecting ABA
coupled syngeneic spleen cells subcutaneously into naive mice (3). DTH
immunity is elicited five days after priming by challenging one footpad
with the chemically reactive diazonium salt of ABA. Twenty-four hours
after challenge immunity is assessed by measuring the thickness of the
challenged foot pad versus the unchallenged one. The characteristics of
of the inflammatory response are typical: the swelling reaches its maximum at 24 hours; the infiltrate is predominantly lymphocytic and mononuclear; and immunity can be transferred with immune T cells but not with
immune serum. The immune cells are I-A restricted, Lyt1 T cells (T_{DH}).
(3). CMC is analyzed by restimulating spleen or lymph node cells,
from animals primed one week previously, with ABA coupled cells in vitro.
After five days in these secondary cultures, CMC is assessed in a standard ^{51}Cr- release assay.

An animal can be made tolerant to ABA by injecting syngeneic haptenated spleens cells intravenously. The tolerazing signal is quite potent and can be given before, at the time of or after subcutaneous
priming to induce nonresponsiveness. In addition to inducing a tolerant
state, the intravenous administration of hapten coupled cells also induces transferable suppressor cells. The cells are thy1.2+, Lyt1+2-3-
and I-J+. (3, 14). The cells are antigen specific in their ability to
transfer suppression. Similarly, the intravenous injection of tumor
cells, or tumor cell membranes, or trinitrophenyl coupled cells (a hapten not known to produce a predominant idiotype) also induces a state of
tolerance and generates antigen specific Ts.

With the use of idiotypic and anti-idiotypic reagents related to the
CRI, it has also been shown that the Ts induced by ABA coupled cells bear
idiotypic determinants on their surface which are similar to those present on CRI+ serum antibody (18). Thus these cells can be lysed with
anti-CRI and complement. Alternatively these Ts can be induced in vivo
by injection of anti-CRI antibodies and can be enriched by adsorption to
antigen coated dishes. Furthermore while the Ts and their products are
not functionally restricted by the major histocompatability complex,
they are restricted to loci linked to the heavy chain allotype. This
observation implies that ligand induced, first order Ts(Ts1) may communi-
cate in an allotype restricted manner with other idiotypic or anti-
idiotypic cells to achieve suppression.

The Ts1 has been found to produce a soluble suppressor factor
(TsF1). TsF1 is I-J+ and CRI+. Careful serological analysis of TsF1
reveals that its idiotypic determinants are encoded by heavy chain

variable region (V_H) genes has been detected (19). This differs from serum idiotype which requires an appropriate heavy chain encoded by V genes linked to the Igh-$_1$ locus on chromosone 12 as well as certain Kappa V_L genes located on chromosone 6. TsF1 is H-2 nonrestricted yet functionally allotype restricted.

The target of Ts1 or TsF1 is a second order suppressor T cell (Ts2). This cell is thy 1.2+, Lyt 1+2+3+,I-J+ and anti-idiotypic. It is induced by the interaction of its receptors (anti-CRI) with the complementary CRI+ structures of TsF1 (8). Ts2 also produces a soluble factor (TsF2) which has H-2 encoded determinants is anti-idiotypic, antigen specific and both H-2 and allotype restricted. The relevant H-2 region(s) which determine the restriction elements have not yet been mapped. Ts2 can be readily isolated on idiotype coated dishes. Anti-idiotypic Ts cells can also be induced by the intravenous injection of CRI chemically coupled to syngeneic spleen cells. While Ts2 are allotype restricted in function, they can be <u>induced</u> in <u>any</u> strain irrespective of its heavy chain allotype (14). However, the Ts2 so induced can only function in strains possessing the same allotype as the donor of Ts1 (or TsF1). Thus Ts2 can be induced with CRI+ TsF1 in a CRI- strain and can transfer suppression to a CRI+ strain. This implies that the expression of an idiotype in a strain is a result of V genes coding for idiotypic and not anti-idiotypic receptors, and that idiotypic structures are antigenic at the level of regulatory networks in both idiotype positive and negative strains.

An initial assumption was that Ts2 was the final effector . However, the inability to demonstrate CRI on activated T_{DH} made it difficult to understand how the anti-idiotype Ts2 could interact with the T_{DH} and mediate suppression. The earlier critical observations of Sy et al (16), which showed that a cyclophosphamide sensitive cell was induced at the same time and by the same protocol as the T_{DH} and was necessary for the expression of suppression, led to a search for a similar cell in our own system. It now appears that subcutaneous immunization induces not only the T_{DH} but also primes another Ts subset termed Ts3. The Ts3 is thy 1.2+, Lyt 1-2+3+ and CRI+ (18). The Ts3 interacts with TsF2 to become fully activated. This interaction is H-2 restricted, although it is not known whether the restriction is one of the Ts2 for H-2 elements on the Ts3 or vice versa. Once activated specifically, the Ts3 suppresses DTH reactions in an antigen nonspecific manner. At present we postulate that the Ts3 suppresses reactions via an interaction with antigen bearing nacrophages and not T_{DH}. Indeed a similar notion was previously suggested in work by Asherson and Zembala (2).

In summary, a CRI+Ts1 induces an anti-idiotype Ts2. The Ts2 provides an activational signal to a primed Ts3 which is the effector suppressor. These communicative interactions are allotype restricted and only the latter Ts2-Ts3 interaction is H-2 restricted. Most of the cells and factors in this regulatory pathway are I-J+. The region(s) which dictate H-2 restriction are not yet known; neither is the precise mode of action of the Ts3. It is not clear if the suppressor factors

interact directly with their targets or if they are presented via other
cell types. Clearly though it is naive to speak of a single suppressor
cell. The suppressor cell population is quite heterogeneous and contains cells from all Lyt subsets. This may work to the advantage of those
trying to manipulate suppressive influences: in a system with multiple
steps, the chances of finding ways to intervene in one of those steps or
to influence several steps simultaneously are increased.

As an approach to manipulation of suppression, we have been studying
various influences on the induction of Ts. It is quite clear that hapten
coupled membranes (13),especially derivatized MHC molecules on those membranes, are the most efficient inducers of Ts; while haptenated soluble
proteins are generally unable to readily induce Ts. It is also significant that the soluble factors which induce Ts bear H-2 determinants.
These observations must be reconciled with the fact that Ts1 bear idiotype and can readily bind to free hapten without H-2 elements or that Ts2
bear anti-idiotype and bind to free idiotype. Perhaps there is an initial requirement for recognition of H-2 plus antigen by Ts1 or Ts2.
Alternatively there may be another cell involved in the induction of Ts.
For Ts2 this is probably the Ts1; but the inducer for Ts1, if any, is not
yet isolated.

This latter possibility is supported by very recent data. In these
series of experiments Ts1 and Ts2 can be induced by two separate unlinked
signals. One signal is a low or suboptimal dose of antigen, anti-CRI,
TsF1, etc. which is incapable of inducing the relevant cell type by itself. The second signal is an I-J specific allogeneic effect. The allogeneic effect is delivered by a radioresistant Lyt1 T cell to the Ts
precursor(4). If the allogeneic effect is to be taken as a reflection
of normal physiologic interactions then high or optimal doses of antigen,
anti-CRI, TsF1, etc. must induce Ts1 or Ts2 with the help of another T
cell subset. Our data is supported by a number of other reports (5,15,20)
in which I-J allogeneic effects or recognition of allogeneic I-J determinants are important in the induction of specific suppression. The
ubiquitous presence of I-J determinants on Ts and their factors may turn
out to hold the key to manipulation of the suppressor network. Indeed,
anti-I-J antisera given in vivo functions to abrogate suppression (7).

Cell Mediated Cytotoxicity and Antibody Responses

The suppressor network described above has been delineated for suppression of the DTH response. In addition the same cell populations and
factors are also able to suppress the generation of CMC by cytotoxic T
cells (Tc). The available data make it likely that the suppressors do
not interact with Tc or their precursors. Rather it is more likely that
Ts inhibit or otherwise influence the delivery of signals from helper T
cells (T_H) necessary for the induction of Tc (6). How Ts and T_H interact is currently not known, however, the lack of idiotypic markers on T_H
could mean that Ts3 suppress T_H in a manner similar to the way in which
T_{DH} are suppressed. The interaction of Ts with T_H rather than Tc also
serves to explain the finding that intravenous inoculation of haptenated

cells can simultaneously lead to the induction of Tc and suppression of T_{DH} (6). Obviously there are several phenomena occurring by the intravenous route and the kinetics of each will determine the final outcome.

This idiotypic network also has relevance for the suppression of antibody responses. Idiotypic or anti-idiotypic Ts could interact with idiotype positive or negative or anti-idiotypic T_H, as above, or B cells could be suppressed direcly by anti-idiotypic T cells. We have examined the latter interactions with the IgA myeloma, MOPC 315 (1). Ts which suppress the secretion of antibody by the myeloma can be generated by intravenously injecting spleen cells chemically coupled with the myeloma protein. The Ts so generated are anti-idiotypic and presumably interact directly with myeloma cells (1). It is important to realize that in this situation suppression can be used to regulate and impede the function of tumor cells directly. Therefore, in the case of certain lymphoid malignancies the suppressor network could be activated in order to initiate immunotherapy. This is in contrast to other malignancies where activation of the suppressor network probably interferes with the induction of immunity against the tumor (7).

The nature and organization of the suppressor network which regulates myelomas is not fully understood. The anti-idiotypic Ts which interacts with the myeloma may be a Ts2 as described for the DTH system since it is induced by an idiotypic signal. However, because it suppresses the myeloma directly, it may also ressemble the true effector suppressor, i.e. the Ts3. If this is the case, then we could also predict that an alternative pathway of regulation occurs in which Ts1 is anti-idiotypic, Ts2 is idiotypic and Ts3 is anti-idiotypic. This myeloma protein coupled cells could induce an anti-idiotypic Ts1. The network continues with the generation of complementary idiotypic Ts2 and finally an anti-idiotypic Ts3. Such Ts3 could interact directly with a myeloma cell. This hypothesis - that there are parallel sets of regulatory networks - preserves a restricted and defined function for the individual cells of the network: Ts1 induce Ts2; Ts2 activate Ts3; and Ts3 are the final effector suppressors. It is not known if Ts3 are able to suppress different cell types and immune responses in different ways or if the same signal serves to suppress all reactivities. Formal proof for parallel sets is lacking in our own work. The exhaustive studies of Lynch and Rohrer (11) on the control of secretion by and growth of myeloma cells by Ts are compatible with the existence of this parallel regulatory network.

Nonidiotypic Immune Responses

As mentioned previously, activated suppressor networks may be of direct value to the therapy of lymphoid malignancies. Furthermore because of the clonality of these tumors, idiotypic - anti-idiotypic interactions are certainly quite relevant to the study of the control of their growth and differentiation. For neoplasms which are likely to be more susceptible to immunological control by positive effector functions rather than by suppression (e.g., nonlymphoid maligancies), the question of the relevance of idiotypic interactions and network regulation in the control of the immune response toward them is important. Both the work of Claman and his associates (12,13,16,17) and our own have shown that tolerance to and suppression of DTH and contact sensitivity to haptens which are not under the control of a predominant idiotype are mediated by mechanisms very similar to those operative in the ABA system. Thus hapten coupled cells administered intravenously generate a set of antigen specific, H-2 nonrestricted Ts. To fully function these Ts require the presence of an auxiliary T cell which is most likely the equivalent of the Ts3. The interaction between the initial Ts and the auxiliary Ts in this system is not fully appreciated. It might involve antigen bridging. Perhaps the lack of a predominant idiotype for these antigens may be more apparent than real, in which case the existence of a common or germ-line idiotype (9,17) would permit Ts1-Ts2-Ts3 interactions, as is apparent in ABA responses. The shared nature of a common germ-line idiotype makes its detection difficult.

I-J mediated signals are also undoubtedly important to these nonidiotypic suppressor systems. The reports quoted previously examined DTH, cytotoxic, proliferative and graft rejection responses to MHC alloantigens. Our own studies with the I-J allogeneic effect have involved not only ABA but also the hapten trinitrophenyl and the male alloantigen (H-Y). Therefore the signaling and recognition processes which take place among suppressor cells may well be independent of the importance of idiotypic regulation in the response to that antigen. This implies that a well designed intervention into the suppressor network could be applied to any antigen.

In the S1509a tumor system a number of reports from this laboratory have shown that antigen specific suppressor cells are responsible for maintaining tumor growth and interfering with the induction and function of positive effector mechanisms. The Ts are generated by tumor antigens in the same way haptenated cells generate antigen specific suppressors (e.g., intravenous injection) and manipulations which interfere with the effective presentation of antigen (e.g., anti-I-A antisera, ultraviolet irradiation) influence in the same manner the induction of Ts for haptens or tumor antigens. Ts specific for S1509a are I-J+, produce a TsF which induces second order Ts, and most importantly anti-I-J antisera interfere with these Ts in vivo (7). This latter observation suggests that the development of rational cancer therapies may follow from a thorough understanding of regulatory interactions which are relevant to the immune response.

Conclusions

A detailed understanding of the induction, elicitation and function of specific Ts will permit a coherent manipulation of immune regulation and permit ways to enhance suppression in the case of some lymphoid tumors and abrogate suppression to certain other neoplasms. A knowledge of the molecular structure of the products of specific Ts and how these molecules function; identification of the product(s) of the Ts3; and an increased understanding of the role of I-J in suppressor signals are current issues which need to be resolved. With their resolution may come the ability to direct much of immune responsiveness at will.

1. Abbas, A.K., Burakoff, S.J., Gefter, M.L., and Greene, M.I. (1980): J. Exp. Med., 152:969-978.

2. Asherson, G.L. and Zembala, M. (1974): Eur. J. Immunol. 4:804-807.

3. Bach, B.A., Sherman, L., Benacerraf, B., and Greene, M.I. (1978): J. Immunol. 121:1460-1468.

4. Bromberg, J.S., Benacerraf, B., and Greene, M.I. (1981): J. Exp. Med. 153:437-449.

5. Czitrom, A.A., Sunshine, G.H. and Mitchison, N.A. (1980): Immunogenet. 11:97-102.

6. Fujiwara, H., Levy R.B., Shearer, G.M. and Terry, W.D. (1979): J. Immunol.. 123:423-425.

7. Greene, M.I. (1980): Contemporary Topics in Immunobiology, edited by Warner, D, pp. 81-110. Plenum Press, New York.

8. Hirai, Y. and Nisonoff, A. (1980): J. Exp. Med. 151:1213-1231.

9. Ju, S-T, Benacerraf, B. and Dorf, M.E. (1978): Proc. Natl. Acad. Sci. 75: 6192-6196.

10. Kuettner, M.G., Wang, A-L., and Nisonoff, A. (1972): J. Exp. Med. 135:579-595.

11. Lynch, R.G., Rohrer, J.W., Gebel, H.M., and Odermatt, B. (1980): In: Progress in Myeloma, edited by M. Potter, pp. 129-150. Elsevier North Holand, Inc., New York.

12. Miller, S.D., Sy,M-S., and Claman, H.N. (1978): J. Exp. Med. 147: 788-799.

13. Miller, S.D., Conlon, P.J., Sy, M-S., Moorhead, J.W., Colon, S., Grey, H.M., and Claman, H.N. (1980): J. Immunol. 124:1187-1193.

14. Nisonoff, A. and M.I. Greene (1980):In: Proc. 4th Intl. Congress, edited by M. Fougerau, J. Dausset, pp 57-80. Academic Press, New York.

15. Streilein, J.W. (1979): Immunological Rev. 46:125-146.

16. Sy, M-S, Miller, S.D., Moorhead, J.W., and Claman, H.N.(1979): J. Exp. Med. 149:1197-1207.

17. Sy, M-S, Moorhead, J.W., and Claman, H.N. (1979): J. Immunol. 123: 2593-2598.

18. Sy, M-S., Nisonoff, A., Germain, R.N., Benacerraf, B., and M.I. Greene. (1981): J. Exp. Med. 153: 1415-1425.

19. Sy, M-S., Brown, A., Benacerraf, B. Gottlieb, P., Nisonoff, A. and Greene, M.I. (1981): Proc. Natl. Acad. Sci (USA) 78: 1143-1147.

20. Zinkernagel, R.M. (1980): Immunogenet:10:373-382.

AUDIENCE DISCUSSION

Dr. Fathman: When an anti-idiotypic suppressor cell sees an idiotypic T cell, how can it tell whether this idiotypic T cell is a helper T cell or a suppressor T cell?

Dr. Greene: Well, in the first case, although I did not show data about it, the anti-idiotypic suppressor cell generated in this manner is both H-2 restricted and idiotypically restricted. It may be that the particular H-2 restriction is very critical in determining the nature of the interaction between the TS2 subset and the TS3 subset. That does not mean, however, that the TS2 is not capable of interacting with idiotypic TS1 or idiotypic T helper cells, because we see the same effect when we look at the immune response at the antibody level. And that response clearly must involve helper cells, both of an idiotypic and anti-idiotypic sort.

Dr. Bach: You base the existence of the TS3 cell on the fact that you can eliminate suppression by the anti-idiotypic suppressor.

Dr. Greene: Yes.

Dr. Bach: Is it possible that you are subdividing two populations of helpers, a population that carries idiotype and one that does not, and that there's some compensatory mechanism to allow the cross-reactive idiotype-negative population to proliferate more, to give more help? This would argue for some other kind of regulatory mechanism.

Dr. Greene: That's an interesting notion but no. When we activate TS3, we see suppression not only of the response but of every other response in the vicinity. That is, we can suppress in an antigen and idiotype nonspecific way. So we would have to account for loss of a helper cell population and at the same time an antigen-induced idiotypic helper cell population which is important for all responses. This seems unlikely.

Dr. Bach: Why?

Dr. Greene: The help of all responses would still have to go through an idiotype positive helper cell. I showed that the TS3 cell, once activated by a TSF2 is capable of suppressing responses in an antigen and idiotype nonspecific way. How would you account for that data by your hypothesis of differential helper cells?

Dr. Fernandez-Cruz: Are the Lyt 1^+2^- cells that inhibit S15092 tumor growth Ia positive?

Dr. Greene: They are Ia negative.

Dr. Warner: Is there no possibility that the TS3 which acts in a nonspecific function is of the monocytic macrophage lineage? Where do you fit some of the nonspecific immunosuppressive factors if that is an Ly 2-bearing cell.

Dr. Greene: The TS3 is an Ly 2-bearing Thy 1.2 positive cell. That cell could make a particle which interacts with a monocytic cell -- I think that's the way the system works. But that TS3 cell itself is definitely a T cell.

Matheson: You showed that at the idiotype level there was a difference between cellular response and the antibody response. Where does that fit in terms of the subsets of cells that you have right now? In terms of your suppression?

Dr. Greene: When you couple idiotypes to cells, this allows you to generate very potent anti-idiotypic T cells, either TS1 or TS2 cells. Also in this case, the TS3 cell would be anti-idiotypic. That TS3 cell itself is apparently capable of leading to the suppression of the expression of the cross-reactive idiotype. So if that cell is analogous to the cells we have typed -- and I see no reason why it shouldn't be, it will turn out to be a Ly 1^+2^+ and that leads to the suppression of the antibody responses.

Dr. Doug Green: Do you have any information on the antigen binding of the TS3? Is it like an AB3 in that it's idiotype positive, but seems to be somewhat antigen nonspecific or antigen undirected?

Dr. Green: It's activated in a specific way by antigen, so it definitely would be idiotype positive and not, as you say, antibody 3 in the network, which would be anti-anti-idiotypic. So there really wouldn't be a formal analogy. These experimental data suggest that the network is not an open-ended one, but very symmetrical and closed.

Dr. Doug Green: Are you doing any experiments in which you put anti-idiotype onto a spleen cell and inject that? Will you get a TS1 that doesn't bind and doesn't interact with antigen?

Dr. Greene: We did those experiments and found that when you administer anti-idiotype, it will induce a population of a TS1-like cell. And if you administer it by another route, you will generate a population of cells which at the effector level is entirely idiotype positive. We've not looked at the interactions of that kind of signal.

[Unidentified]: You described the thymus factor 4678 and factors, TSF1, TSF2 and TSF3. Do you know anything about the chemical nature of these molecules? Are they similar?

Dr. Greene: The TSF1 has been now characterized; we have characterized the crude supernatant and we now have stable hybridomas over a period of 8 months from which we've also characterized the molecule. These hybridomas were produced and characterized by Blake Whitaker, Muneo Takoaki and Jerry Nepom at Harvard. The basic features of the suppressive factor of TS1 cells are the molecular weight is approximately 62,000 daltons as determined by chromotography and SDS polyacrylomide gel. It can be affinity purified on an anti-idiotypic column or an anti-IJ column.

[Unidentified]: What was thymus factor 4678?

Dr. Greene: That's a TSF1.

Dr. Fathman: Why does the mouse look at the idiotype as it's presented as an antibody coded onto a lymphocyte any differently than it looks at ABA? Why doesn't it generate a TS1 in response to that as an immunogen instead of shifting immediately to the TS2 pathway?

Dr. Greene: We have done experiments which show that it does generate TS1 cells; we can generate anti-idiotypic TS1 cells. Idiotype coupled cells provide signals which allow entry to the pathway at all points in which the anti-idiotypic cell population is represented. It can be at the TS1 or the TS2 stage. There is no reason that idiotype on a cell surface cannot be a signal for TS1 cells. However, we would never be able to observe their function, because there's a complementary interaction between three-cell subsets. Then idiotype-coupled cells induce anti-idiotypic TS1 cells, the path would be anti-idiotypic, idiotypic and anti-idiotypic, and the TS3 would be anti-idiotypic and it would have to interact with an immune cell which had a recognizable idiotypic specificity. Remember the TS3 cell is activated coincidentallly with immune cells. In order to resolve this we had to do an experiment using

the myeloma system. We generated an anti-idiotypic TS1, and made a
factor from it. We then transferred anti-idiotypic factor (TSF1) into
another animal and immunized that animal with idiotype coupled cells.
We then took the TS3 cells that were generated in that animal and examined them in vitro and we found very potent suppression of the myeloma
response. These experiments were done with Abbul Abbas.

The Potential Role of T Cells in Cancer Therapy,
edited by A. Fefer and A. Goldstein,
Raven Press, New York © 1982.

Contrasuppression: Its Role in Immunoregulation

Douglas R. Green

Department of Pathology, Yale University School of Medicine, New Haven, Connecticut 06510

Much of modern immunoregulatory research is concerned with the un-complicated idea that for each positive immunological response there is an equal and opposite negative response. This notion, stated by Gershon (8) as the "Second Law of Thymodynamics" can be more simply phrased:

What goes up,
must come down,

meaning <u>suppression</u>. The process by which immune responses are brought into check is an active one. The cells and cell free factors which interact to produce active suppression have been described extensively (4,6) and will not be further discussed here. Instead, I would like to turn to another conceptually simple notion which may be considered a corollary of the above "Second Law". That is,

What goes down,
must come up,

meaning <u>contrasuppression</u>. As in negative regulation, the positive process by which down regulated immune states regain responsiveness is an active one. "Contrasuppression" is a regulatory phenomenon which modulates the responsiveness of the immune system to suppressor cell signals (9), rendering the targets of suppression resistant to such inhibitory effects. In this discussion, the immunoregulatory T cell circuit which effects contrasuppression will be reviewed. In addition, I will present a pot pourri of systems in which contrasuppression can be demonstrated. This assembly attests to the pervasiveness and importance of this regulatory phenomenon.

THE CONTRASUPPRESSOR CIRCUIT

The T cell subsets which interact to produce contrasuppression have been described (9). As in other regulatory T cell circuits the phenom-enon of contrasuppression involves an interaction of an inducer cell and a transducer cell which converts the induction signal into an effect (via an effector cell). This scheme is shown in Figure 1.

The <u>contrasuppressor inducer</u> was first identified in cultures containing <u>in vitro</u> generated suppressor T cells (9). This inducer cell correlates with a cell surface phenotype of $Ly-1^-, 2^+; I-J^+$. The I-J encoded determinant is recognized by a monoclonal anti-I-J reagent (D-7) which distinguishes this I-J product from that found on cells of the suppressor circuit (23) (although neither this nor the "suppres-sor circuit I-J" has been identified on the Ly-2 suppressor effector cell for the sheep red blood cell response (9)).

A cell free product of the contrasuppressor inducer cell has been isolated which bears an I-J encoded determinant, binds antigen, (but with a different cross reactivity pattern than similar suppressor factor) and reproduces the effects of the inducer cell (21).

The contrasuppressor transducer is required if one is to observe the action of either the inducer cell or its product. This cell correlates with the phenotype Ly-1$^+$,2$^+$; I-J$^+$ (9,21) and again this I-J product is recognized by D-7 (23). Removal of this cell population can effectively quench the contrasuppressor circuit, such that suppression can become dominant in situations where none was previously observed (21,12).

The contrasuppressor effector was first recognized in six day cultures of spleen cells from neonatal animals aged approximately 7-14 days (11). These cells are Ly-1$^+$,2$^-$; I-J$^+$ (recognized by D-7 (23)), adhere to the Vicia villosa lectin, and are dependent upon Ly-2$^+$ cells for their generation (as predicted by the circuit). In addition, these cells do not appear in cultures of spleen cells of B cell deficient (μ-suppressed) neonatal animals (16). With the exception of the Ly phenotype, all of these characteristics distinguish the contrasuppressor effector from conventional helper T cells.

These effector cells, or their cell free factor (14), act to render helper T cells resistant to suppressor cell signals. The target, then, of the contrasuppressor circuit appears to be the helper T cell (not the suppressor cell). The helper T cell has been shown to be a target of the effector cell of the suppressor cell circuit as well (10), (see Figure 1).

Evidence for the action of contrasuppressor effector cells on T helper cells comes from experiments utilizing the "intermediate culture" system, shown schematically in Figure 2 (11). Basically, partially purified populations of Ly-1.1 helper T cells, Ly-2 suppressor T cells, and Ly-1.2 contrasuppressor T cells were allowed to interact in culture for 48 hours following which they were treated with both anti-Ly-2 and anti-Ly-1.2 plus complement to remove all but the helper cell population. Following this isolation, the helper cells were added to B cells (anti-Thy-1 plus complement treated spleen) under conditions for in vitro plaque forming cell (PFC) responses to sheep red blood cells (SRBC).

Results of such experiments are shown in Table 1. T helper cells added to B cells gave a good response (group b, column I) which was suppressible when fresh suppressor cells were added to the B cell assay cultures (group b, column II). If the T helper cells had spent 48 hours in the presence of suppressor T cells which were then removed, only minimal helper activity was recoverable (group c).

On the other hand, helper T cells cultured in the presence of both suppressors and contrasuppressors not only retained their activity (group d, column I), but were resistant to further suppressor cell signals (group d, column II) as compared with the controls in group b.

If instead of recovering helper T cells we recovered suppressor cells from these contrasuppressed cultures, the suppressors retained their activity, thus indicating that they themselves had not been targets of the contrasuppressors (results not shown). Use of suppressor factors in place of cells in these experiments has further confirmed the idea that suppressor cells do not act as the target of contrasuppression.

In addition to the activity in vitro, the contrasuppressor effector cell can be shown to function in vivo. Animals can be tolerized for contact sensitivity by intravenous injection of haptenated peritoneal exudate cells (PEC) (17). Contrasuppressor effector cells can block this tolerogenic signal and allow immunity to dominate (18). Thus, animals which received both haptenated PEC and contrasuppressor effector

Figure 1

THE CONTRASUPPRESSOR CIRCUIT

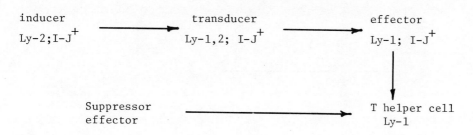

Table 1

THE INTERMEDIATE CULTURE SYSTEM

(see Figure 2)

Cells in intermediate culture	Cell type recovered after 48 hrs	Response (assay culture)	
		Column I B cells	Column II B cells + Ts
a) none	none	−	−
b) T_H	T_H	++	−
c) T_H + Ts	T_H	−	−
d) T_H + Ts + Tcs	T_H	++	+

abbreviations: T_H = helper

Ts = suppressor effector

Tcs = contrasuppressor effector

Figure 2

THE INTERMEDIATE CULTURE SYSTEM

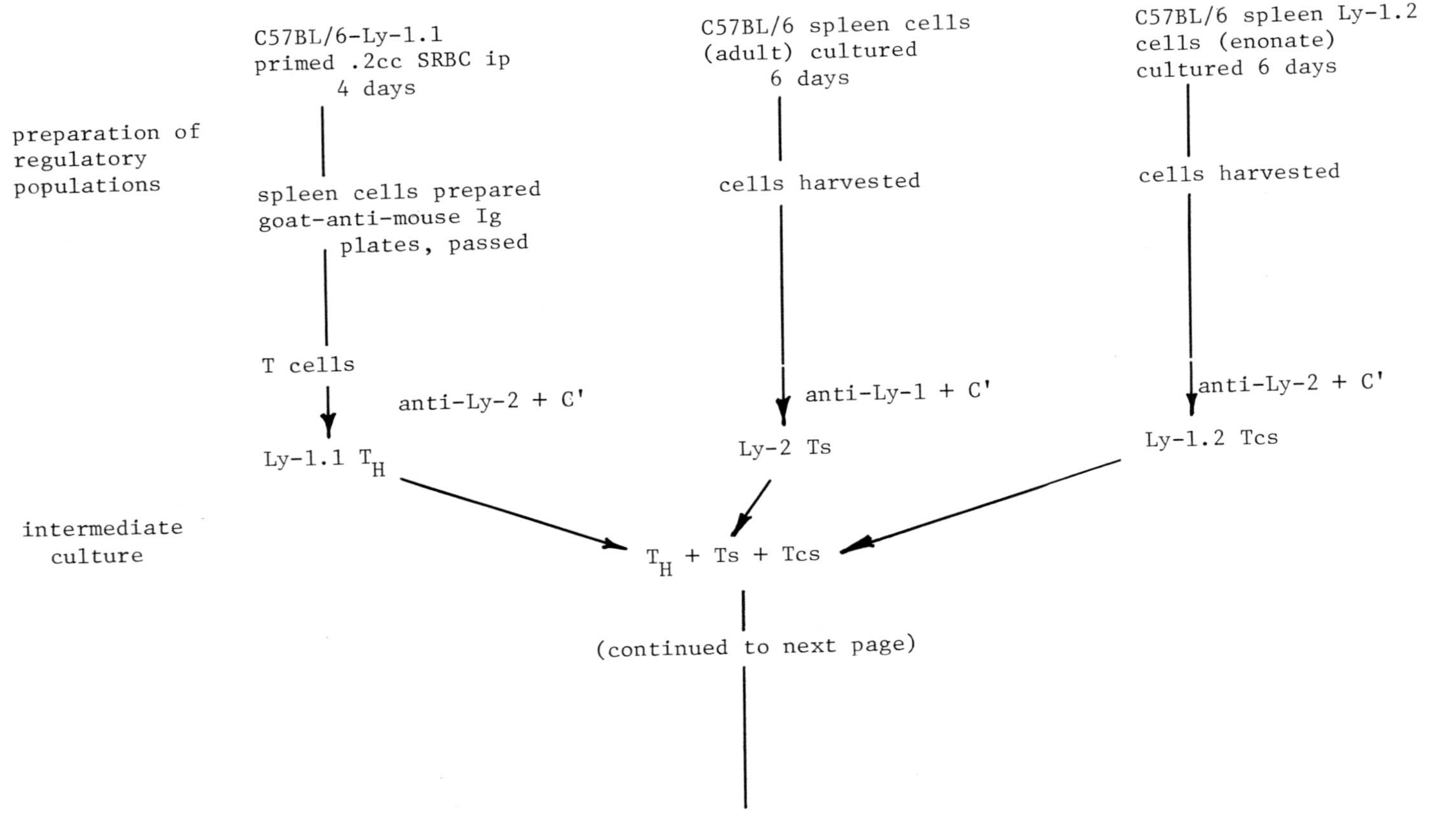

preparation of
regulatory
populations

C57BL/6-Ly-1.1
primed .2cc SRBC ip
4 days

→

spleen cells prepared
goat-anti-mouse Ig
plates, passed

→

T cells

anti-Ly-2 + C'
→

Ly-1.1 T_H

C57BL/6 spleen cells
(adult) cultured
6 days

→

cells harvested

anti-Ly-1 + C'
→

Ly-2 Ts

C57BL/6 spleen Ly-1.2
cells (enonate)
cultured 6 days

→

cells harvested

anti-Ly-2 + C'
→

Ly-1.2 Tcs

intermediate
culture

T_H + Ts + Tcs

(continued to next page)

(Continuation of Figure 2)

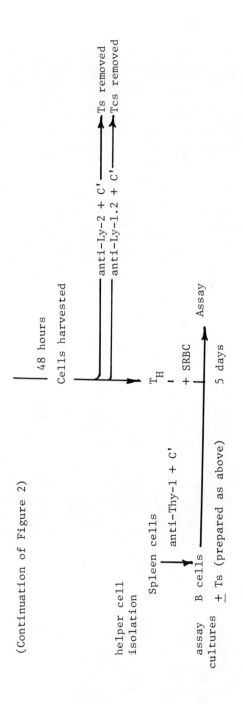

48 hours
Cells harvested

anti-Ly-2 + C' → Ts removed
anti-Ly-1.2 + C' → Tcs removed

helper cell isolation

Spleen cells

anti-Thy-1 + C'

B cells

assay cultures + Ts (prepared as above)

T_H

+ SRBC

Assay

5 days

Abbreviations: T_H = helper cell

Ts = suppressor cell

Tcs = contrasuppressor cell

cells were not only <u>not</u> tolerant, they were potently sensitized to the hapten. This phenomenon requires that the antigen be presented by both an immunogenic and a tolerogenic presenting cell, in which case the contrasuppressors can effect the transformation of the dominant tolerogenic signal to a dominant immunogenic one.

Whether contrasuppression functions under normal physiological conditions to influence the dominance of immunity over tolerance will be considered in the next section.

For the remainder of this discussion, other sources of contrasuppressor effector cells will be described, some of which might be considered to be more "physiological" than the cultures of normal spleen cells from neonatal animals.

THE ADOPTIVE TRANSFER OF IMMUNITY

The theme of adoptive transfer of immunity is a prevalent one in experimental approaches to cancer therapy. Actively immune lymphocytes and now highly enriched active T cell clones can be injected intravenously into animals to produce systemic immunity (c.f. this volume). However, most forms of immune transfer require that the recipient be treated with low doses of irradiation or cyclophosphamide (5,7). The role of suppression in preventing transfer into unrelated recipients has been demonstrated (see, for example, R. North, this volume).

There are several exceptions to this requirement for treating the recipient prior to transfer. The transfer of contact sensitivity responses is particularly noteworthy. Splenic lymphocytes from skin painted animals will confer specific immunity if injected intravenously into normal, untreated recipients (2). What is special about this response that it can be so easily transferred?

Table 2 shows an approach to answering this question (from an experiment by G.M. Iverson). Ly-1 T cells (anti-Ly-2 plus complement treated, goat anti-mouse Ig plate passed splenocytes) from skin sensitized animals are capable of transferring immunity into both normal and low dose cyclophosphamide treated recipients (groups a and c). Removal of an $I-J^+$ subpopulation from the Ly-1 set (with anti-I-J plus complement) had no significant effect on the ability of these cells to transfer immunity into the cyclophosphamide treated group (group d). When this Ly-1; $I-J^-$ population was injected into normal recipients, however, no immunity was adoptively transferred (group b).

In considering these results several points may be made: A) Of the two T cell populations, the Ly-1; $I-J^-$ subset must contain the cells responsible for immunity, as this population confers immunity upon cyclophosphamide treated, antigenically naive animals. On the other hand, B) the Ly-1; $I-J^+$ subset functions to allow transfer of the effects of the immune Ly-1; $I-J^-$ cells into normal animals. C) The effect of a low dose (20mg/kg) of cyclophosphamide is to disrupt the suppressor cell circuit such that suppressor effector cells are not generated (3). Therefore, D) the Ly-1; $I-J^+$ subset is capable of interferring with the action of a cyclophosphamide sensitive suppressor system on immune Ly-1; $I-J^-$ cells such that immunity is transferred.

While other interpretations may be possible, this interpretation is compatible with the action of contrasuppression in the adoptive transfer of contract sensitivity. This is strongly supported by the surface phenotype of the second subset; contrasuppressor effector cells correlate with a profile of Ly-1; $I-J^+$.

Table 2

REQUIREMENT FOR THE PRESENCE OF I-J$^+$; Ly-1 CELLS TO ALLOW THE
ADOPTIVE TRANSFER OF CONTACT HYPERSENSITIVITY BY I-J$^-$; Ly-1 CELLS
UNLESS THE RECIPIENT SUPPRESSOR CIRCUIT IS INACTIVATED

Adoptive immunity transfered with (donor cells)	Treatment of recipient	24 hour ear swelling
a) Ly-1 cells	none	++
b) I-J$^-$,Ly-1 cells	none	-
c) Ly-1 cells	20mg/kg cyclophosphamide	++
d) I-J$^-$,Ly-1 cells	20mg/kg cyclophosphamide	++

If supported by additional evidence, this finding will not only show
a physiological induction of contrasuppression (via skin painting) but
may point the way to new approaches to immunotherapy.

CONTRASUPPRESSION AND HYPERIMMUNITY

The suggestion that systems in which immunity can be transferred
into normal recipients may employ contrasuppression led to another
series of experiments in which contrasuppressors are activated in vivo.
Whereas secondary antibody responses cannot be readily transferred with
immune cells into normal, untreated recipients (5), cells from hyperimmune animals are effective (13).

In order to study the potential activity of contrasuppressor cells
in hyperimmunized animals, a modification of the intermediate culture
system was employed (Figure 3). SRBC primed Ly-1 cells or naive Ly-1
cells serving as the helper cell population were placed in the lower
chamber of a periscopic double Marbrook culture. Nonspecific, culture
generated Ly-2 suppressor cells were placed in the upper chamber,
separated from the lower by a 0.1 μ pore size nucleopore membrane. In
some groups, T cells from animals which had received six or more weekly
injections of SRBC (and which showed serum hemagglutination titers of
ten doubling dilutions or better) were also added to the upper chamber.
After 48 hours the helper T cells were recovered from the lower chamber
and tested for activity by adding them to B cells (anti-Thy-1 plus
complement treated spleen) under conditions for in vitro PFC response
to SRBC.

Typical results are summarized in Table 3. Ly-2 suppressor cells
were capable of inactivating Ly-1 helper T cells across the membrane
(group c). In the presence of T cells from hyperimmunized animals,
however, no inactivation took place (group d). When fresh Ly-2 suppressor cells were added to the B cells (column II) the group which had
interacted with the hyperimmune cells (across the membrane) could be
seen to be resistant to suppressor cell signals (group d, column II).
The cell population in the hyperimmune spleen responsible for both
interferring with suppression (column I) and rendering helper cells

Figure 3

DOUBLE MARBROOK MODIFICATION

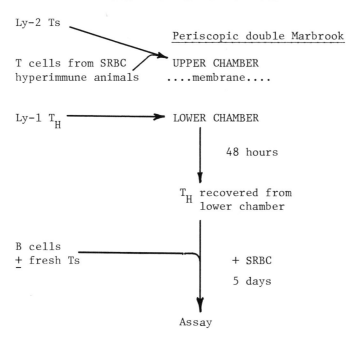

resistant to further suppressive signals (column II) was sensitive to treatment with either anti-Ly-1 or anti-I-J plus complement (groups e and f). Both by function (infectious resistance to suppression) and surface profile (Ly-1$^+$; I-J$^+$) the evidence is in agreement with the activation of contrasuppressor effector cells in the course of hyper-immunization.

In contrast to the contrasuppressor effector cell derived from cultured neonatal cells, the Ly-1; I-J$^+$ cells in the spleens of hyper-immune animals show a degree of antigen specificity in that helper cells for SRBC but not burro red blood cell responses can be contra-suppressed (rendered resistant to suppression) by cells from mice hyperimmune to SRBC (not shown).

The appearance of cells with the phenotype and function of contra-suppressor cells in the spleens of hyperimmune animals helps to explain two paradoxes of this immune state. While hyperimmunized animals are obviously immune, the serum of these animals is potently immunosuppres-sive (13). Recently, Iverson (13) has demonstrated high concentrations (approximately 1mg/ml) of T cell derived suppressor factor in such serum. Others have found that such immunization procedures which are optimal for immunization are also optimal for production of suppressor factors (19,22). The two questions, then, are: Why do hyperimmunized animals produce such quantitites of suppressive material and how do they then maintain immunity in the face of this suppression?

The answer to both of these questions may involve contrasuppression. Both helper T cells and feedback inducers of suppression are known to be targets of the suppressor effector cell (10). By suppressing its own

Table 3

HYPERIMMUNE SPLEEN CELLS HAVE CONTRASUPPRESSIVE ACTIVITY

Intermediate culture		T_H cells recovered from lower chamber and added to:	
Upper chamber	lower chamber	B cells	B + Ts
a) none	none	-	-
b) none	T_H	++	-
c) Ts	T_H	-	-
d) Ts + T_{HI} (T_{HI} treated with with C')	T_H	++	++
e) Ts + T_{HI} (T_{HI} treated with anti-Ly-1+C')	T_H	-	-
f) Ts + T_{HI} (T_{HI} treated with anti-I-J+C')	T_H	-	-

Abbreviations: T_H = helper cell

                       Ts = suppressor cell

                       T_{HI} = T cells from animals hyperimmunized to SRBC

inducer, the suppressor effector essentially turns itself off which results in relatively small amounts of detectable suppressor factor. The helper T cell can be contrasuppressed such that no inactivation of this cell will occur, allowing immunity to dominate in hyperimmune animals. If, in addition, feedback inducers of suppression are simultaneously contrasuppressed, the effect will be a constant activation signal from the suppressor inducer to the suppressor effector. The result of such interactions would be: a) a suppressor "pump" which secretes large quantites of suppressor factor and b) a contrasuppressed helper system which "ignores" this factor. This is exactly what is observed in animals hyperimmunized with sheep red blood cells.

CONCLUSION: LEVELS UPON LEVELS

Experimental evidence of the sort described in this brief discussion led us to the theory of contrasuppression, but a question which often comes to mind is, "Do we really need so much immunoregulation?" The answer is a resounding, "YES".

The immune system is faced with the profound task of making responses which maximally damage invaders while only minimally damaging self tissues. This is not to say that damage to self is accidental; it is, instead, often a decision made by the system as a necessary aspect of the removal of a more immediately harmful foe (1). As we increase our knowledge of immunoregulatory interactions, such heuristic power can be granted to the immune system.

The effect of these considerations is to open the way to an understanding of levels of regulation. The interaction of antigen with helper T cells raises the system from a ground state to "level one", in which immunity can be suppressed by "level one suppressors" of the sort described in the feedback suppression circuit of Gershon and colleagues (4). Contrasuppressors can elevate the system to "level two" such that these suppressors are ineffectual. We may then postulate another form of suppression ("level two suppression") which can inactivate contrasuppressed helper T cells. The suppressor circuit described by Tada, et al (20) might in fact be an example of such level two suppression. Experiments are in progress to test these notions.

In any case, our aim is not to try to trivialize the decision making operations of the immune system, but to dissect and explore their intricacies. A view of immunoregulation can be pictured in which the T helper cell stands center stage. Down regulation is mediated via a T cell interaction with the helper which results in suppression, up regulation by a similar interaction resulting in contrasuppression. Contrasuppression, then, may serve as an essential component of immune processing. Insights into such processing may aid our understanding of why the immune system may sometimes fail in the rejection of neoplasms or other undersirable invaders. In addition, in a field in which active immunity rather than inhibition is most often the desired effect of immunengineering, contrasuppression may prove a powerful clinical tool - more so, perhaps, than suppression.

REFERENCES

1. Asherson, G.L. (1968): Progr. Allergy, 12:192-245.
2. Asherson, G.L. and Ptak, W. (1968): Immunology 15:405-417.
3. Askenase, P.W., Hayden, B.J., and Gershon, R.K. (1975): J. Exp. Med. 141:697-702.
4. Cantor, H., and Gershon, R.K. (1979): Fed. Proc. 38:2058-2064.
5. Celada, F. (1966): J. Exp. Med. 124:7-14.
6. Eardley, D.D., Murphy, D.B., Kemp, J.D., Shen, F.W., Cantor, H., and Gershon, R.K. (1980): Immunogenetics, 11:549-557.
7. Eardley, D.D., and Gershon, R.K. (1975): J. Exp. Med. 142:524-529.
8. Gershon, R.K. (1974): In: The Immune System: Genes, Receptors, Signals, edited by E. Sercarz, A. Williamson, and C.F. Fox, pp 471-484. Academic Press, New York.

9. Gershon, R.K., Eardley, D.D., Durum, S., Green, D.R., Shen, F.W., Yamauchi, K., Cantor, H., and Murphy, D.B. (1978): J. Exp. Med. 153:1533-1546.
10. Green, D.R., Gershon, R.K. and Eardley, D.D. (1981): Proc. Natl. Acad. Sci (U.S.A.) 78:3819-3823.
11. Green, D.R., Eardley, D.D., Kimura, A., Murphy, D.B., Yamauchi, K., and Gershon, R.K. Eur. J. Immunol., "(in press)".
12. Green, D.R., Gold, J., St. Martin, S., Gershon, R., and Gershon, R.K. J. Exp. Med. "(submitted)".
13. Haughton, G. (1971): Cell. Immunol. 2:567-582.
14. Horowitz, M.C., Green, D.R., Murphy, D., and Gershon, R.K. (1981): J. Supr. Mol. Struct. Sup. 5:189 (Abstract).
15. Iverson, G.M., Eardley, D.D., Durum, S.K., Kaufmann, S.H., (1981): J. Supr. Mol. Struct. Sup. 5:172 (Abstract).
16. Janeway, C.A., Broughton, B., Dzierzak, E., Jones, B., Eardley, D.D., Durum, S.K., Yamauchi, K., Green, D.R., and Gershon, R.K. In: Immunoglobulin Idiotypes and Their Expression, edited by C. Janeway, E. Sercarz, H. Wigzell and C.F. Fox, Academic Press, New York, "(in press)".
17. Ptak, W., Rozycka, D., Askenase, P.W., and Gershon, R.K. (1980): J. Exp. Med. 151:362-375.
18. Ptak, W., Green, D.R., Durum, S.K., Kimura, A., Murphy, D.B., and Gershon, R.K. Eur. J. Immunol., "(in press)".
19. Tada, T., Okumura, K. (1979): Adv. Immunol. 28:1-87.
20. Tada, T., Taniguchi, M., Okumura, K. (1979): J. Supra. Mol. Struct. Sup. 3:236 (Abstract).
21. Yamauchi, K., Green, D.R., Eardley, D.D., Murphy, D.B., and Gershon, R.K. (1981): J. Exp. Med. 153:1547-1561.
22. Yamauchi, K., Murphy, D.B., Cantor, H. and Gershon, R.K. Eur. J. Immunol, "(in press)".
23. Yamauchi, K., Taniguchi, M., Green, D.R., and Gershon, R.K. Immunogenetics, "(submitted)".

AUDIENCE DISCUSSION

[Unidentified]: The suppressor-contrasuppressor system must be very inefficient.

Dr. Green: It is indeed. There are helper cells not only for B-cells, but for suppressor cells. It is conceivable that once contra-suppression is activated, it contra-suppresses the helper cells for suppressor cells. The suppressor circuit becomes resistant to its own feedback regulation. Suppressor cells can inactivate their own helper cells. Perhaps contra-suppressors can block that inactivation as well and so you essentially develop a suppressor pump -- the suppressor cells are pushed into overproduction, just like the helper cells are pushed into causing B cells to overproduce.

[Unidentified]: The IJ you are detecting is detected by Tanaguchie's monoclonal?

Dr. Green: Yes.

[Unidentified]: But also by many IJ sera?

Dr. Green: Yes.

[Unidentified]: Some of the IJ sera also inactivated suppressors but the monoclonal does not?

Dr. Green: That's right. That's true of the freeback inducer the LY1 cell that induces suppression and the LY1-2 cell. We've never found an IJ that could kill suppressor effector cells. Tanaguchie's reagent, called D7, doesn't touch any of the cells of the feedback suppressor circuit -- the LY1 inducer, the LY1-2 transducer of the effector cell -- it hits every cell of the contra-suppressor circuit.

[Unidentified]: In regards to restriction of this contra-suppressor, what do you know about idiotype or MHC region restriction?

Dr. Green: There is no indication of MHC restriction. There may be idiotype restriction, although it isn't actually VH. There is a restriction that seems to be mapping somewhere in the IG complex.

[Unidentified]: Can that cell be removed on an antigen monolayer?

Dr. Green: No. We were unsuccessful removing it on antibody, but if we can obtain the T cell idiotype, this might be directed at that idiotype. But now that we've actually isolated the T cell factor which is sheep red blood cell specific and bears a unique idiotype, we're testing that possibility.

Dr. Whisnat: In your modified intermediate culture system, is it necessary to have two suppressors in the upper chamber? Have you ever done the experiment with only the two contra-suppressors?

Dr. Green: If they are the neonatal contra-suppressors, the answer is yes. With the hyperimmune cells, the answer seems to be no.

Dr. Whisnat: Have you tried putting those cells in separate chambers and then transferring the contra-suppressor cells?

Dr. Green: No, I have not. We shall.

Dr. Bach: In the system where you showed that the I-J negative LY1 positive cells showed a differential response depending on pretreatment of the recipient animal and hypothesized therefore that an I-J positive cell was involved, since you can select for those by panning of FACS? Have you actually done the mixing experiment showing that effect?

Dr. Green: We have had no success in either panning or FAC sorting with the I-J.

Dr. Bonavida: What happens to the T helper cells that have been suppressed by the factor in the lower chamber? Do they remain for a long time suppressed? Can you revert them or are they completely eliminated in terms of function?

Dr. Green: Diane Erdly at Harvard is pursuing those studies. She says that if instead of culturing helper with suppressor cells for 48 hours, we culture just 24 hours, there is a marginal inhibition of the helper cells. If those cells are then allowed to culture for another 48 hours without any suppressor cells, they do recover their activity.

Subject Index

Subject Index